Lung Cancer: Causes and Prevention

verlag
chemie
international

Lung Cancer:

Causes and Prevention

Proceedings of the International Lung Cancer Update Conference, held in New Orleans, Louisiana, March 3-5, 1983

Edited by

Merle Mizell and **Pelayo Correa**

verlag
chemie
international

Merle Mizell, PhD
Professor and Director
Laboratory of Tumor Cell Biology
Department of Biology
Tulane University
New Orleans, Louisiana 70118

Pelayo Correa, MD
Department of Pathology
Louisiana State University Medical Center
New Orleans, Louisiana 70112

Library of Congress Cataloging in Publication Data

International Lung Cancer Update Conference (1983 : New
Orleans, La.)
Lung cancer.

(Biomedical advances in carcinogenesis ; v. 1)
Includes bibliographical references and index.
1. Lungs—Cancer—Etiology—Congresses. 2. Lungs—
Cancer—Prevention—Congresses. 3. Tobacco—Physiological
effect—Congresses. 4. Lungs—Cancer—United States—
Congresses. I. Mizell, Merle, 1927- . II. Correa,
Pelayo. III. Title. IV. Series. [DNLM: 1. Lung neo-
plasms—etiology—congresses. 2. Lung neoplasms—pre-
vention & control—congresses. W1 BI853T v. 1 /
WF 658 I61L 1983]
RC280.L8I55 1983 616.99′424071 84-10362
ISBN 0-89573-135-5

Printed in the United States of America.

ISBN 0-89573-135-5 Verlag Chemie International, Deerfield Beach
ISBN 3-527-26148-6 Verlag Chemie GmbH, Weinheim

Contents

Chapter 1	**Keynote Address: The Control of Lung Cancer** *Richard Peto and Richard Doll*	*1*
Chapter 2	**Lung Cancer in Scandinavia: Time Trends and Smoking Habits** *Lyly Teppo*	*21*
Chapter 3	**Trends in Lung Cancer Incidence and Mortality in the United States** *Susan S. Devesa, John W. Horm, and Roger R. Connelly*	*33*
Chapter 4	**Lung Cancer and Occupational Exposures** *William J. Blot*	*47*
Chapter 5	**Air Pollution and Lung Cancer** *Carl M. Shy*	*65*
Chapter 6	**The Causes of Lung Cancer in Louisiana** *Pelayo Correa, Linda Williams Pickle, Elizabeth Fontham, Nancy Dalager, Youping Lin, William Haenszel, and William D. Johnson*	*73*
Chapter 7	**The Causes of Lung Cancer in Texas** *Patricia A. Buffler, Linda Williams Pickle, Thomas J. Mason, and Charles Contant*	*83*
Chapter 8	**Recent Case - Control Studies of Lung Cancer in the United States** *Linda Williams Pickle, Pelayo Correa, and Elizabeth Fontham*	*101*
Chapter 9	**The Epidemiologic Meaning of Histology in Lung Cancer** *John W. Berg*	*117*

Chapter 10 **Lung Cancer in Nonsmokers and Low-Risk Populations** *131*
Joseph L. Lyon, Electra D. Avlon, and John W. Gardner

Chapter 11 **Ecogenetics of Lung Cancer: Genetic Susceptibility in the Etiology of Lung Cancer** *141*
John J. Mulvihill and Allen E. Bale

Chapter 12 **Trends in Histologic Types of Lung Cancer, SEER, 1973-1981** *153*
Constance Percy, John W. Horm, and Thomas E. Goffman

Chapter 13 **Screening for Lung Cancer: The Mayo Lung Project** *161*
Robert S. Fontana and William F. Taylor

Chapter 14 **Lung Cancer in Japan: Effects of Nutrition and Passive Smoking** *175*
Takeshi Hirayama

Chapter 15 **Nutritional Status and Chemoprevention in Relation to Lung Cancer** *197*
Peter Greenwald and William D. DeWys

Chapter 16 **Vitamin A and Lung Cancer in Louisiana** *211*
Barbara Y. Legardeur, Alfredo Lopez-S, and William D. Johnson

Chapter 17 **Prevention of Smoking in Adolescents: Current Perspective on a Social–Behavioral Intervention** *219*
Richard I. Evans

Chapter 18 **The Biology of Lung Cancer vis-à-vis the Emerging New Biotechnology** *229*
Merle Mizell

Chapter 19 **Transforming Genes of Human Lung Carcinomas** *239*
Geoffrey M. Cooper

Chapter 20 **In Vitro Studies of the Biology of Lung Cancer** *247*
Desmond N. Carney, Adi F. Gazdar, Francis Cuttitta, and John D. Minna

Chapter 21 **Radioactivity and Cigarette Smoke** *263*
Thomas H. Winters and Joseph R. DiFranza

Chapter 22 **Lung Cancer Incidence and Type of Cigarette Smoked** *273*
Peter N. Lee

Chapter 23 **Smoking Cessation Programs and Lung Cancer** *285*
Ellen R. Gritz

Chapter 24 **Cancer Prevention and the Smoking, Tobacco, and Cancer Program of the National Cancer Institute** *297*
Joseph W. Cullen

Chapter 25 **Lung Cancer and Smoking: Reflections and Unresolved Issues** *313*
Ernst L. Wynder and Marc T. Goodman

Subject Index *325*

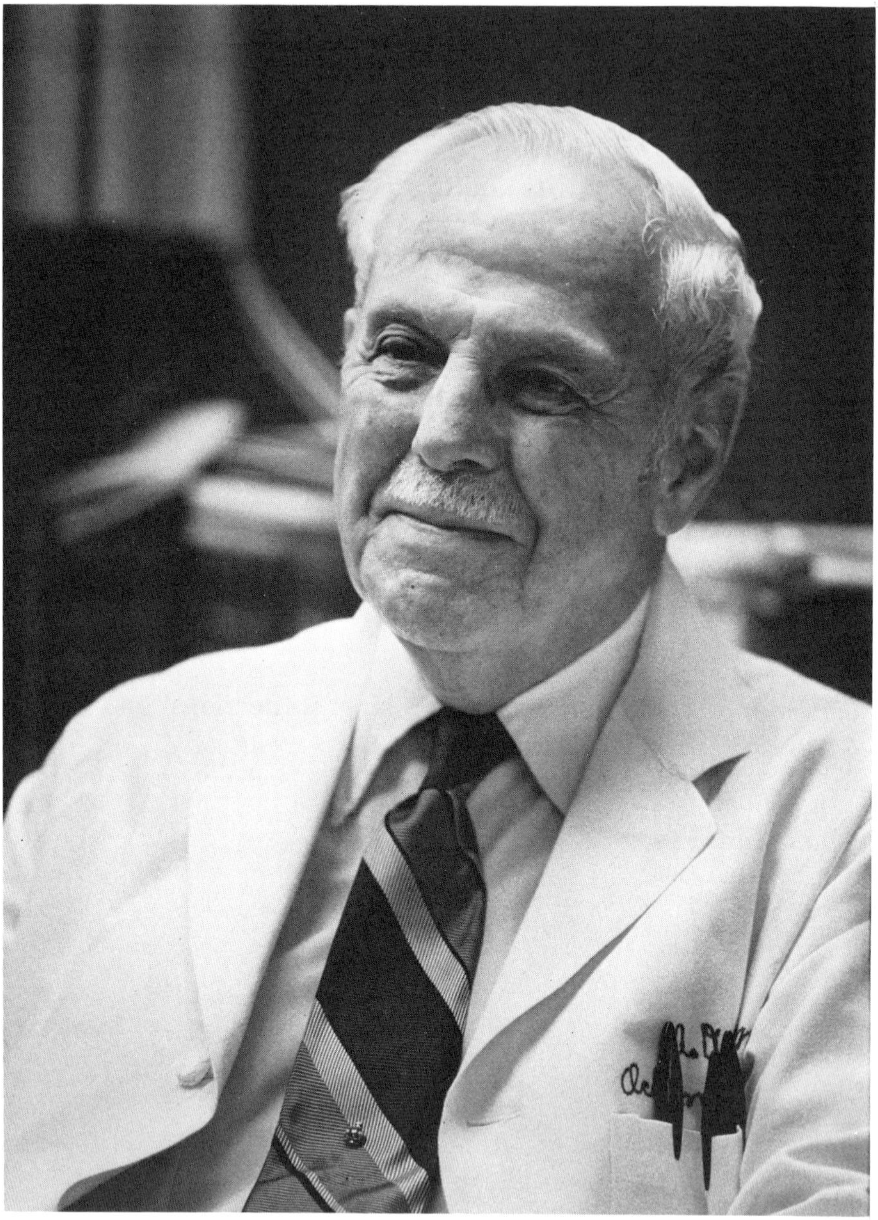

". . . I have probably seen and operated upon more cancer of the lung than anyone else, a condition of which I am not proud because I wish I had never seen a case, as the outlook is still pretty bad." . . . New Orleans, May 29, 1981, Alton Ochsner (1896-1981).

To

Alton Ochsner, MD

It is fitting that this conference is dedicated to my father, Alton Ochsner, since at one time he stood alone in the belief that smoking was a cause of carcinoma of the lung. It was a stand from which he never swayed, despite the criticism he suffered from his colleagues.

My father fought furiously for that which he believed and yet was willing to change if proved wrong. In looking through his bibliography the other day, I came across an editorial he wrote in 1937 in Surgery, Gynecology & Obstetrics, *entitled "Empiricism in Medicine." In this editorial he stated that Galen's teaching that "pus was laudable" was observed empirically for centuries before doctors realized that pus was not laudable. Because of the adherence to Galen's teaching, many died unnecessarily and others bore pain, suffering, and disfiguration beyond belief. The editorial emphasized to me that my father always taught that one must learn and change with time. He first suggested in 1936 that smoking was a cause of cancer of the lung and championed this hypothesis for years, despite the fact that he was ridiculed by some of his peers: at a particular national meeting when he projected a slide which showed the incidence of carcinoma of the lung and sales of cigarettes having a parallel graph, another surgeon imposed on his slide the sales of brassieres to mock his theory.*

Dr. Evarts Graham, his Professor of Surgery at Washington University and who later became as adamant as my father as an antismoking crusader, told my father, "You are going to crucify yourself if you continue to say there is a relationship between cancer of the lung and smoking. The medical profession will think you are nuts." Many years later when Dr. Graham developed cancer of the lung, he wrote to my father and stated that he wished he had listened to him, for had he done so, he would certainly have lived longer.

Although my father was dogmatic in certain spheres, his mind was flexible enough to change when statistics proved him wrong. He championed pneumonectomy as the treatment for cancer of the lung, feeling that in order to have an adequate cancer operation, one had to remove the entire organ. He felt this so strongly that if he performed a minor resection of a lung tumor which at surgery appeared to be benign and yet on histological examination proved to be malignant, he would return the patient to the operating room and do a radical pneumonectomy. When the statistics of Dr. William Overholt showed that treatment of cancer of the lung was equally as good with lobectomy as with pneumonectomy, Dad was prompt in changing his teaching and accepted lobectomy as the principal means of eradicating cancer of the lung.

People remember this man as a scholar, innovator, teacher, and exceptional civic leader.

John Ochsner, MD, Chairman
Department of Surgery
Ochsner Clinic

Preface

The main cause of lung cancer is cigarette smoking; about that the scientific work reported in this book leaves no doubt. Approximately 90% of the deaths from lung cancer and almost one-third of the deaths from cancer of all kinds can be traced directly to smoking. In 1982, about 129,000 Americans died from smoking-related cancers, according to estimates from the Office of Smoking of the U.S. Department of Health and Human Services. But cancer is not the only disease smokers have to fear: the habit also causes elevated rates of heart disease.

According to research reported in this volume, about one in four regular cigarette smokers will be killed before their time by the habit. And the magnitude of the problem is greater than usually is realized. Of every 100 healthy young male smokers in England, statistics predict that one will die a victim of violent crime, two will be killed in traffic accidents, and 25 will die from a disease brought about by cigarettes. Similar proportions of deaths will occur in the United States. Women are quickly gaining equality with men in the lung cancer arena: in 1982, lung cancer surpassed breast cancer as the leading cause of cancer deaths among women in eight states. The pattern, which is believed to be nationwide, is attributed to an increase in smoking which began among women 30 years ago.

The cost for smokers is high in terms of dollars as well as health. In Louisiana, where 2,100 persons die every year from lung cancer, more than $300 million annually are spent on the purchase of cigarettes and medical costs and loss of earnings account for approximately $586 million per year. The state—especially its southern area—has one of the highest cancer rates in the nation, and many of the studies in this volume look at some of the reasons.

Several papers demonstrate that smoking no longer can be considered a personal habit concerning only smokers. Passive smoking—smoke inhaled from nearby smokers—increases the lung cancer rate. Research conducted in Japan has demonstrated that nonsmoking wives of heavy smokers suffer a lung cancer risk at least twice as great as nonsmoking wives of nonsmoking husbands. Research has also shown that radioactive materials are a common component of cigarette smoke. Other studies in the book explore the relationships of nutrition, smoking, and lung cancer: a precursor of vitamin A that comes from green and yellow vegetables can perhaps lower cancer risks. Smoking can work synergistically with occupational exposure to cancer-inducing agents to increase dramatically the risk of lung cancer. Studies have shown that some individuals may have genetic factors that make them more susceptible to certain environmental carcinogens.

Cigarette smoking is a form of drug dependence because nicotine is an addiction-causing drug. And cigarette smoking is *known* to cause cancer. The addiction to this toxic drug produces many times more deaths than addictions to marijuana, morphine, and cocaine combined. Yet those drugs are illegal. Why then, one may ask, are cigarettes advertised and sold all over the world? When cigarette addiction began about 60 years ago, its deleterious effects on health were not known because smoking-induced cancers can take as long as 30 years to develop. Now, cigarettes are a multibillion dollar industry with extremely well-organized lobbies and advertising efforts. Well over $1 billion each year are spent on efforts to promote this addictive and deadly drug; that sum is more than the total budget of the National Cancer Institute.

What can be done? Some of the research in this volume explores the alternatives. Abolishing smoking, of course, is unrealistic, but other efforts hold promise. Reducing tar in cigarettes may, over the years, reduce cancer rates, but in absolute numbers, lung cancer deaths are likely to go on increasing well into the twenty-first century due to saturation marketing efforts and increases in absolute numbers of smokers. Public education efforts about the deadly effects of smoking are inadequate at the present time and could be made much more effective. And legislation—with higher taxes—can make a difference. In Finland ambitious new laws were enacted in 1977: these laws prohibited advertising and sales promotion of cigarettes; forbade smoking in all public places except in designated areas; outlawed the sale of tobacco products to persons under 16 years of age; reserved money from tobacco tax revenue for developing health-oriented government tobacco policy; and made the government responsible for establishing the limits of harmful components in tobacco products. Finland now leads the world in reducing lung cancer deaths, especially in younger individuals.

The best way to change smoking patterns, which would automatically affect lung cancer occurrence, is to convince young people never to begin smoking. Parents must be aware of their responsibilities as role models and schools should make a health education program emphasizing the hazards of smoking a part of instruction from kindergarten through college.

The college students from Tulane's Chapter of Alpha Epsilon Delta, recognizing the hazards of smoking, helped with various phases of the conference and continue to sponsor antismoking activities. In fact, plans for this book began when Alton Ochsner became an honorary member of AED (the National Pre-Medical Honor Society). We were seated around a banquet table in a New Orleans garden district restaurant when the International Lung Cancer Update Conference was first discussed. Dr. Ochsner planned to present a short history of lung cancer at the conference, for as he told us ". . . . . this disease has grown up with me. It did not exist when I was a medical student." Unfortunately Alton Ochsner died before the conference convened, so this volume lacks his historical perspective. Nevertheless, this book is dedicated to the memory of Alton Ochsner and we were pleased to have his son, John Ochsner, participate in his stead. We gratefully acknowledge the continuing aid of the student members of AED and their antismoking efforts; as well as the help of Diana Pinckley, Director of Tulane University Relations, and her efficient staff for their aid in cover design and various aspects of production. The organizers of the conference are especially indebted to Lorraine Mizell, whose untiring work helped make the meeting a success and whose continuing efforts and administrative expertise helped produce this monograph.

The conclusion is clear: cigarette smoking causes lung cancer. If scientists and concerned citizens can communicate that simple message to the public, the cigarette advertising salvos and lobbying efforts may all be for naught. There will then be hope of controlling this disease.

Merle Mizell, PhD
Pelayo Correa, MD

Acknowledgments

I speak on behalf of Tulane Medical Center when I say that we are pleased and proud that Tulane University has served as one of the cosponsoring universities of this International Lung Cancer Update Conference.

It is fitting that this monograph be dedicated to the memory of Alton Ochsner, MD, an honorary alumnus of Tulane School of Medicine. He served on the Tulane faculty for many years as professor and chairman of surgery, prior to establishing along with four other Tulane department heads what has become the Alton Ochsner Medical Foundation. Dr. Ochsner, an internationally known surgeon, dedicated his life to the elimination of lung cancer.

We have come far in the battle against lung cancer, but there is still much more we can learn about the etiology, prevention, treatment, and ultimately the elimination of lung cancer as a significant cause of human suffering. It is through participation in cooperative efforts such as this international conference that we hope to provide an exchange of information which will lead to even more answers about lung cancer.

John J. Walsh, MD, Chancellor
Tulane University Medical Center

I am glad to acknowledge the success of the joint efforts of our institutions: Louisiana State University, Tulane University, Cancer Association of Greater New Orleans, and the Board of Regents in organizing and carrying out the International Lung Cancer Update Conference.

The conference addressed an issue of great importance to our community and provided up-to-date presentations by some of the best international experts in the field. The conference has already stimulated important discussions in our scientific community and has established an objective scientific basis to approach the lung cancer problem in our state. I hope the impetus provided by the conference will continue until a strategy for prevention is developed.

Paul F. Larson, MD, Dean
Louisiana State University
School of Medicine in New Orleans

The Louisiana Board of Regents and its Advisory Committee on Research and Development are pleased to have had the opportunity to sponsor the International Lung Cancer Update Conference. The state of Louisiana, its citizens, and its institutions of higher learning are all beneficiaries of this meeting.

As a result of bringing the world's authorities on lung cancer research together in New Orleans to present and exchange research findings about the state of the art in this field, the world has seen that Louisiana is seriously concerned about this dread disease and intends to promote scientific research in order to address this problem. Therefore the state's image with the scientific community has been enhanced worldwide.

Louisiana's citizens have benefited from this conference because they received the most current and reputable advice from the foremost experts in the field about what they can do to enhance their chances of living lung-cancer-free lives. They learned that this disease is largely self-inflicted.

Finally the scholars, scientists, and medical practitioners in Louisiana's institutions of higher learning, as well as the scientific community outside our colleges and universities, have benefited from the opportunity to exchange information with, ask questions of, and interact with the experts who participated in this conference.

The International Lung Cancer Update Conference was a tremendous success, and we at the Board of Regents are extremely pleased to have been a part of it.

William Arceneaux, PhD
Commissioner of Higher Education
Louisiana Board of Regents

Sponsoring a conference is an uncommon event for the Louisiana Board of Regents' Research and Development Program. Generally only research projects which address issues that are of particular concern to the state (eg, hazardous waste, economic development, wetlands, the state's high incidence of cancer) are supported with these state-appropriated funds. Since one of the goals of this program, however, is to upgrade the quality of research in Louisiana's institutions of higher learning, the Board of Regents and its Advisory Committee on Research and Development decided that sponsorship of this conference not only was appropriate, but also would be a decided investment in the future of quality cancer research in the state.

In sponsoring this conference, the state provided its scientists a rare and perhaps unique opportunity to learn from and exchange ideas with the world's foremost authorities in the lung cancer field in a convenient location and forum. The knowledge and information the state's scientists gleaned as a result of this conference should stimulate interest in this area, as well as promote the submission of research applications to the R&D Program that are at the forefront of knowledge in this field.

The response to this conference from the Louisiana scientific and medical communities was overwhelmingly positive. The Board of Regents was fortunate that the organizers of the conference were responsible and talented individuals who undertook this task in a serious and dedicated manner. Their hard work and combined talents, in conjunction with the outstanding speakers and excellent scientific presentations, made the conference an unequivocal success. On behalf of the Board of Regents and its Advisory Committee on Research and Development, we thank these individuals for their contributions not only to the R&D Program but also to the continued advancement of knowledge in this state.

Priscilla Kilcrease, PhD, Director
Research and Development Program
Louisiana Board of Regents

The Board of Directors and staff of the Cancer Association of Louisiana, Inc, and the Cancer Association of Greater New Orleans, Inc, a United Way agency, are very proud to have been involved in the planning and coordination of the International Lung Cancer Update Conference held March 3-5, 1983.

Many of the papers presented in the monograph reviewed the smoking habits and the epidemiologic trends in lung cancer incidence and mortality in the United States, Europe, and Japan. They all repeatedly emphasized the importance of cigarette smoking as the major causative factor in lung cancer.

Environmental hazards (eg, air pollution and asbestos) and host factors (eg, genetics and nutrition) play a small role in the overall etiology of lung cancer. The most important conclusion of the International Lung Cancer Update Conference is that an international emphasis should be placed on smoking cessation programs aimed not only at high-risk adult populations but more importantly at all adolescents.

The only rational approach is to prevent lung cancer by getting individuals to either stop smoking or never to start to smoke cigarettes.

Robert G. Weilbaecher, MD, President
Cancer Association of Greater New Orleans, Inc
Cancer Association of Louisiana, Inc

With the high incidence of lung cancer in Louisiana, it was very appropriate for New Orleans to be selected as the host city for the International Lung Cancer Update Conference. The Cancer Association of Louisiana and the Cancer Association of Greater New Orleans are glad to cosponsor a conference that brings together some of the world's lung cancer experts.

Personally, I have appreciated the opportunity to be involved in a program that could help resolve some of the health problems of Louisiana's citizens.

Ruth A. Sherwood, Executive Director
Cancer Association of Greater New Orleans, Inc
Cancer Association of Louisiana, Inc

Contributors

Electra D. Avlon
Department of Family and Community Medicine
The University of Utah
50 North Medical Drive
Salt Lake City, Utah 84132

Allen E. Bale
Clinical Epidemiology Branch
National Cancer Institute
Landow Building 5A21
Bethesda, Maryland 20205

John W. Berg, MD
Department of Pathology
University of Colorado School of Medicine
4200 East Ninth Avenue
Denver, Colorado 80262

William J. Blot, PhD
Environmental Epidemiology Branch
National Cancer Institute
Landow Building C309
Bethesda, Maryland 20205

Patricia A. Buffler, PhD
Epidemiology Research Unit
The University of Texas
Health Science Center at Houston
P.O. Box 20186
Houston, Texas 77025

Desmond N. Carney, MD
National Cancer Institute
Navy Medical Oncology Branch
Naval Hospital
Bethesda, Maryland 20814

Roger R. Connelly, MSc
Biometry Branch
National Cancer Institute
Landow Building 5C19
Bethesda, Maryland 20205

Charles Contant, MS
Epidemiology Research Unit
The University of Texas Health Science Center at Houston
School of Public Health
P.O. Box 20186
Houston, Texas 77025

Geoffrey M. Cooper, PhD
Dana-Farber Cancer Institute
and Department of Pathology
Harvard Medical School
Boston, Massachusetts 02115

Pelayo Correa, MD
Department of Pathology
Louisiana State University Medical Center
New Orleans, Louisiana 70112

Joseph W. Cullen, PhD
Division of Resources, Centers and Community Activities
National Cancer Institute
Building 31, Room 4A32
Bethesda, Maryland 20205

Francis Cuttitta, PhD
National Cancer Institute
Navy Medical Oncology Branch
Naval Hospital
Bethesda, Maryland 20814

Nancy Dalager
Environmental Epidemiology Branch
National Cancer Institute
Landow Building 3C15
Bethesda, Maryland 20205

Susan S. Devesa, PhD
Biometry Branch
National Cancer Institute
Landow Building 5C19
Bethesda, Maryland 20205

William D. DeWys, MD
Division of Cancer Prevention and Control
National Cancer Institute
Bethesda, Maryland 20205

Joseph R. DiFranza, MD
Department of Family and Community Medicine
University of Massachusetts Medical Center
55 Lake Avenue North
Worcester, Massachusetts 01605

Sir Richard Doll, FRS, FRCP
ICRF Cancer Epidemiology and Clinical Trials Unit
Radcliffe Infirmary
Oxford, OX2 6HE
United Kingdom

Richard I. Evans, PhD
Social Psychology/Behavioral Medicine Research and Graduate Training Group
University of Houston
Houston, Texas 77004

Robert S. Fontana, MD
Department of Medicine
Mayo Medical School
Rochester, Minnesota 55905

Elizabeth Fontham, PhD
Department of Pathology
Louisiana State University Medical Center
New Orleans, Louisiana 70112

John W. Gardner, MD, Dr PH
Department of Family and Community Medicine
The University of Utah
50 North Medical Drive
Salt Lake City, Utah 84132

Adi F. Gazdar
National Cancer Institute
Navy Medical Oncology Branch
Naval Hospital
Bethesda, Maryland 20814

Thomas E. Goffman, MD
Biometry Branch
National Cancer Institute
Landow Building 5B06
Bethesda, Maryland 20205

Marc T. Goodman
American Health Foundation
320 East 43rd Street
New York, New York 10017

Peter Greenwald, MD
Division of Cancer Prevention and Control
National Cancer Institute
Bethesda, Maryland 20205

Ellen R. Gritz, PhD
Macomber-Murphy Cancer Prevention Program
Division of Cancer Control
Jonsson Comprehensive Cancer Center
University of California
Los Angeles, California 90024

William Haenszel, DrPH(Honr)
Illinois Cancer Council
36 Wabash Avenue
Chicago, Illinois 60603

Takeshi Hirayama, MD
Epidemiology Division
National Cancer Center Research Institute
Tsukiji 5-chome, Chuo-ku
Tokyo 104, Japan

John W. Horm, MSc
Biometry Branch
National Cancer Institute
Landow Building 5C19
Bethesda, Maryland 20205

William D. Johnson, MS
Department of Biometry
Louisiana State University Medical Center
New Orleans, Louisiana 70112

Peter N. Lee, MA
Independent Consultant in Statistics and Epidemiology
25 Cedar Road
Sutton, SM2 5DG
United Kingdom

Barbara Y. Legardeur, MPH
Department of Medicine
Louisiana State University Medical Center
New Orleans, Louisiana 70112

Youping Lin
Department of Pathology
Louisiana State University
Medical Center
New Orleans, Louisiana 70112

Alfredo Lopez-S, MD, PhD
Department of Medicine
Louisiana State University
Medical Center
New Orleans, Louisiana 70112

Joseph L. Lyon, MD, MPH
Utah Cancer Registry
Department of Family and
Community Medicine
The University of Utah
50 North Medical Drive
Salt Lake City, Utah 84132

Thomas J. Mason, PhD
Environmental Epidemiology
Branch
National Cancer Institute
Landow Building 3C15
Bethesda, Maryland 20205

John D. Minna, MD
National Cancer Institute
Navy Medical Oncology Branch
Naval Hospital
Bethesda, Maryland 20814

Merle Mizell, PhD
Laboratory of Tumor Cell Biology
Biology Department
Tulane University
New Orleans, Louisiana 70118

John J. Mulvihill, MD
Clinical Epidemiology Branch
National Cancer Institute
Landow Building 5A21
Bethesda, Maryland 20205

Constance Percy, MS
Biometry Branch
National Cancer Institute
Landow Building 5B06
Bethesda, Maryland 20205

Richard Peto, MA, MSc
Cancer Studies Unit
Radcliffe Infirmary
Oxford, OX2 6HE
United Kingdom

Linda Williams Pickle, PhD
Population Studies Section
Environmental Epidemiology
Branch
National Cancer Institute
Landow Building 3C15
Bethesda, Maryland 20205

Carl M. Shy, MD
Department of Epidemiology
School of Public Health
The University of North Carolina
at Chapel Hill
Chapel Hill, North Carolina 27514

William F. Taylor, PhD
Department of Biostatistics
Mayo Medical School
Rochester, Minnesota 55905

Lyly Teppo, MD
Finnish Cancer Registry
Liisankatu 21 B
SF-00170 Helsinki 17,
Finland

Thomas H. Winters, MD
Department of General
Internal Medicine
University of Massachusetts
Medical Center
55 Lake Avenue North
Worcester, Massachusetts 01605

Ernst L. Wynder, MD
American Health Foundation
320 East 43rd Street
New York, New York 10017

CHAPTER 1

Keynote Address: The Control of Lung Cancer[1]

RICHARD PETO and RICHARD DOLL

Cancer Studies Unit, Radcliffe Infirmary, Oxford OX2 6HE, Great Britain
ICRF Cancer Epidemiology and Clinical Trials Unit, Radcliffe Infirmary, Oxford OX2 6HE, Great Britain

ABSTRACT

During the 1980s, about 1 million Americans and 2 million Europeans are likely to die of tobacco-induced lung cancer, and there is increasingly heavy marketing of manufactured cigarettes in developing countries. This will produce large increases in lung cancer in the next century. These increases are inevitable, just as the increases in United States cigarette usage 40 and more years ago are responsible for the large increases in United States lung cancer rates today. This increased usage overwhelms the beneficial effects of cigarette tar level reductions. By contrast, in Britain and Finland male lung cancer rates in middle age had already stabilized before the large tar reductions began, and in early middle age the male lung cancer death rates have already halved, and are still dropping fast. Unless recent tar reductions have implausibly large adverse effects on vascular or respiratory disease, they have perhaps been underrated as practical public health measures. (United States and United Kingdom tar reductions still can be accelerated, and at present many other countries lag well behind.)

Although the control of fossil fuel combustion products, ionizing radiations, asbestos, and other occupational factors is certainly worthwhile, it cannot avoid any substantial fraction of lung cancer deaths, and although substantially protective nutritional modifications may exist, none has yet been reliably identified. Meanwhile, recent European experience shows that governments can, if they wish, achieve substantial reductions in both tar deliveries and cigarette usage without materially affecting personal freedoms, and unless one or both of these are achieved in many different countries there is little prospect of avoiding any substantial fraction of the many millions of lung cancer deaths that threaten to occur over the next few decades.

Key Words: **Lung cancer prevention, cigarette sales trends, cigarette tar reduction, lung cancer trends, smoking duration, quantitative information, cigarette-lung cancer international correlation, cigarette taxation, tobacco price increases**

[1]This article is expanded from a report prepared for the WHO Cancer Unit, but it does not necessarily reflect the views of the WHO or of its Cancer Unit.

Lung Cancer: Causes and Prevention.

For the control of each type of cancer, three strategies are available—prevention, screening (early detection), and treatment. Over the past few decades cancer research has produced (or suggested) some important results in all three areas. These include, for example, the effects of hepatitis B virus on the risk of liver cancer, of lower tar cigarettes on the risk of lung cancer, of screening on the prognosis of cervical cancer, and of cytotoxic drugs on the treatment of Hodgkin disease. It therefore is reasonable to be optimistic about, but impossible to predict reliably, what cancer research will produce over the next few decades.

If, however, we consider the promise not of what future research may one day offer but of what present-day knowledge can already offer, then the most practicable, and cost-effective, opportunities for avoiding premature death from cancer probably involve not screening or improved treatment, but prevention, and this is particularly true of lung cancer.

This conclusion does not involve the unrealistic assumption that tobacco can be eliminated: instead, it merely assumes that cigarette sales can be somewhat reduced (eg, by politically realistic price changes, or by the type of education that already appears to have had a substantial effect on white-collar cigarette usage), that the tar delivery per cigarette can likewise be somewhat reduced, and that gross occupational exposures (eg, to levels of asbestos far higher than are nowadays permissible in, for example, the United States) can be avoided. Nor does this conclusion involve the assumption that lung cancer is already a major health problem everywhere, for it applies not only in countries where cigarette smoking has been widespread for decades (eg, the United States, where lung cancer already accounts for some 25–30% of all cancer deaths) but also in countries in which cigarette smoking has become widespread only in recent decades (eg, China, where lung cancer as yet accounts for only about 5–10% of all cancer deaths). This is because the main rise in lung cancer produced by cigarettes may take as much as half a century to materialize, so countries where cigarette smoking is only now becoming or has only recently become widespread can expect large increases in lung cancer during the 1990s or early in the next century unless effective action against the health effects of tobacco can be achieved.

The reasons that the prevention of lung cancer is of such overwhelming importance are, first, that the disease is extremely common[2]; second, that it is

[2]The types of cancer that cause most deaths worldwide are cancers of the lung and of the stomach. Recent International Agency for Research on Cancer/WHO joint estimates (1) suggest that by 1975 the annual number of new cases of lung cancer was already about 0.6 million (developed "west," 0.3 million; developed "east," 0.1 million; China and rest of "third" world, 0.2 million), a total similar to that for stomach cancer. For both diseases, about 90% of affected patients are likely to die. However, whereas in most countries stomach cancer rates are either steady or decreasing, lung cancer rates are (with a few interesting exceptions that may result from cigarette tar delivery reductions) either steady or increasing. So, during the 1980s lung cancer will account for more deaths than any other type of cancer; indeed, the annual number of lung cancer deaths is probably already, in the early 1980s, about two-thirds of a million, and it may well exceed a million by the end of the century.

[3]Even with expensive high-technology support, current surgical management of lung cancer cures only about 10% of all cases, and although this percentage is sufficient to justify the widespread use of surgery (at least in developed countries), it is small, has shown little change in recent decades, and is hardly improved at all by the addition of any other current modes of therapy.

generally incurable[3]; third, that effective preventive measures are already reliably known[4]; and last, that implementation of these measures will also have a substantial impact on many other diseases[5].

Consequently, what will follow is a description not of early detection or treatment, but only of the preventability of lung cancer, where chief emphasis must inevitably be on the effects of smoking, either alone or in combination with other causative factors. There already have been many excellent reviews of the effects of tobacco on lung cancer (and, of course, on many other diseases), and of the prospects of controlling the smoking epidemic (2). Therefore, the present text is intended not as a balanced (and repetitious) account of the whole problem, but as a discussion centering on those particular aspects of the relationship between smoking and lung cancer that commonly engender important misunderstandings, and of those particular aspects of prevention that commonly are underemphasized.

For a comprehensive review of the overall health effects of tobacco, the U.S. Surgeon-General's 1979 report (3) may be consulted [although for a description of the effects of tobacco just on cancer the Surgeon-General's 1982 report (4) is much to be preferred]. For a review of the overall epidemiology of cancer in developed countries, the report of Doll and Peto (5) may be consulted, especially as Appendix E reviews in some detail the effects of past changes in tobacco usage and recent changes in cigarette tar deliveries on lung cancer trends. Finally, for reviews of practical steps toward the avoidance of smoking, in addition to the United States Surgeon-General's 1979 report (3), the UICC (6), World Health Organization (2) and Ontario Council on Health (7) reports are invaluable.

Epidemiology of Smoking and Lung Cancer

The Need for Prolonged Exposure

There are a few key features of the effects of tobacco on lung cancer that are slightly counterintuitive, and these are discussed at some length by Doll and Peto (5). Chief among them, and the key to any proper understanding of tobacco carcinogenesis, is the extraordinary relevance of the *duration* of smoking to lung cancer onset rates. For example, after 45, 30, and 15 years of cigarette smoking, the excess annual incidence rates of lung cancer may be about 0.5%, 0.1% and under

[4]The most effective step is to avoid increases, or to produce decreases, in cigarette consumption, but changes in the harmfulness of cigarettes also may help. There may be considerable political difficulties in taking any actions that will affect cigarette consumption substantially, but it is nevertheless likely that some such actions will be practicable in at least some countries over the next few years. Moreover, substantial decreases in the sales-weighted mean tar deliveries of manufactured cigarettes are likely to be politically practicable in many countries, as they have little economic impact on governments, growers, manufacturers, advertisers, media, retailers, or consumers.

[5]Tobacco is also an important cause of various less common types of cancer, eg, of the mouth, pharynx, larynx, and esophagus, and probably also of the pancreas and urinary tract. More importantly, at least in developed countries such as Britain, tobacco probably kills more people from respiratory and vascular disease than from cancer.

0.01%, respectively (Table 1). The annual lung cancer incidence rates to be expected among smokers may be estimated by adding up a background (nonsmoker) rate, which, like the onset rates of many other types of cancer, depends strongly on age (but not, of course, on tobacco exposure), plus an excess rate, which depends

Table 1. Approximate[a] effects of various durations of cigarette smoking on annual incidence of lung cancer

Years of cigarette smoking	Annual excess incidence: Moderate smokers %	Annual excess incidence: Heavy smokers %
15	0.005	0.01
30	0.1	0.2
45	0.5	1
(60)	(1.5?)	(3?)

[a]Estimated from data reported by Doll and Peto (8) for male British doctors. The cumulative risks would be far greater than these annual risks, of course, so an eventual total of over 10% of regular cigarette smokers may die of tobacco-induced cancer, depending on the number and type of cigarettes smoked.

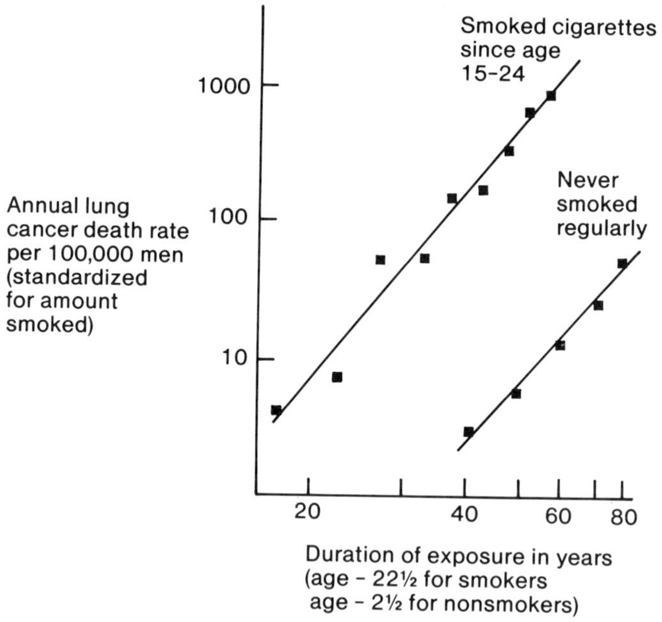

Figure 1. Background and excess risks: lung cancer death rates among (a) non-smokers (lower line) in relation to age, and (b) regular cigarette smokers (upper line) in relation to approximate years of smoking. From Ref. (9). These two lines can be used directly to indicate the approximate background and excess risks, for in middle and old age the lung cancer incidence rates among people who have smoked cigarettes throughout adult life greatly exceed the rates among nonsmokers of similar age. (This might not, however, be true for people who did not begin to smoke substantial numbers of cigarettes until middle age, for the background and the excess annual risks per 100,000 men indicated by these lines are, respectively, approximately 10^{-6} times the fourth power of years of age 10^{-4} times the fourth power times years of regular cigarette smoking.)

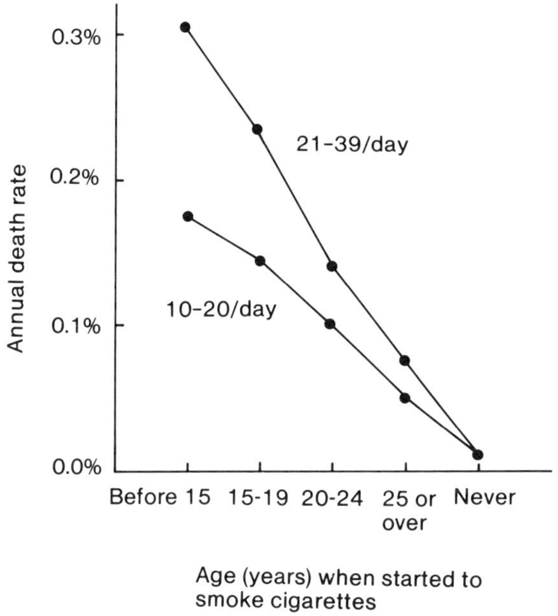

Figure 2. The relevance of smoking in early adult life: relationship, in prospective survey data of regular smokers, between the age when regular cigarette smoking began in early adult life and lung cancer death rates at age 55-64 (mean = age 60) for United States males. From Ref. (5). Data are presented separately for heavy and for moderate smokers.

strongly on duration of regular tobacco exposure (but not otherwise, at least to a first approximation, on age). Typical background and excess rates for males are depicted in Figure 1 (9), and those for females may be about two-thirds as great.

The most surprising consequence of the overwhelming effects of the duration of smoking is illustrated, using real data[6], in Figure 2, which shows how strongly the annual excess risk of death from lung cancer at 60 years of age depends on whether men started smoking at 15 or at 25 years of age (ie, on whether by the age of 60 they had smoked for 45, or for only 35, years). Failure to appreciate the relationship illustrated in Figure 2 has led to a variety of unjustifiable conclusions, eg, that cigarettes do not cause lung cancer or, less perversely, that low-tar cigarettes have at least as great an effect as high-tar ones (10); that air pollution is of comparable importance to tobacco [see, however, Cederlöf et al (11)]; or that new causes of lung cancer (rather than the delayed effects of past changes in tobacco usage) are chiefly responsible for the rapid increases in lung cancer in recent years. In each case the point that often is overlooked is that current patterns of lung cancer mortality rates in late middle age or in old age depend strongly not only on current patterns of tobacco usage, but also on the patterns of cigarette usage among young adults as much as half a century ago.

[6]The data utilized are from the third largest prospective survey yet reported and are similar to the findings in the larger two surveys; the corresponding results from all three of these surveys are presented in the U.S. Surgeon-General's 1982 report (4).

Therefore, current trends, current urban/rural differences, and current international differences in lung cancer reflect, among other things, past trends, past urban/rural differences, and past international differences in cigarette usage by young adults. Consider, for example, the extent to which current trends in United States lung cancer mortality rates among men now aged 70 may be affected by the large trends in cigarette consumption 50 years ago among people then aged 20 (5). (For details, see Appendix E of Doll and Peto, (7). In 1930, United States cigarette consumption was increasing rapidly among young men, and national sales rose from 1 cigarette per adult a day in 1915 to about 10 per adult a day in 1945. The effects of those increases are only now becoming fully apparent, and largely as a very long delayed result of them, United States male lung cancer rates in late middle and old age are still rising steeply, despite the fact that cigarette sales per adult have remained at approximately 10–12 a day ever since 1945, and that tar levels per cigarette have fallen substantially (Figure 3). Contrary to various suggestions, the "discrepancy" that has been seen for the past 25 years in the United States between rising lung cancer rates (see Figure 4) and falling tar levels does not imply, or even suggest, that Americans are exposed to increasing levels of carcinogenic pollutants other than tobacco, or, as the recent (10) National Academy of Sciences–National Research Council (NAS–NRC) report suggested, that tar level reductions in cigarettes have been ineffective. Indeed, but for tar-level reductions, the current increases in United States lung cancer mortality rates probably would be appreciably more rapid.

Likewise, in many countries the smoking of manufactured cigarettes by young adults was a habit that tended to become established first in the towns before it spread to the surrounding countryside, rather than the converse. Consequently,

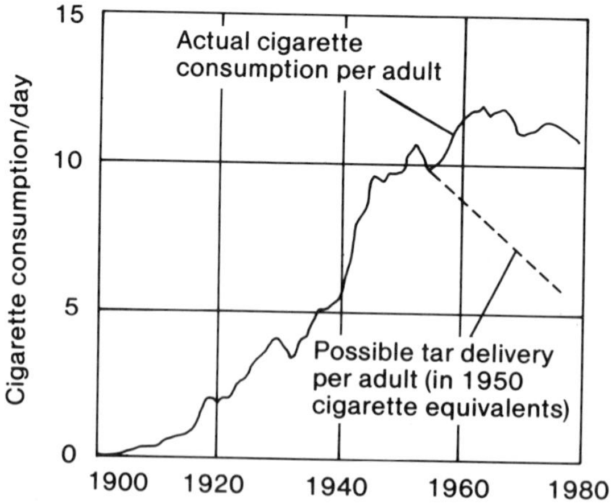

Figure 3. Trends in United States consumption: mean daily sales of manufactured cigarettes per United States adult aged over 18 years, together with a crude estimate of tar yield per adult. From Ref. (5). The estimate of tar yield allows approximately for decreases since the 1950s in tar yield per cigarette smoked in a standard manner, but not for any systematic changes in the manner in which cigarettes are smoked.

half a century ago cigarette smoking was probably more prevalent among young men in towns than among young men in the country. Disparities in recent years between urban and rural lung cancer rates among today's old smokers therefore may result chiefly not from air pollution but from a delayed effect of past urban–rural differences in cigarette usage among the people who were then young but who are now old.

Finally, it is wholly wrong to suggest that the poor international correlation between current smoking habits and current lung cancer rates indicates that smoking is not the chief determinant of worldwide lung cancer mortality. For, such a correlation effectively relates the lung cancer rates of the grandparents to the smoking habits of their grandchildren. If instead the national lung cancer rates for one generation are related to national cigarette consumption rates when that generation were young adults, a moderately close relationship does emerge (Figure 5).

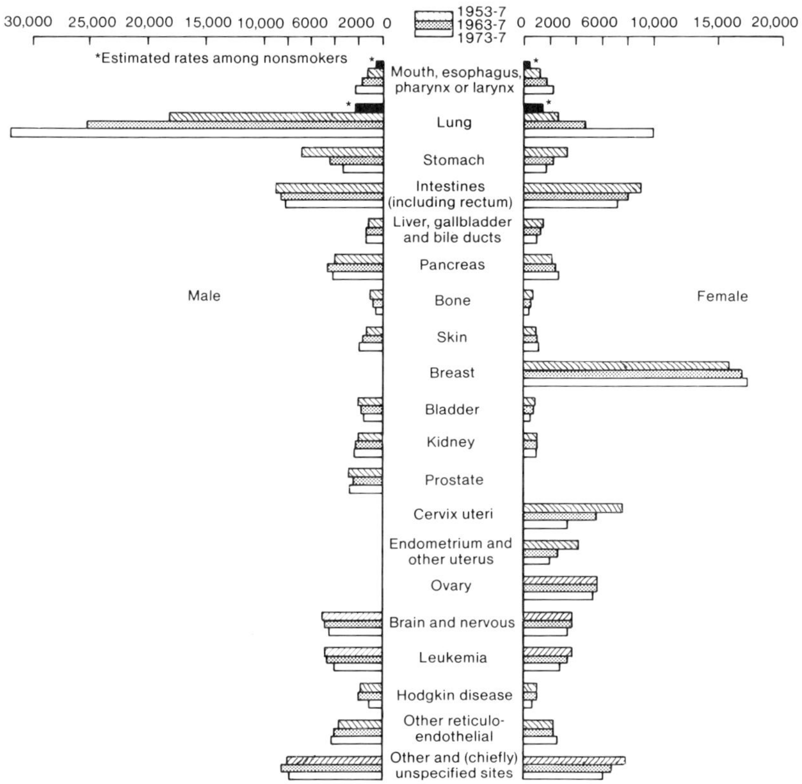

Figure 4. Recent trends in United States cancer mortality rates: age-standardized death certification rate (per 100 million people aged under 65) in the 1950s (top bar), the 1960s (middle bar) and the 1970s (bottom bar) for various types of cancer in the United States. From Ref (5). For cancers of the lung and upper respiratory and digestive tracts, estimated rates for lifelong nonsmokers are also given (asterisked bar, above the rates for the 1950s).

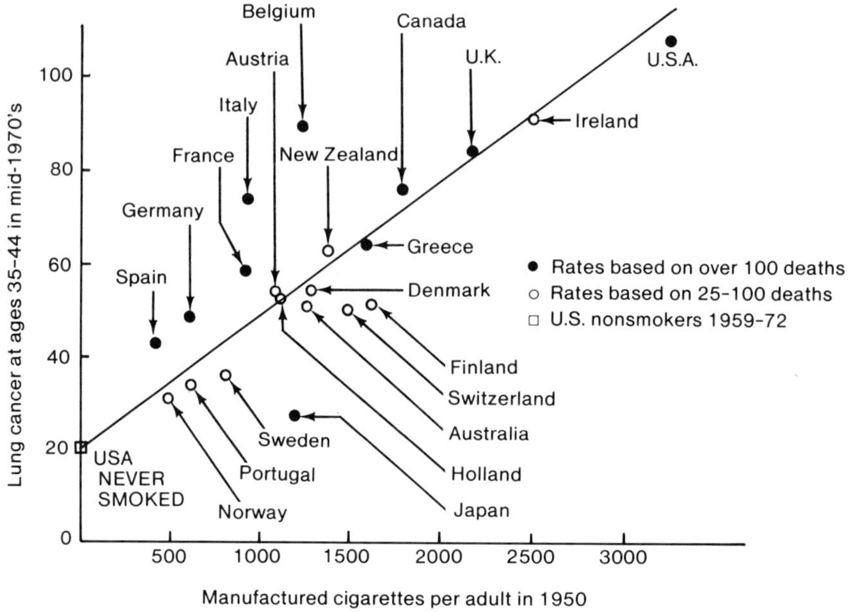

Figure 5. Lung cancer and smoking in the same generation: relationship between lung cancer mortality (mean of male and female rates) for one generation in early middle age with manufactured (excludes handrolled cigarettes in Belgium and smuggled cigarettes in Italy) cigarette consumption when that generation of people were in early adult life: data for various countries, and for US non-smokers estimated by fitting a power-law relationship to the prospective survey data reported by the American Cancer Society (25).

Other Features

Dose-Response Relationships

In Table 1, it may be seen that doubling the dose may approximately double the excess risk at each age. Partly because of difficulties of dosimetry[7], it is not really known whether, as Doll and Peto have tentatively suggested (8), a doubling of the true dose rate produces an approximately fourfold increase in the age-specific effect, or whether, as is suggested by much other data, it merely produces a twofold increase. Whatever the exact truth, however, it is clear that two packs a day for 20 years is far less hazardous than one pack a day for 40 years, so any reports based on inappropriate concepts such as "pack-years" should be treated warily.

Effects of Stopping Smoking

When smoking ceases, the annual excess risk remains roughly (perhaps to within a factor of two) constant thereafter. Referring to Table 1, it may be seen that the annual excess risk after 30 years of smoking is about 0.1%, so if a smoker stops

[7]The effective dose may not be simply proportional to the number of cigarettes smoked per day, for the CO uptake per cigarette appears to be less for heavy than for moderate smokers. Also, because the chief target area is the main airways, rapid inhalation may deposit less on them than slow inhalation does. This suggestion is reinforced by reports (12) that in some, although not all, studies heavy smokers who describe themselves as "not inhaling" get *more* lung cancer than do comparably heavy smokers who "do inhale"!.

after 30 years, then approximately this annual excess risk may persist indefinitely. Thus, for example, 15 years later the annual excess risk may still be about 0.1% instead of the 0.5% that it would have been had smoking continued, so about 80% of the excess risk is being avoided. It is not true, however, that the annual absolute excess risk decreases substantially, and still less is it true that it decreases to zero after 10 years; only one prospective study has suggested that, and the others clearly refute it. But, the large increases in risk that would otherwise happen are avoided by stopping smoking.

The Importance of Cigarettes as Opposed to Pipes

In Britain and the United States, cigarettes appear to have a far greater effect than pipe or cigar tobacco did, and so the switch earlier this century from pipes to cigarettes has produced vast increases in lung cancer. The reasons for this difference are not adequately known, especially as the smoke from pipes and cigars is about as carcinogenic as that from cigarettes for laboratory animals. One suggestion is that the difference depends chiefly on the greater alkalinity of the smoke from pipes and cigars, which may both make inhalation less pleasant and facilitate the transport of nicotine across the oral mucosa, thereby obviating the need to inhale (13, 14). This suggestion may not be difficult to test and, if confirmed, may point to an important way of diminishing the hazards of cigarettes, but at present this remains speculative[8]. A related suggestion is that the "air-cured" tobacco of, for example, certain French cigarettes somewhat resembles pipe tobacco and is therefore substantially less carcinogenic than the "flue-cured" tobacco typical of British and American cigarettes, but the international differences in lung cancer on which this suggestion rests owe so much to differences in duration of cigarette smoking that it is still unclear whether there are also any material differences in the hazards of the various cigarettes. (During the 1930s and 1940s, for example, British cigarette consumption was four times that in France.)

Interaction with Other Causative Factors

A variety of other causative factors for lung cancer are known, of which the best studied are asbestos, ionizing radiations, and urban air pollution. All these have a far greater absolute extra effect on smokers than on nonsmokers (illustrated for asbestos in Table 2), as may various other causative factors. Some of the benefits of control of certain other causes of lung cancer therefore may be attainable indirectly by reducing tobacco exposure. However, because effective tobacco exposures are currently increasing in many countries (and even where they are decreasing, the immediate decreases are unlikely to be enormous), the theoretical possibility of avoiding tobacco exposure clearly does not justify inaction where other substantial causes of lung cancer can be reduced materially[9].

[8]In the study of Cederlöf et al (15) in Sweden, pipe smokers had the same tenfold excess of lung cancer that cigarette smokers had, which rather suggests that the smallness of the effects in Britain or the United States may result more from traditions about how pipes are smoked than from the pharmacology of the smoke—and it is unlikely that such traditions will themselves be wholly determined by pharmacologic factors.

[9]Apart from smoking, asbestos, ionizing radiations, and combustion products of fossil fuels, the other reliably established causes of lung cancer are bis(chloromethyl)ether (BCME), mustard gas, and certain compounds or oxidation states of As, Cr, and Ni (5).

Table 2. Multiplicative effects of heavy asbestos exposure and of smoking on lung cancer risks[a]

	Relative risk of lung cancer for:	
	Nonsmokers	Smokers
No known asbestos exposure	1 (reference category)	11
Heavy asbestos exposure (prolonged employment as a lagger before 1968 United States dust controls were introduced)	5	53

[a]Data from Selikoff (16). Note that although such heavy asbestos exposure is no longer permitted in many countries, places where heavy occupational exposures do still occur may offer excellent opportunities for limited disease prevention, because even if the workers do not smoke (so the excess risk of bronchial carcinoma is low), the risk of mesothelioma, which does not depend on synergy with tobacco, will still be high.

Miscertification of Lung Cancer Deaths

People, and especially old people, dying of lung cancer may never have their disease recognized and may be miscertified as dying of some other condition. Progressive rectification of such errors produces large, purely artifactual, increases in lung cancer death certification rates. In middle age such effects were substantial during the first half of the century, even in developed countries—for example, when diagnostic radiology was introduced during the 1920s, it produced about a threefold increase in British lung cancer death *certification* rates—but in middle age such effects are now limited chiefly to underdeveloped countries. In old age, however, large (eg, twofold) artifactual increases have continued to occur since 1950, even in various developed countries, whereas among old people in many underdeveloped countries lung cancer death certification rates are still grossly unreliable [as are "age-standardized" lung cancer death certification rates, unless standardization is to the truncated age range 35–64 recommended by the International Agency for Research on Cancer (IARC), (17) to circumvent such difficulties.]

Tar Deliveries

The effects of changes in tar deliveries need to be properly understood by anyone concerned with the avoidance of cancer, for at least in developed countries they may offer one of the more important cancer control strategies. Between the 1930s and the 1970s there have been reductions of more than 50% in the mean (ie, sales-weighted) tar delivery per cigarette in the United States, Britain, Scandinavia, and a few other places. These changes were small until the late 1950s and then they suddenly became rapid, with decreases from 30-odd mg per cigarette in the mid-1950s down to approximately 15 mg per cigarette by the 1970s. The changes are not expensive and involve the use of filtertips, porous paper (or even, as an extreme measure, "ventilated" filters that allow air to enter into the side of the filter to dilute the smoke) and modified types of tobacco (which may in some instances actually be less expensive than unmodified tobacco). There is, of course, a reduction not only in the unwanted components of the smoke but also in those substances (eg nicotine?) to which some smokers are addicted, and when such reductions occur many smokers are likely to compensate, either by smoking more cigarettes[10] or, perhaps more commonly, by taking in more smoke per cigarette[11]. It appears, however, that the latter form of compensation is not always sufficient to outweigh the reduction in tar (19), in which case the net result will be inhalation of less tar into the lung. This conclusion is suggested both by common sense and by observation, but even if it is accepted it does not prove that the hazards will be correspondingly reduced, for despite some 30 years of laboratory research the importantly carcinogenic factors in cigarette smoke have not yet been identified reliably. Moreover, it is difficult to predict how changed patterns of inhalation will change what is deposited on the main target areas—which, for lung cancer, are not the peripheral tissues, but in the large airways—as the smoke streams past them.

Consequently, it is necessary to discover by direct epidemiologic observation whether the risks of lung cancer are materially reduced by the widespread switch to lower tar cigarettes. Unfortunately this is not easy to do, for not only are smokers of low-tar brands self-selected but also, just as it is only after some decades of smoking that the full risks materialize, so perhaps it is only after some decades of using low-tar cigarettes that the full benefits will materialize. Therefore, even if the effects in late middle age will one day be substantial, they may not yet be. Any substantial effects that are going to materialize in *early* middle age should be beginning to be evident by now in Britain, however, for although the tar reductions of the 1950s were only moderate, those of the 1960s were substantial in Britain, North America and Scandinavia. Thus, a 40 year old in 1980 will have been smoking from about 1960 to 1980, throughout most of which time tar levels were substantially lower than in previous decades.

Two main pieces of epidemiologic evidence are currently available, the first being the results from classical case-control or prospective surveys. Unfortunately, such data as are currently available are limited by the fact that they relate chiefly to late middle or old age, when most of the lung cancers occur, and even recent

[10]In principle, tar reductions could either increase or decrease the number of people who smoke (by making it less of an ordeal for nonsmokers to acquire the habit or by making the habit less addictive) and could either increase or decrease the number of cigarettes one individual smoker consumes (by increasing the number needed to achieve a given dose or by decreasing the satisfaction per cigarette). In practice, however, the patterns of cigarette consumption in different countries do not appear to be influenced consistently in either direction by changes in cigarette consumption.

[11]Surprisingly, there appears to be little reliable information on which of the many characteristics of the cigarette (eg, nicotine, draw resistance, taste) importantly affect "compensation." If these could be identified and modified (eg, by increasing the nicotine delivery, draw resistance, or whatever of low-tar cigarettes), then maybe the intake of many toxins could be decreased simultaneously. Such compensation presumably underlies the recent disappointing finding by Kaufman et al (18) that the risks of myocardial infarction are not materially different among smokers of different types of cigarette.

studies relate chiefly to people who have smoked low-tar cigarettes for only a fraction of their smoking lives. This difficulty is exacerbated in studies performed during the 1960s (or early 1970s) by the fact that the tar reductions then available for study were not only more recent, but also less extreme, than those currently available. A related source of difficulty is that as overall tar levels decrease, the higher tar levels simply cease to exist, so direct concurrent comparison of people now on low-tar cigarettes can be only with people on moderate-tar cigarettes, and not with the old very high tar brands. Despite these difficulties, when Lee and Garfinkel (20) reviewed all the case-control and prospective studies then available they concluded that:

> a reasonably clear picture has emerged. This is that smokers of filter (or low tar/nicotine) cigarettes have a lower mortality than smokers of plain (or high tar/nicotine) cigarettes for those diseases most strongly associated with smoking . . . . These reductions in mortality have been seen in those who have smoked the more modern types of cigarette for only a small part of their smoking lives. The fact that those who have smoked them for longer show even greater reductions in mortality suggests that the overall picture will improve even more in years to come.

Because of difficulties of self-selection, of comparing the new with the old concurrently, and of characterizing individuals' recent lung cancer rates in early middle age (ie, the rates among people who have smoked low-tar cigarettes for much of their adult lives), the case–control and prospective survey data can be supplemented usefully by a second type of epidemiologic data, ie, the study of national trends in early middle age. However, for reasons that already have been discussed, it is not advisable to use for this purpose data (such as those from the United States) in which any downward trends caused by tar reductions are likely to be diluted or even reversed by upward trends resulting from the delayed effects of past increases in tobacco consumption. Instead, it is better to use the British data. For by the 1950s (when the rapid tar decreases began) British male lung cancer rates in early middle age had already approximately stabilized (Table 3). Table 3 also describes their subsequent evolution, and the reductions are extremely impressive. They are most unlikely to result from changes in air pollution, for not only are any effects of air pollution likely to be far smaller than this (11), but also similar halvings in early middle age have been seen over the last 20 years in unpolluted Finland. Moreover, both in Finland and in Britain the changes appear, if anything, to be accelerating downward, so if this pattern carries on into late middle age during the next decade or two, then at least in these two countries (where the male death rates are at present uniquely high) lung cancer may some day decrease for a few years[12] as fast as it once increased.

A final piece of human evidence that tends indirectly to confirm the reality of these changes is provided by a comparison of histologic sections from American

[12]It will not decrease to anywhere near non smoker rates, however, unless there is widespread abandonment of cigarette smoking. Similarly, in those other populations where lung cancer rates have not yet completed their rise, even a tar-level reduction that halves the carcinogenicity of cigarettes may merely slow, rather than reverse, the progressive increase of the disease over the next few decades.

Table 3. Recent trends in England and Wales male lung cancer death certification rates in early middle age[a,b]

	Death certification rates per million men from cancers of the respiratory tract, excluding larynx			
Age (yrs)	**1951–55 (a)**	**1956–60 (b)**	**1980 (c)**	**Ratio (c#b)**
30–4	38[c]	37[c]	13	0.3
35–9	101[c]	95[c]	45	0.5
40–4	253[c]	256[c]	134	0.5
45–9	589[c]	597[c]	378[d]	0.6

[a]Note *both* the approximate constancy before tar deliveries began to be greatly reduced *and* the large decrease thereafter.

[b]Note: (1) These trends are not materially affected by changes in curative treatment of the disease. (2) Sales-weighted tar levels started to fall rapidly only at the end of the 1950s but are now less than half of what they then were. (3) Mean cigarette consumption per British male aged 30-50 did not change greatly until the past few years and in 1955, 1965 and 1975 was respectively, 10.5, 9.9, and 10.2 (21): the 10-20% decrease in consumption that existed in the second half of the 1970s is too small and too late to be chiefly responsible for the large decreases in lung cancer mortality rates in the 1970s. (4) In unpolluted Finland, where male cigarette smoking also began so long ago that the trends had nearly flattened out by the late 1950s, male lung cancer rates in early middle age have likewise been approximately halved over the past 20 years, and in both countries the decreases appear, if anything, to be accelerating. (In Finland, as in Britain, no large changes in cigarette consumption were evident before the mid 1970s.)

[c]High mean tar intake throughout smoking history.

[d]High intake only in first decade or so of smoking history.

autopsies in the 1950s and in the 1970s (22). In the 1950s smokers had a high, dose-related prevalence of what were thought to be preneoplastic lesions, whereas by the 1970s such lesions were an order of magnitude less common among smokers. The exact biologic significance of these lesions, however, remains obscure, especially because their prevalence decreased so sharply during a period in which lung cancer rates were rising. (They may be indicators not so much of the extent to which the main neoplastic endpoints are occuring, but of the extent to which one of the "stages" of carcinogenesis is occurring.)

Practical Action: Discouraging Sales and Decreasing Tar Levels

Sales

A variety of WHO and UICC expert reports have been prepared on how voluntary organizations and governments can decrease cigarette consumption, and these deserve careful scrutiny for they contain much well-judged advice. There are, however, two important respects in which they may be somewhat deficient. The first is that tax increases may not be sufficiently emphasized. Because many governments derive large tax yields from tobacco sales, all but this one of the strategies that may be considered for reducing cigarette sales, will also, if effective, reduce tax revenues. Although in principle governments may believe they act only for the good of their citizens, in practice they may tend to decide that what is

Table 4. Elasticity: Predicted change in cigarette sales per 10% increase in real price

Country studied	Estimates in 9[a] different papers of the change in annual cigarette sales associated with a 10% price increase (%)
United States	−5, −8, −4, −4
Canada	−7
United Kingdom	−6, −5
Switzerland	−8
Finland	−3[b]

[a]Between 1950 and 1968 no studies of the elasticity of cigarette demand were published, but since 1968 at least ten have been. All are cited except for that of Atkinson and Skegg (1974), which is superseded by the reanalysis by J Peto (1974) of the identical data. For references, see Ontario Council of Health (7).

[b]This estimate of only 3% was published in 1974 and would have been more extreme if it had been possible to include the subsequent large increase in price and decrease in consumption that took place in Finland in the mid-1970s.

economically easiest for the government is best for the citizens. Consequently, the one strategy—increasing the tax on tobacco—that increases rather than decreases tax revenues perhaps deserves more emphasis than it usually gets, especially because it is one of the few strategies for which there is clear, direct evidence of effect. In 1981, for example, increases by a total of about 20% in British cigarette prices produced decreases that, although substantial, were less than 20% in cigarette sales, so the tobacco manufacturers complained of unemployment in the industry while the government collected more tax. The same thing happened in Finland in the mid-1970s. Several reports during the past 15 years have examined more formally the quantitative relationship between price and consumption in these and various other countries with remarkably consistent findings (Table 4). At least for the subsequent year or two, a 10% increase in price appears to produce about a 5% decrease in consumption. If such a decrease were largely permanent, then it would in the long term prevent about 10,000 tobacco-induced deaths per million cigarette smokers. It is more difficult to produce a reliable estimate of the extent to which these year-to-year changes in consumption, produced by price changes, persist over longer periods, for so many other factors also may be involved. Despite this, however, some direct evidence for the commonsense notion that price does affect long-term, as well as short-term, consumption is afforded by the general tendency for cigarette consumption to be high in many countries where the price is low (7). In view of such data, the promise of deliberate shifts of taxation from other goods to tobacco may deserve greater emphasis than it often receives.

A second deficiency of emphasis is that there may have been insufficient stress on the long-term advantages of getting quantitatively informative material across about the total risks from tobacco, and the extent to which, at least in developed countries, these exceed all other reliably known causes of death. The reasons any serious program of cancer prevention must stress the health effects of tobacco are illustrated by Table 5, which has been abstracted from the chapter on Cancer Epidemiology in the *Oxford Textbook of Medicine* (23). This perspective, however, is

Table 5. Reliably established, practicable[a] ways of avoiding the onset of life-threatening cancer in the United States or United Kingdom[b].

	Percentage of all US/UK cancer deaths known to be thus avoidable
Avoidance of tobacco smoke	30
Avoidance of alcoholic drinks or mouthwashes	3
Avoidance of obesity	2
Regular cervical screening and genital hygiene	1
Avoidance of inessential medical use of hormones or radiology	<1
Avoidance of unusual exposure to sunlight	<1
Avoidance of known effects on people of current levels of exposure to carcinogens in:	
Occupational context	<1[c]
Food, water or urban air	<1

[a]Excluding ways such as prophylactic prostatectomy, mastectomy, hysterectomy, oophorectomy, artificial menopause, or pregnancy.
[b]From Doll and Peto (23).
[c]The proportion of current United States cancer deaths that are likely to result from occupational factors was estimated to be about 4% (5). The most important reliably known effect was that of asbestos, for the delayed effects of past exposure to asbestos may well account for 1–2% of all current United States cancer deaths, a figure that is still rising and that eventually may well be 2–3%. However, because the approximate magnitude of the health effects of exposure to asbestos became widely accepted, exposure levels have been greatly reduced and are now in general far lower than the old levels, the delayed effects of which are now materializing. Although further restrictions on current exposure levels could further reduce their future effects, these future effects are unlikely to be as great as the current effects of the heavy past exposures. Consequently, even the abolition of asbestos is likely to produce a decrease in future cancer death rates that is far smaller than 2%, and the same is true of various other occupational carcinogens (eg, benzidine), the delayed effects of which are still appearing, long after substantial reductions in exposure have taken place.

unfamiliar even to most cancer research workers, let alone to most nonmedical people. Indeed, in recent surveys in Britain most people mistakenly imagined that traffic caused more deaths than tobacco; in fact tobacco causes over 20 times as many UK deaths as traffic. Likewise, in the United States recent surveys have indicated that many people believe that background radiation from nuclear power plants is a greater health risk than tobacco (24), whereas in fact tobacco is several thousand times more important. Such gross misperceptions, of course, may have substantial effects on behavior. Indeed, the chairman of R.J. Reynolds, America's largest cigarette manufacturer, reportedly (*New York Times*, April 12, 1981) said to his shareholders that the reason the cancer scare was no longer hitting cigarette sales so hard was that so many things have been linked to cancer that people were "beginning to take a more objective [sic] view of the health evidence"! He may well be right about the effect of the string of reports about new carcinogens, because only a remarkably percipient newspaper reader or televiewer would be able to guess, after reading about one new cancer scare after another, that boring old non-newsworthy tobacco was still causing about one-third of all cancer deaths—an effect ten times as large as the next most important reliably known effect. It is admittedly difficult to communicate risks in a way that will be understood and remembered approximately correctly, especially by people who have no framework of other risks with which to compare them. However, it should be possible as long as the main message is set clearly apart from the lesser messages that qualify it and that may help prevent people from rationalizing it away[13]. After all, the chief message is merely that "ABOUT A QUARTER OF ALL REGULAR CIGARETTE SMOKERS WILL BE KILLED BEFORE THEIR TIME BY THE HABIT," which is considerably less complicated than the mass of quantitative information about house prices, groceries, car prices, etc, that already has become part of the folklore of consumer societies. How exactly this main message should be put over is a matter for experiment; comparisons with other conditions may (especially in Britain) be helpful, eg,

SMOKING IS BRITAIN'S BIGGEST KILLER
Among 1000 young adults who smoke cigarettes regularly,
- about 1 will be murdered
- about 6 will be killed on the roads
- about 250 will be killed by tobacco.

[13]For example, one might follow the main message with a few explanatory notes, such as:

- Some of those killed by tobacco would have died soon anyway, but others might have lived on for 5, 10, 20, 30, or more extra years; the average amount of life lost by them being 10–15 years.
- If you give up before you have got serious heart disease, bronchitis, or cancer, then you avoid most of the risk of death from smoking.
- Damage to the body from smoking accumulates, so those who start in their teens will be at the greatest risk in middle age.

Even in the United States, where road accident death rates are more than double those in Britain and murder rates are about ten times those in Britain, some such comparisons may be helpful (although it may then be advisable to start with only 100 young United States adults, and to threaten about 1, 2, and 25 of them with death).

Whatever format is preferred, however, the central point remains: The reason one wants to prevent smoking is not just because it is dangerous—dozens of things are dangerous—but because it is *so* dangerous. This indicates getting some sort of quantitative information over, both about the effects of smoking itself on mortality and, perhaps at least as importantly, about how much smaller all reliably known other carcinogenic effects are. Such information may in the short term make only a few people give up, but over a few years wide acceptance of such a perspective may have substantial effects, either on individual behavior or on making other actions politically acceptable.

Tar Levels

The foregoing epidemiologic evidence (especially that on trends in lung cancer mortality among English men in early middle age) strongly suggests that, even without any substantial changes in cigarette sales, practicable reductions in sales-weighted tar deliveries may well reduce the lung cancer mortality from smoking substantially. There was, moreover, in Lee and Garfinkel's review (20), no evidence that any other disease was aggravated by such changes among smokers of similar numbers of cigarettes[14]. Also, although tar and nicotine decreases do produce some compensation in the manner in which cigarettes are smoked, they do not appear to be important determinants of whether or not people smoke, or of the number of cigarettes that they smoke.

Tar reductions can be implemented with no substantial political problems (especially if they are done centrally, or at least without advertising campaigns that may suggest misleadingly to non- or ex-smokers that low-tar cigarettes are safe), for they do not adversely affect the growers, manufacturers, taxers, distributors or advertisers, and the smokers appear hardly to notice gradual changes in tar deliveries. It is, therefore, unfortunate that while the WHO and UICC have organized several meetings on smoking avoidance, some of which have produced reports listing a variety of practical suggestions for governments or for voluntary groups to consider, no similar reports are available to help governments accelerate tar reductions. The problems are, of course, quite different from one country to another, depending on whether the country is a tobacco grower, a cigarette manufacturer, an exporter, or an importer, on whether cigarette manufacture or distribution is virtually a government monopoly, on whether advertising is allowed, on the current tar levels, and so on. For countries such as Britain, differential taxation (which has already been used once successfully to cut off the highest tar levels) could be used again to cut off the next highest levels, and restrictions could be imposed on the advertising of, for example, all brands delivering more than 10 mg of tar. For countries such as China and Russia, where cigarettes are manufactured and distributed by the state with little or no advertising, and where typical tar levels exceed the upper limit of what is currently sold in Britain, large changes could be produced at little cost and with great benefit to their people early in the next century[15]. However, the practical problems of how to help governments decrease tar levels (without inadvertently encouraging a belief that low-tar cigarettes are safe) is a large question, almost as deserving of carefully thought out, practical reports as the problems of smoking avoidance are.

Ultimately, of course, the aim is to produce circumstances in which very few people choose to smoke, but in a world where cigarette sales are still increasing, rather than decreasing it is not wise to let the perfect be the enemy of the possible.

[14]In view of the extent to which smokers of low-tar cigarettes do "compensate," however, and of the uncertainty as to which smoke components chiefly affect heart disease and chronic obstructive lung disease, there should be no implicit expectation that these diseases will also be avoided, and indeed the large case–control study of Kaufman et al (18) suggests approximate equivalence of the effects on myocardial infarction of the different types of cigarette that are currently available.

[15]During the 1950s, men in Finland still smoked "Russian-style" cigarettes, and in 1960 male lung cancer incidence rates in early middle age were similar in Russia and in Finland. By the early 1980s, however, typical Finnish cigarette tar deliveries had dropped to only 10–15 mg., while typical Russian cigarette tar deliveries were still about 20–30 mg.. Recent Finnish male lung cancer incidence rates in early middle age have decreased by nearly half, while those in Russia have hardly altered.

Table 6. Information for governments on simple measures for the control of lung cancer[a]

Price increases will produce fewer deaths and more revenue (as long as they do not feed back into wage demands).
Tar reductions should be encouraged (especially in countries such as Russia and China where typical tar levels are still of the order of 20–30 mg, which is extremely high).
Advertising could be taxed, restricted, prohibited, or limited to cigarettes delivering under 10 mg tar.
Simple, clear, quantitative information could be communicated effectively to the general population: ABOUT A QUARTER OF ALL REGULAR SMOKERS ARE KILLED BEFORE THEIR TIME BY TOBACCO.

[a]General note: recommendation of these few simple measures (which might have a substantial effect in just a few years on exposures) does not, of course, detract from the need for a wide range of other measures, including many of those suggested by WHO (2), UICC (6), and others.

Tar-level reductions are not the only simple possibility for governments (Table 6), and they may do little for vascular or respiratory disease. But they may well offer one of the more immediately practicable means of avoiding an appreciable proportion of the mass of lung cancer deaths that can otherwise be expected to occur during the first few decades of the next century.

References

1. Parkin DM, Stjernsward J, Muir CS. Estimates of cancer occurrence throughout the world. WHO Bulletin (in press).
2. World Health Organization. Controlling the smoking epidemic: report of the WHO expert committee on smoking control. Technical Report Series 636. Geneva: WHO, 1979.
3. U.S. Surgeon-General. Smoking and health. U.S. Department of Health, Education and Welfare Publ No (PHS) 79-50066. Washington, DC: U.S. Government Printing Office, 1979.
4. U.S. Surgeon-General. The Health Consequences of Smoking—Cancer. U.S. Department of Health Education and Welfare Publ No (PHS) 82-50179. Washington, DC: U.S. Government Printing Office, 1982.
5. Doll R, Peto R. Quantitative estimates of avoidable risks of cancer in the United States today. JNCI 1981. 66:1191-1308.
6. Gray N, ed. Lung Cancer Prevention: Guidelines for smoking control. Geneva: Union Internationale Contre le Cancer, 1977.
7. Ontario Council of Health. Smoking and health in Ontario: a need for balance. Report of the Task Force on Smoking of the Ontario Council of Health. Toronto: Ontario Government Bookstore, 1982.
8. Doll R, Peto R. Cigarette smoking and bronchial carcinoma: dose and time relationships among regular smokers and lifelong non-smokers. J Epidemiol Community Health 1978; 32:303-13.
9. Doll R. The age distribution of cancer: implications for models of carcinogenesis (with discussion). J R Statist Soc A 1971; 134:133-6.
10. National Academy of Sciences-National Research Council. Reduced tar and nicotine cigarettes: smoking behavior and health. Washington, DC: National Academy Press, 1982.
11. Cederlöf R, Doll R, Fowler B, Frieberg L, Nelson N, Vouk V. Air pollution and cancer: risk assessment methodology and epidemiological evidence. Environ Health Perspect, 1978; 22:1-12.
12. Doll R, Peto R. Mortality in relation to smoking: 20 years' observations on male British doctors. Br Med J, 1976; 2:1525-36.
13. Wald N, Doll R, Copeland G. Trends in tar, nicotine, and carbon monoxide yields of UK cigarettes manufactured since 1934. Br Med J 1981; 1:763-5.

14. Wald N, Idle M, Boreham J, Bailey V, Van Vunakis H. Serum cotinine levels in pipe smokers; evidence against nicotine as a cause of coronary heart disease. Lancet 1981; ii:775-7.
15. Cederlöf R, Friberg L, Hrubec Z, Lorich U. The relationship of smoking and some covariables to mortality and cancer morbidity. Stockholm: Karolinska Institute, 1975.
16. Selikoff IJ. Constraints in estimating occupational cancer mortality. In Peto R, Schneiderman MA, eds, Quantification of occupational cancer. New York: Cold Spring Harbor Publications, 1981.
17. International Agency for Research on Cancer. Cancer incidence in five continents, Vol III. Geneva: World Health Organization, 1976.
18. Kaufman DW, Helmrich SP, Rosenberg L, Miettinen OS, Shapiro S. Nicotine and carbon monoxide content of cigarette smoke and the risk of myocardial infarction in young men. N Engl J Med 1983; 308:409-413.
19. Wald N, Idle M, Boreham J, Bailey A. Inhaling habits among smokers of different types of cigarette. Thorax 1980; 35:925-8.
20. Lee PN, Garfinkel L. Mortality and type of cigarette smoked. J Epidemiol Community Health 1981; 35:16-22.
21. Lee PN. Statistics of smoking in the United Kingdom. Research Paper No 1, London: Tobacco Research Council, 1976.
22. Auerbach O, Hammond EC, Garfinkel L. Changes in bronchial epithelium in relation to cigarette smoking 1955-1960 versus 1970-1977. N Engl J Med 1979; 300:381-6.
23. Doll R, Peto R. (1983). Epidemiology of cancer. In: Oxford Textbook of medicine. Weatherall DJ, Ledingham J, Warrell DA, eds., Oxford: Oxford University Press, 1983: 4.51-4.79.
24. Upton A. The biological effects of low-level ionizing radiation. Sci Am 1982; 246(2):29-37.
25. Garfinkel L. Cancer mortality in nonsmokers: Prospective Study by the American Cancer Society. JNCI 1980; 65:1169-1173.

CHAPTER **2**

Lung Cancer in Scandinavia: Time Trends and Smoking Habits

LYLY TEPPO

Finnish Cancer Registry, Liisankatu 21 B, SF-00170, Helsinki 17, Finland

ABSTRACT

According to the Scandinavian population-based nationwide cancer registries (which have been in operation for 25–40 years), the incidence rate of lung cancer in males is highest in Finland (74.4/100,000 in the mid-70s), followed by Denmark (51.8), Norway (25.4), Sweden (23.8), and Iceland (16.3 in 1964–1972). In females, the variation is smaller, from 12.1 in Denmark to 5.4 in Norway.

In the 1950s and 1960s, the incidence of lung cancer was on the increase in all five Scandinavian countries. In about 1970, the trend curve for males in Finland leveled off and has since been showing a slight decrease. In Sweden the rate turned to a decrease in 1976. In the remaining countries the incidence continues to increase. The female rates are increasing in all the Scandinavian countries.

The variation in the incidence of lung cancer in the Scandinavian countries reflects the variation in the smoking habits some 30–40 years earlier. Only little variation exists in the current prevalence of smoking.There was considerable variation in the risk of lung cancer among males between different occupational groups in Finland, the standardized incidence ratio (SIR) being highest (2.08) among miners and lowest (0.18) in religious work. More than 90% of the variation in the SIR of lung cancer between the main occupational categories can be explained by variation in the prevalence of smoking.
Key Words: **Lung cancer; incidence; trends; smoking; occupation**

In this presentation Scandinavia refers to the five Nordic countries—Denmark (population 5.1 million), Finland (4.8 million), Iceland (0.2 million), Norway (4.1 million), and Sweden (8.3 million). The total population of these countries is about 22.5 million. In addition to being located in northern Europe these countries have

Lung Cancer: Causes and Prevention.

much in common as regards their climate, history, culture, religion, and everyday way of life. Close contacts are maintained on many levels: employment, travel, trade, education, etc. The standards of living and the medical care systems and resources are similar. However, there are some differences, and these may be relevant to cancer epidemiology. For instance, the population of Finland is ethnically different from that of the other Nordic countries, the Finns, according to the current theory, being of Baltic origin with some eastern elements. Similarly, the Finnish language is totally different from the languages spoken in the other Nordic countries.

Each of the five countries keeps a population-based nationwide cancer registry. Cancer registration started in Denmark in 1942, in Finland and Norway in 1952, in Iceland in 1954, and in Sweden in 1958. Similarities between working practices of the cancer registries and the health care systems of the countries result in comparable cancer statistics. Furthermore, the long period of cancer registration permits construction of time trends in incidence rates (1). All the incidence rates and other cancer data (published or unpublished) given here are from the respective cancer registries.

Variation in the Incidence

There is marked variation in the incidence of lung cancer in Scandinavia (Table 1). The rate among males is by far the highest in Finland (74 per 100,000), where it is about 50% higher than that in Denmark and three times that in Norway and Sweden. Iceland has a very low rate. Among females, the rate is highest in Iceland and Denmark (about 12 per 100,000). In the remaining three countries the rate is only half that and does not differ appreciably between the countries. The rate among males in Finland is one of the highest in the whole world and is comparable with the well-known high rates in Great Britain. On the other hand, the rate among females is not exceptionally high in Finland and is, in fact, one of the lowest in Scandinavia. Consequently, the male–female ratio of the rates is high (Table 1). In Iceland, the situation is reversed: a low rate in males is accompanied by a relatively high rate in females, resulting in a low male–female ratio.

In Finland, cancer of the lung is the leading cancer type among males, some 30% of all new cancers being located in the lungs. Cancer of the lung is the leading

Table 1. Age-adjusted ("world standard population") incidence rates (per 100,000 person-years) of lung cancer in Denmark (2), Finland (2), Iceland (3), Norway (2) and Sweden (2), by sex, and the male–female ratios of the rates

Country	Years	Males	Females	M/F
Denmark	1973–1976	51.8	12.1	4.3
Finland	1971–1976	74.4	5.8	12.8
Iceland	1964–1972	16.3	11.0	1.5
Norway	1973–1977	25.4	5.4	4.7
Sweden	1971–1975	23.8	5.7	4.2

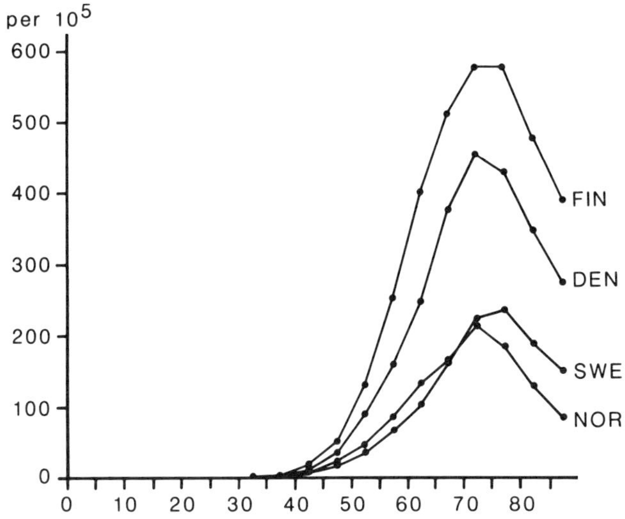

Figure 1. Age-specific incidence rates (per 100,000 person-years) of lung cancer in males in Denmark, Finland, Norway, and Sweden (for the years covered see Table 1). Reproduced with permission from Ref (2).

type of cancer in Denmark, too, but in Sweden and Norway it occupies second place after prostatic cancer, and in Iceland third place after cancers of the prostate and stomach (4).

In spite of the marked differences in the total incidence of lung cancer among males, the age-specific incidence curves run a similar general course: the peak incidence occurs around the age of 70, and in all these countries the incidence decreases toward the oldest age groups (Figure 1).

There is a marked geographic variation in the incidence of lung cancer within Finland, Sweden, and Norway. The lowest rate in the Finnish provinces is higher than the highest rate in Sweden or Norway.

In all the Scandinavian countries the rates are higher in urban areas than in rural districts, for both males and females. In Finland, however, the urban–rural ratio of the rates among males is exceptionally low and is decreasing. In 1966–1970 the ratio was 1.24 and 10 years later, in 1979, it was down to 1.05.

Incidence Trends

Trends in the incidence rate among males show that Finland has held the lead for decades, and the same is true for the second position held by Denmark (Figure 2). In general, the trend has been increasing continuously in all five countries. Finland exhibits a somewhat exceptional pattern in that a distinct leveling off, and even a slight decrease in the rate, was observed in the 1970s. This results from a decrease in the rate in urban areas; the rural rate is still increasing, which explains the decreasing urban–rural ratio in Finland referred to above. The incidence among females is increasing in all five countries.

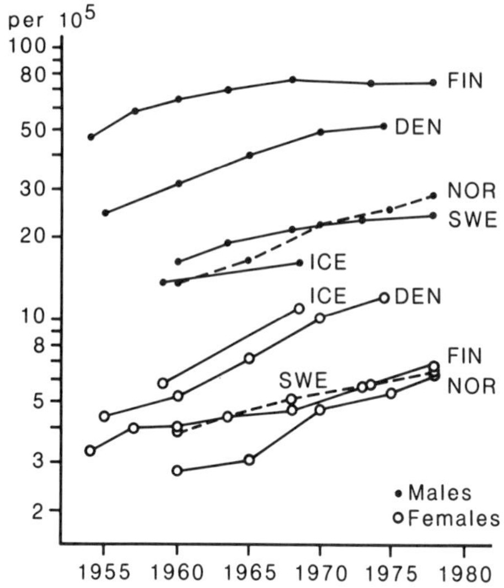

Figure 2. Trends in the age-adjusted ("world standard population") incidence rates (per 100,000 person-years) of lung cancer in Denmark (2, 3, 5, 6), Finland (2, 3, 5–7), Iceland (3, 6), Norway (2, 3, 5, 6, 8), and Sweden (2, 3, 5, 6, 9), by sex.

The trend in the total age-adjusted incidence rates does not tell the whole truth about the changes in the risk of lung cancer. A more detailed picture can be obtained from birth cohort analyses. In Norway, the age-specific incidence rates of each cohort are higher than those of the previous cohort. In Finland, younger cohorts, ie, those born since 1913, are beginning to follow the pattern of the previous cohorts, and the cohort born around 1933 is already experiencing a lower risk of lung cancer than the previous cohort (10).

The ratio of the estimated cumulative lifelong lung cancer risks between two consecutive 5-year birth cohorts shows a decreasing trend among males in all Scandinavian countries (10). In Finland, the ratio among the youngest cohorts is below 1.0; in other words, the risk has started to decrease when compared with older cohorts. The latest ratio is below 1.0 in Denmark and Sweden, too, suggesting that even in these countries the total incidence rate of lung cancer can be expected to drop when these younger cohorts reach cancer age. The situation is not so favorable for females in Denmark and Norway, where the ratio is still clearly above 1.0 and perhaps is even increasing (10).

Cohort analyses indicate that a change is taking place in the risk of lung cancer for younger males. This change suggests that the future incidence rates will not be as high as would be expected if the observed trend in the total lung cancer incidence were to be extrapolated directly into the future. In Finland, a prediction study was carried out in which the lung cancer risk was forecast up to the year 2000 (11). A logistic model was used, based on the observed age-incidence curves of 5-year birth cohorts and the estimated intercohort incidence ratios. It was shown that the incidence is expected to decrease in males but to increase continuously in females (Table 2).

Table 2. Mean annual age-adjusted ("world standard population") incidence rates (per 100,000 person-years) of lung cancer and mean annual numbers of lung cancer cases in Finland: observed figures in 1973–1977 and predicted figures for 1988–1992 and 1998–2002, by sex[a]

	1973–1977	1988–1992	1998–2002
Incidence			
Males	75.2	69.3	50.9
Females	5.9	10.5	14.6
No of cases			
Males	1961	2064	1778
Females	230	463	681

[a]Reproduced with permission from Ref (11).

The predicted incidence rates can be converted to numbers of cases by taking into account the population forecast by age. Because the mean age of the population is expected to increase, resulting in an increase in the old, high-risk section of the population, the number of cases among males will decrease much more slowly than the incidence rate (Table 2). A similar forecast for females predicts that the annual number of new cases will increase by almost 200% by the year 2000 (Table 2).

Smoking Habits and Lung Cancer in Scandinavia

Smoking was introduced into Finland from Russia in the late 19th century and has been popular ever since, ie, for about 100 years now. People started to smoke much later in the other Scandinavian countries. In the 1920s and 1930s, the annual number of cigarettes smoked per adult in Finland was about 1500 as against 400–500 in Norway, Sweden, and Denmark (12). The consumption of cigarettes increased in Finland in the 1950s and has remained more or less stable ever since. In the other countries, consumption increased further in the 1960s and 1970s, and today it has almost reached that in Finland.

When measured by the proportion of daily smokers, the consumption pattern is different. The frequency is, and has been, highest in Denmark and, somewhat unexpectedly, lowest in Finland. Because there are now no marked differences in the total amount of tobacco smoked, those Finns who smoke are more likely to be heavy smokers than are smokers in the other Scandinavian countries. Present-day smoking habits do not seem to explain the differences between the Scandinavian countries in the risk of lung cancer. However, if the incidence rates are compared with data on smoking some 30–40 years ago, a rather good correlation is observed (12).

The proportion of male smokers in Finland has decreased gradually since the early 1960s (Figure 3). Whereas in the early 1960s 57% of the adult males were daily smokers, the figure was around 45% in the 1970s and as low as 32% in 1982.

This decrease is probably a result of the nationwide antismoking campaigns conducted by the Cancer Society of Finland and other organizations with the backing of the state authorities. A decrease in the prevalence of smoking in the 1960s should result in a change in the trend in the incidence of lung cancer in the 1970s, and this is, in fact, what has happened: the trend curve has leveled off (Figure 4).

There has been a slight increase in the prevalence of daily smokers among women (Figure 3). Accordingly, no change in the course of the lung cancer trend has been noticed, and the incidence is increasing continuously (Figure 4).

New legislation on tobacco was enacted in Finland in 1977. The main provisions of this law are (14):

1. Advertising and sales promotion of tobacco are prohibited.
2. Smoking is prohibited in all public places (offices open to the public, theaters, schools, etc) and public transport facilities except in separate areas especially set aside for that purpose.
3. Sale of tobacco products to persons under 16 years of age is prohibited.
4. A sum corresponding to at least 0.5% of the tobacco tax revenue is to be reserved annually in the state budget for the development of health-oriented tobacco policy (health education, research, and evaluation).
5. The government is responsible for fixing the limits of harmful components of tobacco products (tar, nicotine, and carbon monoxide), and tobacco products can be classified as "very harmful" or "harmful" on the basis of the amounts of harmful constituents.

The present tar limit of 18 mg per cigarette may be lowered to 15 mg. The trend in Finland is toward low-tar cigarettes, and in 1982 the proportion of low-tar cigarettes was already 30%.

The tobacco legislation could well have an effect on the risk of lung cancer in the population, by reducing both the frequency of smoking and the exposure to to-

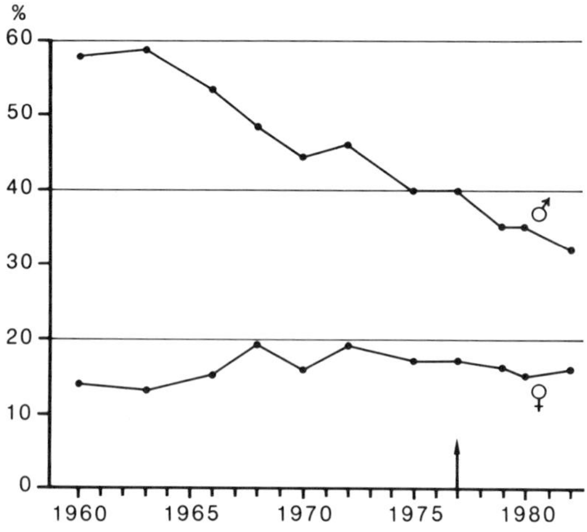

Figure 3. Trend in the percentage of current smokers among the adult population in Finland, by sex. Arrow: new tobacco legislation. Reproduced with permission from Ref (13).

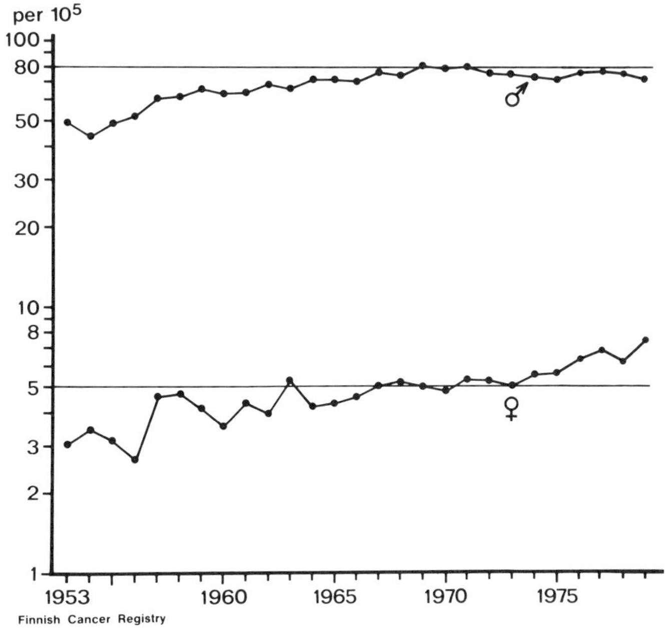

Figure 4. Trend in the age-adjusted ("world standard population") incidence rate (per 100,000 person-years) of lung cancer in Finland in 1953–1979, by sex.

bacco smoke. The immediate effect would be a decrease in the prevalence of smoking. However, no apparent change in the regular course of the trend curves (Figure 3) has been observed so far, and no rapid effects, of course, can be expected in the trend in the long-term adverse effects of smoking, eg, incidence (or mortality) of lung cancer. The Finnish Cancer Registry carefully monitors the situation in the country and in different sections of the population.

The lung cancer situation in Finland and Norway has been analyzed more closely by Pedersen and his co-workers (15). In 1962 about 5000 males in Finland and 5000 males in Norway were interviewed about their smoking and other habits. The study groups consisted of a random sample of males of a certain age from six areas in Finland and six areas in Norway. Urban and rural areas with both a low and a high risk of lung cancer were chosen in each country. For each of the 12 study areas two indices were produced, one describing smoking habits, the other the risk of lung cancer. The smoking index of a given area was constructed on the basis of the frequency of smoking of different quantities of tobacco, and on the estimated risk of lung cancer in each smoking category. The average smoking index within all the 12 study areas was defined as 1.0, and all individual indices were expressed in relation to this. The incidence of lung cancer was calculated in each area and similarly expressed in relation to the mean of all areas, which was defined as 1.0. The incidence rates referred to 1953–1962 and to ages comparable to those included in the interviewed sample.

A slightly higher number of current smokers was found in Norway, but there were many more heavy smokers in Finland than in Norway (15). This means that the smoking indices calculated for each area were, in general, higher in Finland. There was overlapping in the smoking indices between Finland and Norway, but no overlapping whatsoever in the lung cancer risk indices between the countries (Figure 5). Only 55% of the difference in the mean rates between the study areas in Finland and Norway in 1953–1962 can be explained on the basis of the observed variation in smoking habits assessed in 1962.

The time factor must be taken into account. At the time of the original analysis, lung cancer incidence data were available only for the period preceding the interview. Some time has now elapsed, and a reanalysis has been carried out (16). The incidence of lung cancer has been increasing in all six study areas in Norway, whereas in Finland the rates have leveled off or begun to drop. If the area-specific lung cancer risk indices for 1975–1979 are plotted against the original smoking indices for 1962, a better fit is observable. Contrary to the 55% in the previous analysis, 64% of the difference in the risk between Finland and Norway can now be explained on the basis of the observed smoking habits. Hakulinen and Magnus (16) calculated that the ratio of the age-adjusted incidence rates of lung cancer in Finland and Norway (3.5) is reduced to 1.7 after adjustment for smoking habits and further to 1.3 after allowing a 15-year time lag between the interview and risk estimate. One can assume that if the situation were to be reanalyzed after a further 10 or 20 years, an even smaller proportion of the difference would remain unexplained. In other words, the past differences in the smoking habits between Finland and Norway may, after all, be sufficient to explain a large part of the substantial difference found in the incidence of lung cancer.

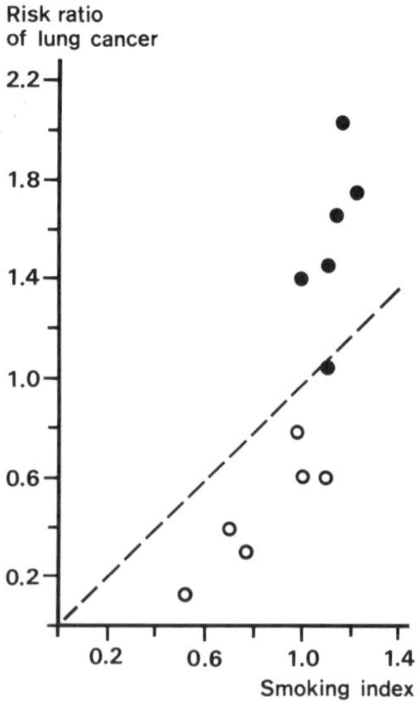

Figure 5. Correlation between the area-specific smoking indices and lung cancer incidence indices (risk ratios) in six areas in Norway (o) and Finland (•). Reproduced with permission from Ref (15).

A further reason for the higher risk of lung cancer in Finland may be that most smokers in Finland smoke cigarettes, whereas in the other Scandinavian countries there is quite a large proportion of pipe and cigar smokers as well.

Occupation and Smoking as Risk Indicators in Lung Cancer

In a study conducted by the Finnish Cancer Registry the risk of lung cancer was analyzed in different occupational categories, and an attempt was made to find out to what extent the variation observed between the different occupational groups might result from differences in smoking habits (17).

The series consisted of all male patients, 35–69 years of age, with lung cancer diagnosed in Finland in 1971–1975 and reported to the Finnish Cancer Registry. The Registry data on these patients were supplemented by an occupation code recorded in the Finnish national census on January 1, 1971, ie, before lung cancer had been diagnosed. The records were linked automatically, using the personal identification code given to each resident in Finland. After some exclusions there were 6700 males with information on their occupations. These cases were tabulated by occupational group and age. The corresponding expected numbers of cases were calculated on the basis of the occupation and age-specific numbers of person-years at risk in 1971–1975 produced by the Central Statistical Office of Finland for the whole Finnish population, and the age-specific incidence rates of lung cancer in the economically active male population. The standardized incidence ratios (SIRs) were estimated as the ratios of the observed and corresponding expected numbers of cases.

There was considerable variation in the SIR of lung cancer between different occupational groups, the difference between the highest and the lowest being over ten-fold (Table 3). The SIR was highest (2.08) in mining and quarrying. Other groups with a high SIR were unskilled construction workers, construction metal workers, forestry workers, and joiners. All these groups do hard physical work, mostly out of doors. Moreover, these workers generally belong to the lower socioeconomic strata. Low SIRs were encountered among priests, lawyers, teachers, physicians, and administrators. In other words, academic professions in which a long education leads to higher socioeconomic strata were associated with a low risk of lung cancer.

Occupational carcinogenic exposures are of course much more prevalent among the above-mentioned high-risk occupations, but in general this refers only to a limited number of workers in the mostly heterogeneous group. The smoking habits of the main occupational categories in Finland were available as the result of an interview study carried out by alcohol researchers in 1968. Two different measures of the smoking habits of an occupational group were applied. One was simply the proportion of current smokers; the other was an index in which the quantities smoked also were taken into consideration. The index was defined as

$$\mathrm{I} = 1 \times N + 5 \times M + 15 \times H$$

in which N is the percentage of nonsmokers, M is the percentage of moderate smokers (fewer than 15 cigarettes per day), and H is the percentage of heavy smokers (15 cigarettes or more per day). The coefficients 1, 5, and 15 indicate the relative risks of lung cancer among nonsmokers, moderate smokers, and heavy smokers, respectively.

The gradient in the prevalence of current smokers and the smoking index between different main occupational categories seems to be similar to that found for the SIR of lung cancer: low prevalence in the low-risk academic professions and high prevalence in manufacturing, in which the risk of lung cancer, too, was high. Hence, a positive association is found between smoking and the risk of lung cancer, and the correlation is almost identical for both smoking indices used. It can be calculated that 92% of the variation observable in the SIR of lung cancer between the main occupational categories can be explained by the variation in the prevalence of smoking.

Three conclusions can be drawn. First, it appears that data on lung cancer risk by occupation or by any other parameter are of only limited applicability if information on smoking habits is lacking. Second, smoking is the most important factor explaining the occupational variation in the risk of lung cancer. Third, if all occupational groups could reduce their smoking to the level found in the academic professions, which is a fairly realistic goal, 52% of the lung cancer cases diagnosed in 1971-1975 in Finland could have been prevented. The result would be much more dramatic if the prevalence among priests could be reached.

Table 3. Observed and expected numbers of male lung cancer cases (35-69 years of age) and standardized incidence ratios (SIR) in selected occupational categories in Finland in 1971-1975[a]

Occupational category	Observed	Expected	SIR
Mining and quarrying	42	20.2	2.08
Unskilled construction workers	126	69.9	1.80
Construction metal workers	119	81.1	1.47
Forestry	168	114.9	1.46
Joiners	264	186.4	1.42
Painting and lacquering work	78	55.1	1.42
Farmers with 10 hectares or more land	325	473.5	0.69
Technical work	92	144.5	0.64
Wholesale and retail dealers	38	59.9	0.63
Chemical, physical and biologic work	11	20.8	0.53
Transport service work	14	29.1	0.48
Administration of establishments and organizations	49	105.5	0.46
Medical work	6	16.4	0.37
Pedagogical work	22	60.4	0.36
Legal work	4	12.9	0.31
Religious work	2	11.0	0.18

[a]Reproduced with permission from Ref (17).

References

1. Ringertz N, ed. Cancer incidence in Finland, Iceland, Norway and Sweden. A comparative study. Acta Pathol Microbiol Scand Sect A 1971;Suppl 224
2. Waterhouse J, Muir C, Shanmugaratnam K, Powell J, eds. Cancer incidence in five continents, Vol IV. International Agency for Research on Cancer Scientific Publ 42. Lyon: IARC, 1982.
3. Waterhouse J, Muir C, Correa P, Powell J, eds. Cancer incidence in five continents, Vol III. International Agency for Research on Cancer Scientific Publ 15. Lyon: IARC, 1976.
4. Teppo L. Epidemiology of cancer in Northern Europe. In: Grundmann E, ed, Cancer campaign, Vol 6, Cancer epidemiology. Stuttgart: Gustav Fischer Verlag, 1982:5–13.
5. Doll R, Muir C, Waterhouse J, eds. Cancer incidence in five continents. A technical report. Berlin: Springer-Verlag, 1966.
6. Doll R, Payne P, Waterhouse J, eds. Cancer incidence in five continents, Vol II. Berlin: Springer-Verlag, 1970.
7. Finnish Cancer Registry. Cancer incidence in Finland 1977, 1978, 1979. Helsinki: 1981, 1982, 1982.
8. The Cancer Registry of Norway. Incidence of cancer in Norway 1977, 1978, 1979. Oslo: 1979, 1981, 1982.
9. National Board of Health and Welfare, the Cancer Registry. Cancer incidence in Sweden 1977, 1978, 1979. Stockholm: 1981, 1982, 1982.
10. Kvale G. Cancer of the larynx and lung. Incidence trends in the Nordic countries. In: Magnus K, ed, Trends in cancer incidence. Causes and practical implications. New York: Hemisphere Publishing, 1982.
11. Läärä E. Development of cancer morbidity in Finland up to the year 2002. (In Finnish, with English summary.) Publications of the National Board of Health, Finland, Series Original Reports 3/1982. Helsinki: 1982.
12. Saxén E, Teppo L, Hakulinen T. Epidemiology of lung cancer in Scandinavia. In: Mohr U, Schmal D, Tomatis L, Davis W. eds, Air pollution and cancer in man. Proceedings of the Second Hanover International Carcinogenesis Meeting held in Hanover, October 22–24, 1975. International Agency for Research on Cancer Scientific Publ 16. Lyon: IARC, 1977:217–28.
13. Rimpelä M. Trends in the smoking habits in Finland in 1949 and 1960–1977. Sosiaalilääketiet Aik-L 1978;15:112–23.
14. The National Board of Health. Legislative and administrative action for control of tobacco-smoking in Finland. Helsinki:1979.
15. Pedersen E, Magnus K, Mork T, et al. Lung cancer in Finland and Norway. An epidemiological study. Acta Pathol Microbiol Scand 1969; Suppl 199.
16. Hakulinen T, Magnus K. Regional differences in the incidence of lung cancer in Norway and Finland. With reference to smoking habits. Symposium of the Nordic Cancer Union "Smoking and Cancer," Oulu, Finland, June 2-4, 1982.
17. Pukkala E, Teppo L, Hakulinen T, Rimpelä M. Occupation and smoking as risk determinants of lung cancer. Int J Epidemiol 1983; 12:290–296.

CHAPTER **3**

Trends in Lung Cancer Incidence and Mortality in the United States

SUSAN S. DEVESA, JOHN W. HORM, and
ROGER R. CONNELLY

Biometry Branch, National Cancer Institute, Landow 5C19, Bethesda, Maryland 20205

ABSTRACT

Increases observed in lung cancer incidence and mortality rates exceed those of any other primary cancer site. Among white males, incidence rates increased more than 200% from the late 1940s to the late 1970s; the corresponding increase among white females was greater than 250%. Rates continue to increase among the older age groups; among the younger groups, the rates of increase are diminishing and some decreases are apparent among males. Rates among nonwhite males, which were lower than those among white males in the past and about equal in the early 1960s, are now substantially higher than those among white males. Geographic patterns have changed over time among white males, as rates in the south have increased more rapidly than in other areas of the country. Lung cancer mortality rates among males were about 30% higher in New Orleans compared to the rest of the country, and incidence rates were the highest of ten reporting areas during the mid-1970s.
Key Words: **Lung neoplasma, incidence, mortality, mesothelioma**

Introduction

The number of deaths in the United States attributed to lung cancer increased from 18,000 in 1950 to 99,000 in 1979, and it is estimated that there will be 117,000 lung cancer deaths during 1983 (Table 1) (1–3). This is more than a six-fold increase during the 33 years. The number of lung cancer deaths among males has been greater than among females at each point in time: in 1950 the male–female ratio was 4.4 and in 1983 it is projected to be 2.4. Whereas there has been a fivefold increase among males, there has been a tenfold increase among

Lung Cancer: Causes and Prevention.

Table 1. Impact of lung cancer[a] in the United States from 1950 to 1983[b]

	Total	Males	Females
Number of deaths			
1950	18,313	14,922	3,391
1960	36,420	31,257	5,163
1970	65,454	53,005	12,449
1979	99,059	73,243	25,816
1983 (estimate)	117,000	83,000	34,000
Number of newly diagnosed cases			
1983 (estimate)	135,000	94,000	41,000

[a]Lung, bronchus, trachea, pleura.
[b]Sources: Refs. (1)–(3).

females. It is estimated that 135,000 cases will be diagnosed during 1983, with about 94,000 occurring among males and 41,000 among females. These increases result from several factors: increases in the size of the population, changes in the age distribution of the population, with increasing proportions in the older age groups which are at higher risk of developing cancer, and increases in the rate of occurrence of lung cancer. The purpose of this report is to present the secular trends in rates of lung cancer incidence and mortality and to consider the variations by sex, race, age group, and geographic area.

Materials and Methods

Although mortality data are available for the entire country, corresponding incidence data, which indicate newly diagnosed cases rather than deaths, are not. The U.S. National Cancer Institute (NCI) has supported several surveys of cancer incidence in selected areas of the country: the first in 1937, the second in 1947 (4), a special survey in Iowa in 1950 (5), and the Third National Cancer Survey (TNCS) in 1969–1971 (6). Since 1973, the NCI-sponsored Surveillance, Epidemiology, and End Results (SEER) program has gathered information regarding cancer incidence, mortality, and survival; the participating population-based registries, which now include five states and four cities, provide information pertaining to more than 10% of the entire United States population (7). However, the same geographic areas were not included in each of the surveys or programs. Finally, the state of Connecticut has supported a tumor registry for many years, and this registry is now a participant in the SEER program (8). The original data from the first survey are not available; the current analysis therefore commences with the late 1940s. Drawing on the above-mentioned sources, we have compiled incidence trend data for five geographic areas (5GA): Atlanta, Detroit, San Francisco–Oakland, Iowa, and Connecticut. The populations in these five areas represented between 6 and 7% of the United States population at each time considered and currently represent about 72% of the SEER population.

All rates are average annual rates per 100,000 population. The 1970 United States population distribution was used as the standard for age adjustment. Incidence trends pertain to a composite of the years 1947–1950, the 3 years 1969–1971 (TNCS), and then 2-year averages from 1975–1976 through 1979–1980 (SEER). Corresponding mortality data are 5-year averages from 1950–1954 through 1965–1969, 1970–1975, and then 2-year averages corresponding to the incidence data for 1975–1976 and 1977–1978, and finally 1979 (1980 mortality data are not yet available).

Mortality trends are shown both for the entire United States and for the same five geographic areas for which incidence trends are presented. The cohort mortality curves are based on every fifth year's rates from 1950 to 1975. Mortality trends by race and sex utilize 5-year average annual rates from 1950–1954 through 1975–1979. The coding of race was not as specific in the earlier incidence reporting as it is currently, so most of the data presented pertain only to whites.

Only invasive malignancies are included; in situ tumors of this site are very rare—less than one per 100,000 per year—and are not included. As malignancies arising in the pleura, lung, and bronchus were not distinguished in the earlier coding systems, pleura is included with lung in all considerations of trends. In addition, those of the trachea, pulmonary, and lung, not specified as secondary, are included in the mortality data. The classification of mesotheliomas not specified as malignant has changed over time: they were reportable but not considered malignant during the TNCS, not reportable during the early SEER years, and since 1977 have been reportable and considered malignant; they are included in the mesothelioma rates for 1969–1971.

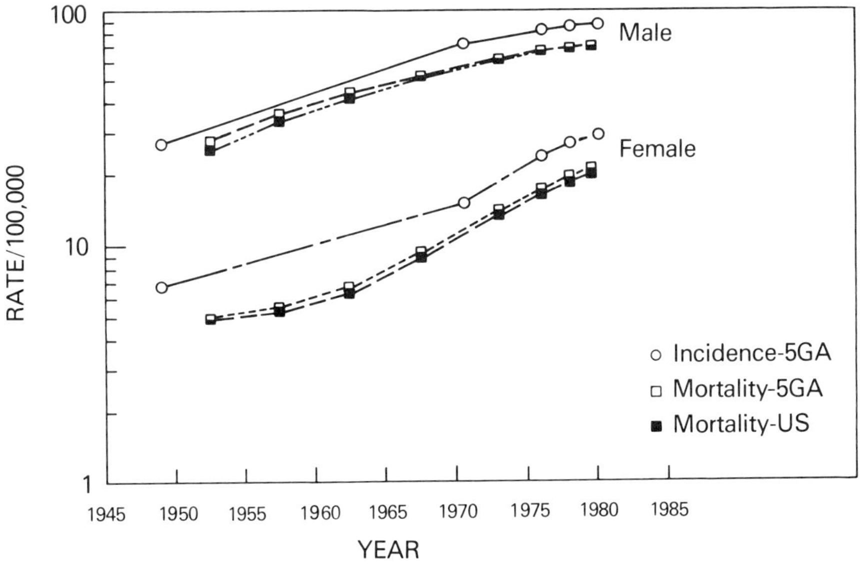

Figure 1. Incidence and mortality trends for lung cancer among whites.

Results

The increases in incidence of lung cancer among white males residing in these 5GA are larger than for any other primary site. The average annual age-adjusted rate increased from 27 to 85 per 100,000 over the 30-year period from the late 1940s to the late 1970s (Figure 1); this was an increase of more than 200%, or 3.5–4% per year. In the past, the lung cancer mortality was slightly higher among white males in the 5GA than in the country as a whole; since the mid-1960s the rates have been quite similar. In recent years there appears to be a change in slope or a decrease in the rate of increase in both incidence and mortality rates.

The increases in incidence of lung cancer among white females also are larger than those for any other primary site. Although the rates are considerably lower than those among males, the proportional increases are larger: more than 250% during the 30 years or about 5% per year. Although we do not have data, the in-

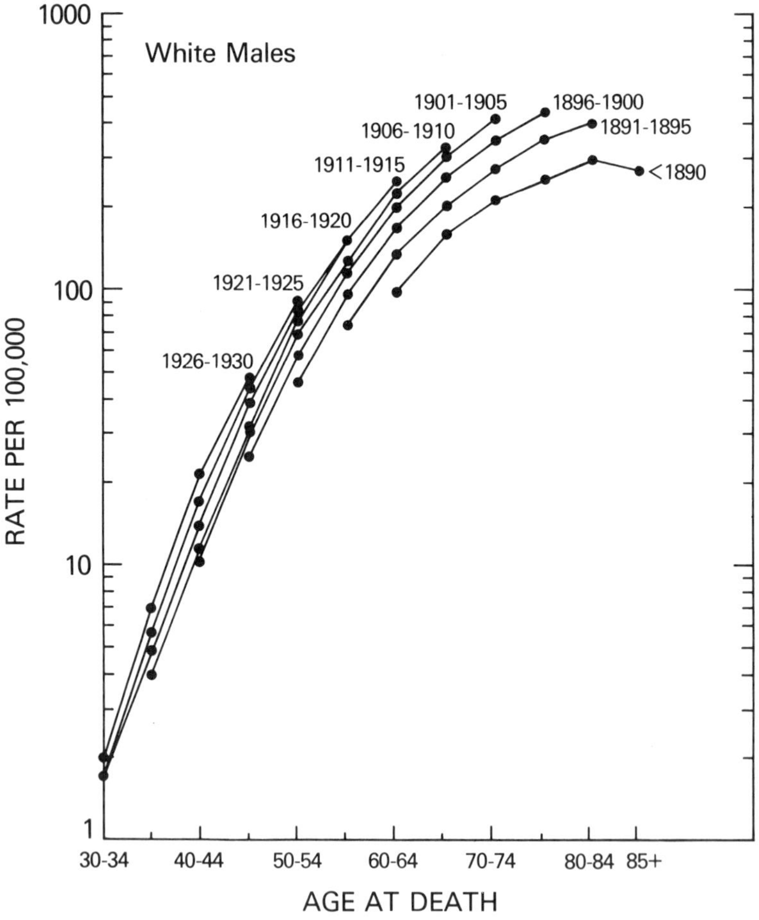

Figure 2. Age-specific United States lung cancer death rates among white males by birth cohort.

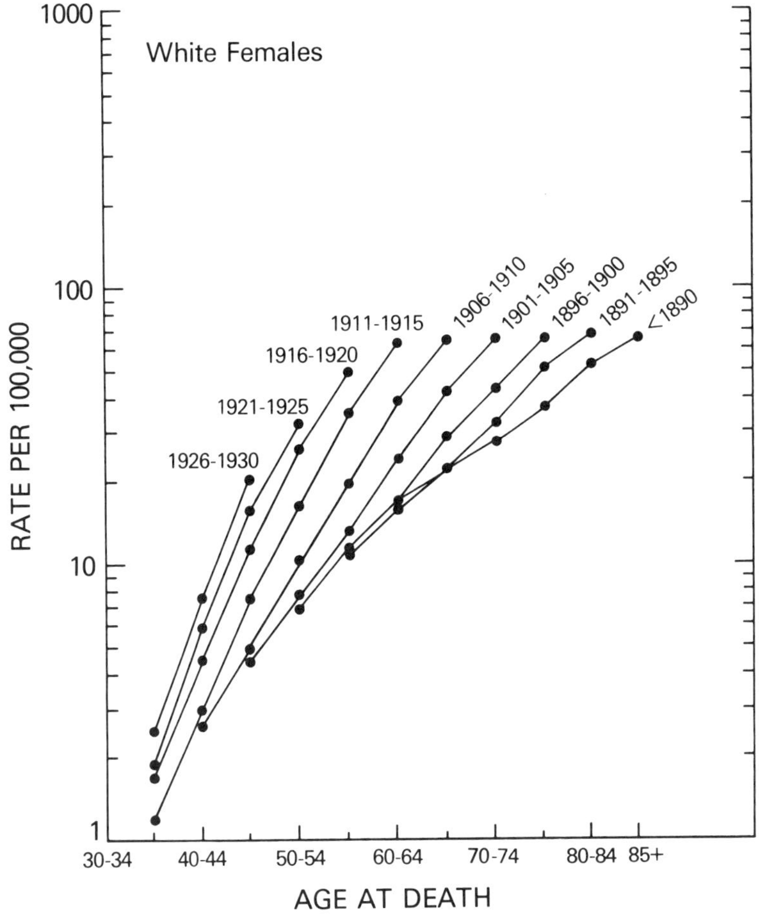

Figure 3. Age-specific United States lung cancer death rates among white females by birth cohort.

cidence curve probably paralleled the mortality curve between the late 1940s and 1969–1971. The increases among females have occurred primarily since the early 1960s; this is considerably later than among males. The mortality rates for the 5GA have been only slightly higher than those for the entire United States at each point in time, and the shapes of the curves are quite similar. There appears to be some moderation in the rate of increase in the late 1970s.

Each successive birth cohort of white males has experienced higher lung cancer death rates through 1975 than the preceding cohort (Figure 2). The rates increase exponentially with age, and it is not clear whether there is a peak in risk prior to the oldest age category. Proportional increases were greater in the earlier compared to later cohorts. The rates also increase exponentially with age among birth cohorts of white females (Figure 3), and there is little evidence of a change in slope with increasing age. Although the rates are much lower, the proportional increases between cohorts are greater among females than among males.

There is variation in the incidence trends by age. Among white males (Figure 4), there has been a very recent downturn for those aged 25–34, although the rates are

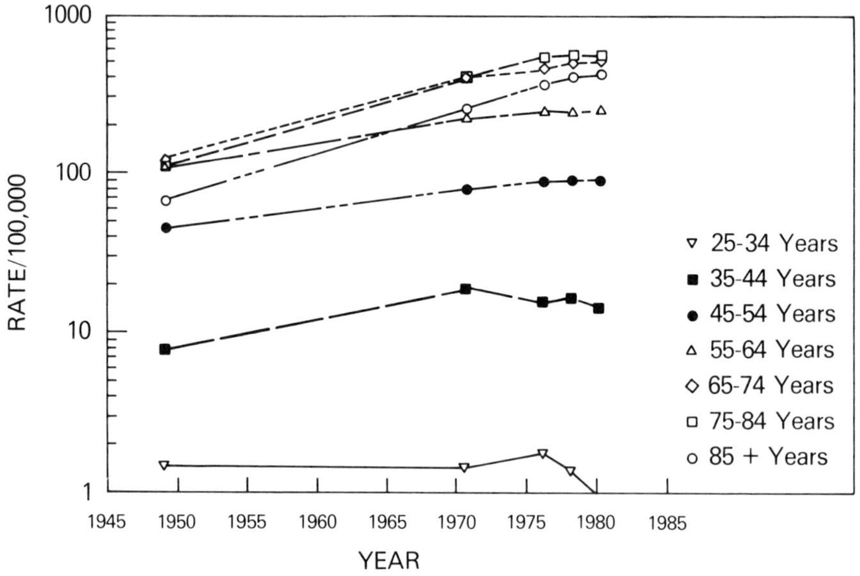

Figure 4. Age-specific incidence trends in five geographic areas for lung cancer among white males.

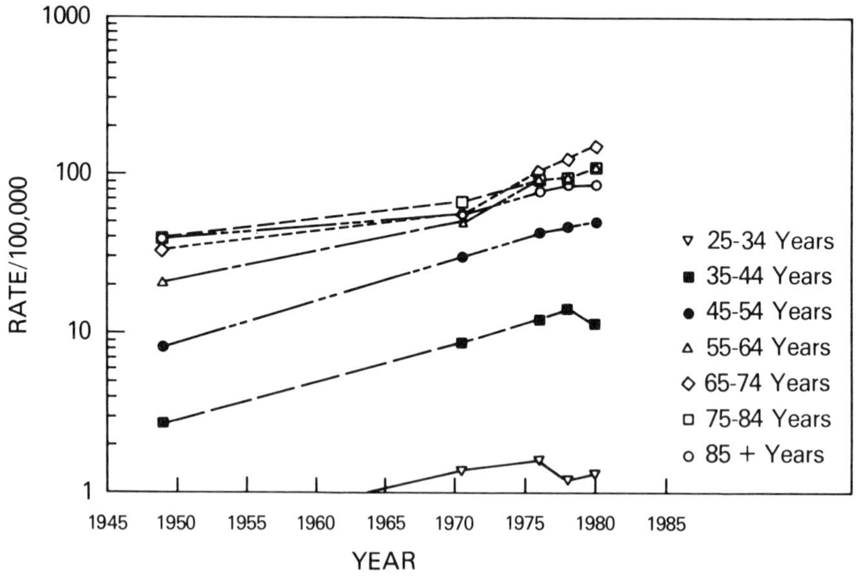

Figure 5. Age-specific incidence trends in five geographic areas for lung cancer among white females.

based on small numbers of cases; the rate for 1979–1980 was 0.95 (not zero). Among those aged 35–44, increases were apparent from the late 1940s to 1969–1971, and decreases have occurred since then. Incidence increased in all the other age groups, with the largest proportional increases occurring among those

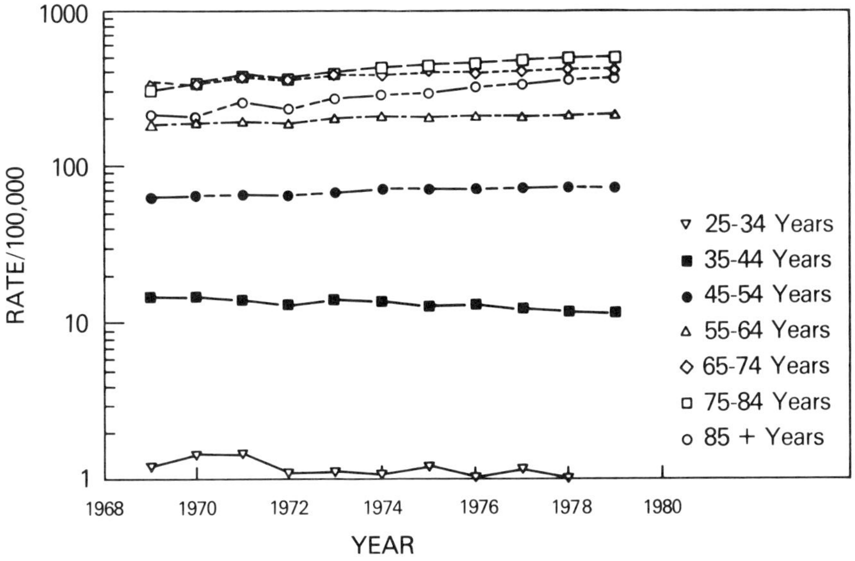

Figure 6. Age-specific United States lung cancer mortality trends among white males.

aged 65 and over. Each of the age groups 45 and older shows moderating increases during the 1970s. In contrast, increases prior to 1970 among white females were more pronounced among those under age 65 than those over age 65 (Figure 5). Since then, the largest increases have been among those aged 65–74. There is some suggestion that the rates may be turning downward among females aged 25–44, although the number of cases is relatively low, particularly under age 35.

In the country as a whole, recent mortality data indicate some downturn in rates among white males aged 35–44 (9); over the period from 1969 to 1979 (Figure 6),

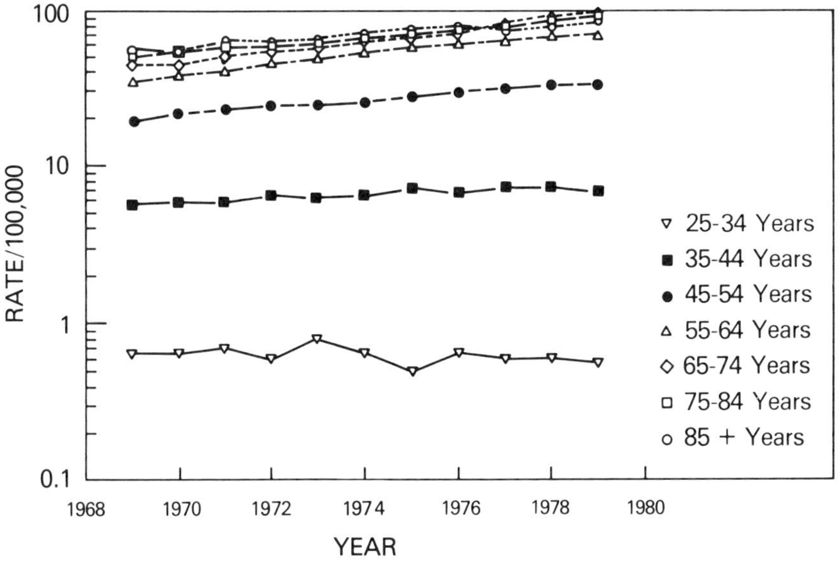

Figure 7. Age-specific United States lung cancer mortality trends among white females.

rates decreased from about 15 to 12 per 100,000 per year. Mortality rates among those aged 45–54 have been fairly stable since 1974, whereas rates among the older age groups continue to increase. Among white females, decreases are suggested only among the very youngest group (under age 35) (Figure 7) (the vertical scale for this figure is different from that used for males to better show the trends). The age group 35–44 shows increases during the early part of the decade, with some indication of leveling off during the latter half of the 1970s. Mortality rates are continuing to increase among all age groups 45 and older.

It has been noted for some time that there is geographic variation in the occurrence of cancer (10). In addition, the patterns have changed over time (11). During the 1950s, the rates were highest in scattered areas around the country, particularly in the northeast and the urban areas. The lung cancer mortality rates were also elevated in a number of Louisiana parishes. Mortality patterns had shifted by 1970–1975, with many of the counties in the southeast having relatively high rates and the rest of the country showing much less variation as urban–rural differences diminished.

The available incidence data support the mortality patterns. The lung cancer rate for Atlanta white males was relatively low in the past (Figure 8) and subsequently has become one of the highest. Increases are apparent in each of the geograpic areas, although increases in Iowa occurred later than in the other areas. Regional differences appear to be diminishing. There is a general change in slope during the 1970s decade.

The incidence rate among white males in New Orleans was higher during the late 1940s than in any other area shown; it was also the highest of the ten cities included in the early survey (4). The New Orleans rate also was high during the

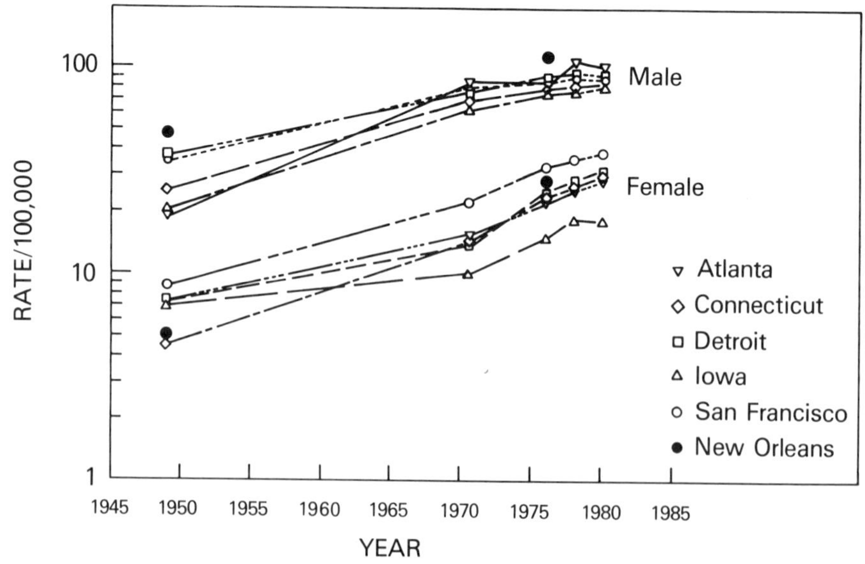

Figure 8. Area-specific incidence trends for lung cancer among whites.

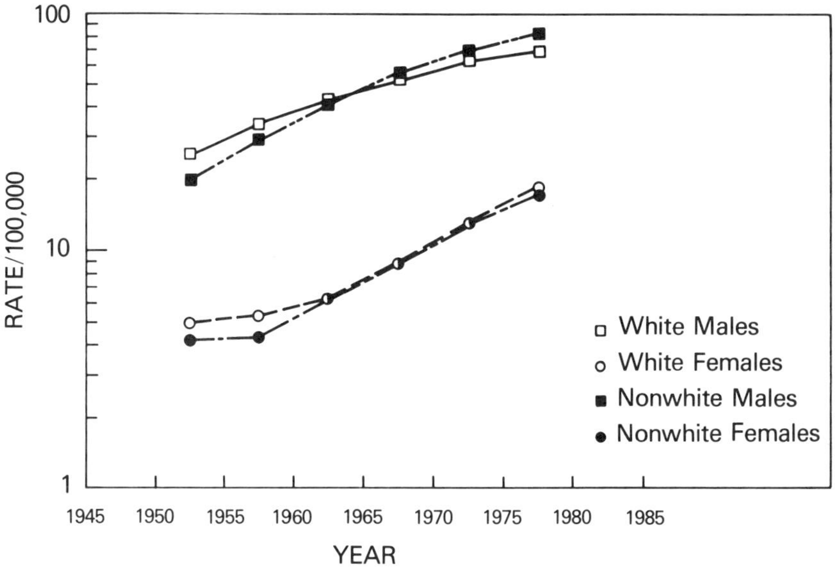

Figure 9. Mortality trends of lung cancer in the United States by race and sex.

1970s. The patterns among white females are somewhat different. The rate in New Orleans was relatively low during the late 1940s and somewhat high during the mid-1970s; the rates in San Francisco-Oakland have been consistently higher than in the other areas; the rate in Iowa showed only small increases from 1950 to 1969–1971, and since then it has increased substantially.

In the early 1950s, lung cancer mortality rates in the total United States were 15–20% lower among nonwhites than among whites of the same sex (Figure 9). By the early 1960s, the rates were quite comparable; rates among females have risen similarly since then. Mortality rates among nonwhite males have continued to rise faster than among white males such that the rate was 18% higher by the late 1970s. The mortality curve, however, does appear to be rising less steeply in recent years. Over the 25-year period shown in Figure 9, the mortality increases among both male and female nonwhites are almost fourfold.

During more recent years, data are available not only for the more diverse group of nonwhites but also specifically for blacks. Between 1969 and 1979, lung cancer mortality rates among black males have increased in all age groups over 55 (Figure 10). Among those aged 45–54, increases were apparent until the late 1970s. Rates among the 35–44 year age group are relatively stable, whereas those for the 25–34 age group suggest some decline. The age-specific mortality trends among black females have been somewhat similar, with larger increases among the older compared to the younger age groups.

There is geographic variation in the lung cancer incidence rates among black as well as white males in the areas participating in the SEER program (Figure 11) (7). The rate for all areas combined was 44% higher among black males than white males (110.0 versus 76.4 per 100,000 per year, respectively). The average annual

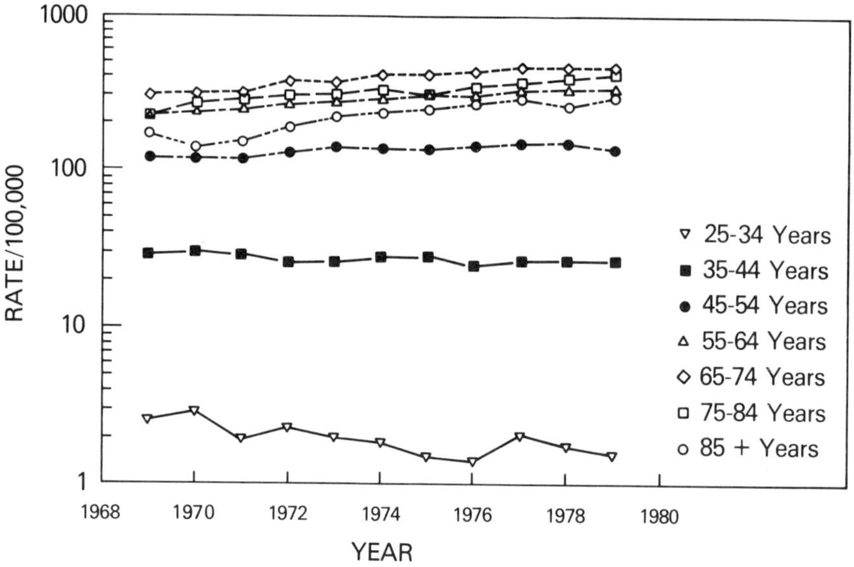

Figure 10. Age-specific United States lung cancer mortality trends among black males.

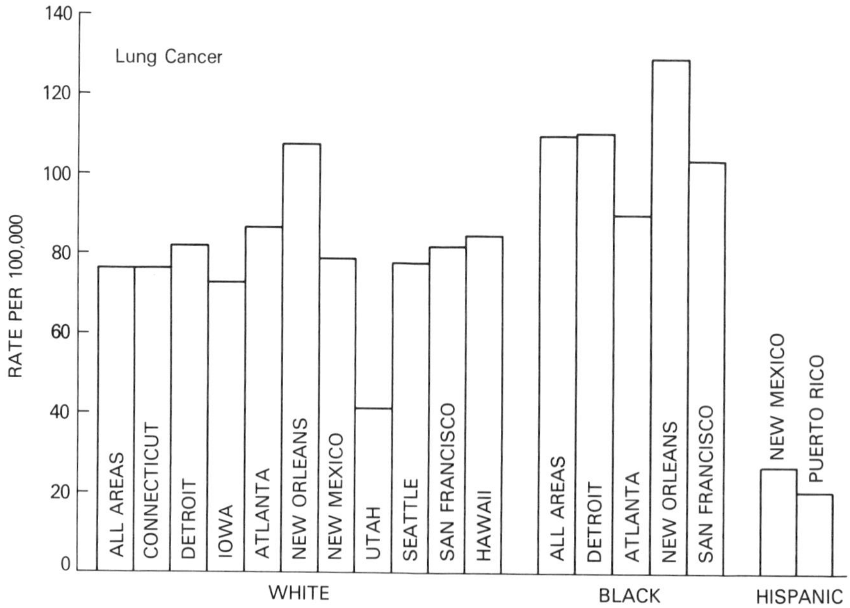

Figure 11. Average annual age-adjusted (1970 United States population) incidence rates for males by race and registry, SEER program, 1973–1977. Courtesy Dr. John L. Young, Jr, NCI.

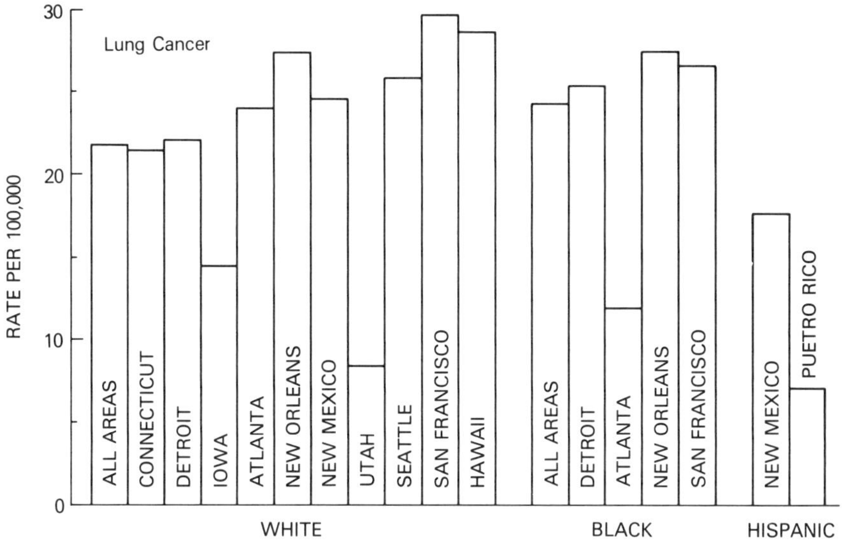

Figure 12. Average annual age-adjusted (1970 United States population) incidence rates for females by race and registry, SEER program, 1973–77. Courtesy Dr. John L. Young, Jr, NCI.

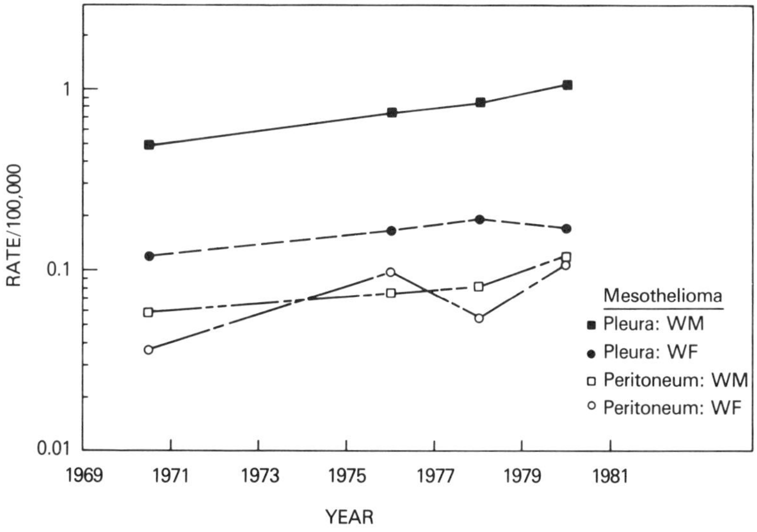

Figure 13. Incidence trends in five geographic areas for mesothelioma among white males and females.

rate for 1973–1977 was highest in New Orleans in both races. The second highest rate among white males was in Atlanta. However, Atlanta black males do not appear to share the excess risk observed among blacks in the other areas. Incidence rates are particularly low among white males in Utah and among Hispanic males in New Mexico and Puerto Rico. Lung cancer incidence among black females is only 11% higher than among white females (24.3 versus 21.8/100,000) (Figure 12). (The scale for this figure also is different from that used for males to better show the patterns.) There is considerable geographic variation within each race. Among white females, rates are relatively high in San Francisco, Hawaii, and New Orleans and relatively low in Iowa and Utah. Among black females, the rate is relatively high in New Orleans and particularly low in Atlanta.

Mesothelioma is a rare type of tumor, accounting for less than 1% of all lung/pleural cancers (7). However, the trends in mesothelioma incidence are of particular interest because of the association between this cancer and asbestos exposure (12). There are difficulties in compiling comparable data because medical diagnosis, terminology, reporting rules, and coding schemes have changed over time. As a result, it is not clear how much of the observed increase in mesothelioma of the pleura from 1969–1971 to 1979–1980 among white males is real and how much is artifact (Figure 13; note that the scale for this figure is 1/100 that of earlier figures). Reported rates among white females are considerably lower than among white males. Mesothelioma also occurs in other sites, primarily the peritoneum; incidence rates for the peritoneum are quite low and are similar for males and females.

Discussion

Large increases have occurred in lung cancer over the past 30 years among both males and females. These increases have affected all age groups and are continuing in the older groups, but there is some suggestion that rates among the younger groups are moderating and possibly actually decreasing. This is very encouraging and we hope to see these trends continue, with the patterns among the younger continuing into the older age groups. Whether these moderations in rates reflect decreases in the prevalence of smoking, which have been greater among males than among females (13), or changes in the chemical composition of cigarettes, with decreases in the tar/nicotine content (14), is not known. Occupational exposures to carcinogens (12) may have diminished as workplace environments have improved. Nevertheless, the lung remains the leading primary site of cancer among men and is second only to colorectal cancer among both sexes combined (7). The geographic patterns of lung cancer incidence and the changes therein suggest areas that may be fruitful for further research.

Acknowledgments

This analysis would not have been possible without the efforts and contributions of many people. These include the staffs of the surveys, registries, and SEER program, throughout the country and at the National Cancer Institute; the programming assistance of the staffs of Geomet and ORI, Inc., in particular Mary Ann Read, Margaret Seldin, Claudette Zaccack, and Janice Chang; the special programing for the mortality data by Frank W. McKay of the Clinical Epidemiology Branch, National Cancer Institute; and the clerical and secretarial support of Josephine I. Davis and Carol A. Ball.

References

1. McKay FW, Hanson MR, Miller RW. Cancer mortality in the United States: 1950–1977. National Cancer Institute Monogr 59, National Institutes of Health Publ 82-2435. Bethesda, Md: National Institutes of Health, 1982.
2. National Center for Health Statistics. Mortality tapes including data through 1979. Hyattsville, Md.: NCHS, 1982
3. American Cancer Society. Cancer facts and figures-1983. New York: ACS, 1982.
4. Dorn HF, Cutler SJ. Morbidity from cancer in the United States: parts I and II. Public Health Monogr 56, Public Health Service Publ 590. Washington, DC: U.S. Public Health Service, 1959.
5. Haenszel W, Marcus SC, Zimmerer EG. Cancer morbidity in urban and rural Iowa. Public Health Monogr 37, Public Health Service Publ 462. Washington, DC: U.S. Public Health Service, 1956.
6. Cutler SJ, Young JL Jr, eds. Third National Cancer Survey: incidence data. National Cancer Institute Monogr 41, U.S. Department of Health, Education and Welfare Publ No (NIH) 75-787. Bethesda, Md: National Cancer Institute, 1975.
7. Young JL Jr, Percy CL, Asire AJ, eds. Surveillance, Epidemiology, and End Results program: incidence and mortality data, 1973–77. National Cancer Institute Monogr 57, National Institutes of Health Publ 81-2330. Bethesda, Md: National Cancer Institute, 1981.
8. Heston J, Meigs JW, Kelly J, et al. Forty-five years of cancer incidence in Connecticut: 1935–1979. National Cancer Institute Monogr in press.
9. Horm JW, Asire AJ. Changes in lung cancer incidence and mortality rates among Americans: 1969–78. JNCI 1982;69:833–837.
10. Mason TJ, McKay FW, Hoover R, Blot WJ, Fraumeni JF Jr. Atlas of cancer mortality for U.S. counties: 1950–1969. U.S. Department of Health, Education and Welfare Publ (NIH) 75-780, Bethesda, Md: U.S. Government Printing Office, 1975.
11. Blot WJ, Fraumeni JF Jr. Changing patterns of lung cancer in the United States. Am J Epidemiol 1982;115:664–673.
12. Fraumeni JF Jr, Blot WJ. Lung and pleura. In: Schottenfeld D, Fraumeni JF Jr, eds: Cancer Epidemiology and Prevention. Philadelphia: WB Saunders, 1982:564–582.
13. U.S. Department of Health and Human Services. The Health Consequences of Smoking for Women—a report of the Surgeon General. Rockville, Md: USDHHS, Office on Smoking and Health, 1980.
14. U.S. Department of Health and Human Services. The Health Consequences of Smoking: The Changing Cigarette—a report of the Surgeon General. Rockville, Md: USDHHS, Office on Smoking and Health, 1980.

CHAPTER 4

Lung Cancer and Occupational Exposures

WILLIAM J. BLOT

Environmental Epidemiology Branch, National Cancer Institute, Landow C309, Bethesda, Maryland 20205

ABSTRACT

Much of what is known about the human carcinogencity of a number of chemical and physical substances comes from epidemiologic studies of respiratory cancer in occupational groups. This review of cancer in the workplace focuses on agents or processes identified or suspected as occupational lung carcinogens. The review summarizes available epidemiologic evidence and offers suggestions for future research to evaluate occupation in the multifactor etiology of lung cancer.
Key Words: **Lung cancer, occupation**

Introduction

Lung cancer is the leading cause of cancer death among males in most western nations. Although smoking is the major determinant of lung cancer risk, other respiratory exposures can induce lung tumors on their own or enhance the carcinogenic effect of tobacco smoke. Most notable among these are certain chemical and physical substances that can be found in the workplace. Knowledge of which occupational agents can cause lung cancer, the magnitude of their effects at differing levels of exposure, and the interactions between on the job exposures and smoking or other risk factors, although far from complete, has increased in recent years. Therefore a review of the epidemiologic evidence regarding occupational lung cancer at this time may be useful in summarizing information and suggesting opportunities for future etiologic research.

Lung Cancer: Causes and Prevention.

History

The first lung cancers recognized as occupational in origin are likely those occurring in underground miners working the metal mines of the mountains in central Europe in the latter part of the 19th century. The likely cause of this "mountain disease" is now thought to be the miners' inhalation of radon and subsequent recurrent exposure of bronchial tissue to α-emitting radon daughters. Lung cancer was a rare disease then and continued to be so into the early part of the 20th century, but as incidence began to rise reports of the cancer in occupational groups appeared. Review of stated occupation on death certificates in England and Wales in the 1920s and 1930s suggested that lung cancer might be associated with the coal carbonization process, and by the 1940s arsenic and chromium compounds were implicated and lung cancer was first reported in workers suffering from asbestosis (1).

When lung cancer began to occur in near-epidemic proportions from the 1950s onwards, the detection of clustering of excess cases among occupational groups (and the separation of the influence of smoking) by means of alert clinical observation became less feasible. The epidemiologic method of study emerged, however, as a systematic way of evaluating occupation as a risk factor for lung cancer and has since become the primary means of identification of occupational hazards. As described below, most of the existing knowledge of workplace lung carcinogens has come from cohort studies of the mortality experience of groups of industrial employees and from case-control studies of lung cancer which retrospectively ascertained detailed occupational histories.

Known Occupational Lung Carcinogens

Among all nonmedicinal substances recognized as human carcinogens, the majority are causes of lung cancer detected through observation of occupational groups (2). Described below are eight agents (or processes) known to have caused lung cancer in man.

Arsenic

Inorganic arsenic had been suspected as carcinogenic to the skin and perhaps other tissues as early as the 1800s, but definitive evidence linking exposure to this substance with lung cancer accrued only by the late 1960s and 1970s (3). In 1969, Lee and Fraumeni showed a threefold excess mortality from lung cancer between 1938 and 1963 among a cohort of 8000 employees of a copper smelter in the western United States (4). The increase was nearly eightfold among men who had worked in areas of the smelter where exposure to arsenic trioxide, a constituent of the ores being smelted, was highest. Updated followup shows that an excess persists through the 1970s, with mortality rates varying in proportion to cumulative arsenic exposures, and that smoking is not responsible (5, 6). Studies of other copper smelters in the United States, Japan, and Sweden have shown similar results. In contrast, no increase was found for zinc refinery workers, where potential for arsenic exposure is minimal, but some suggestion of excess lung cancer was noted in a zinc smelter, where exposures to airborne arsenic are intermediate between those for copper smelters and for the general population (7, 8). Recent data on smelter workers in Sweden suggest that arsenic and smoking may interact in a multiplicative fashion in increasing lung cancer risk (9), but information from American copper smelters provides no evidence of an enhanced risk among workers who are heavy smokers (6, 10). Analysis of the temporal patterns of risk suggest that arsenic exerts its strongest influence at the late stages of carcinogenesis (11, 12).

Arsenic also has been associated with lung cancer in other occupational groups. Workers engaged in the manufacture of arsenical pesticides (mostly pentavalent arsenate compounds) in the United States have been reported within the past decade to have experienced elevated lung cancer mortality rates, consistent with the excess proportionate lung cancer mortality rates noted in British sheep dip preparers in the 1940s (3). Lung tumors also have been found at autopsy among German and French vintners showing symptoms of arsenicism from arsenical pesticide sprays (3).

Therefore, although inorganic arsenic has failed to produce cancers in experimental animals [until recently arsenic and benzene were the only two recognized human carcinogens without supporting evidence of carcinogenicity in animals; arsenic now retains this distinction alone as Zymbal gland carcinomas and several rare malignancies have been induced in benzene-exposed rats (13)], the epidemiologic evidence is considered sufficient to declare it a human carcinogen (2).

Asbestos

Of all known chemical or physical carcinogenic substances, asbestos accounts for the greatest share of occupational lung cancers. Strong evidence that inhalation of asbestos fibers could increase the risk of lung cancer was reported in 1955, when Richard Doll showed a tenfold excess of the cancer among asbestos factory workers (14). Since that time the role of this widely utilized material in inducing tumors has been elucidated by a number of large-scale epidemiologic investigations of various occupationally exposed groups, including miners, millers, and insulation, textile, cement, and shipyard workers.

Although mesothelioma, asbestosis, and alimentary tract and kidney cancers have been reported in asbestos workers, lung cancer is the major asbestos-related disease, resulting in approximately 20% of the deaths among certain exposed cohorts. The percentage of lung cancer is even higher in heavily exposed subgroups, as risk tends to rise with increasing intensity and/or duration of exposure (15). The length of exposure need not necessarily be long, however, as evidenced by the doubled risk of lung cancer 20 years after work for less than 9 months in a United States amostite factory, by the occurrence of excess lung cancers among gasmask manufacturers briefly exposed in the 1940s, and by the current 40–70% excess of lung neoplasms among men in southeast Atlantic coastal areas of the United States who worked in shipyards that operated only during World War II (15–17). Occupational exposures usually are to mixed forms of asbestos, but all fiber types (crocidolite, amosite, chrysotile, anthophyllite) are thought to increase the risk of respiratory cancer. The fibers seem capable of inducing all histologic types of lung cancers. A disproportionate number of lung adenocarcinomas was found in a British autopsy series of patients with asbestosis, but no unusual distribution of cell types has been noted in American asbestos workers, although the tumors appear more often in the lower lobes (15, 18).

A distinctive characteristic of asbestos-induced lung cancer is its synergistic relation with cigarette smoking. A recent survey of 276 lung cancer deaths among insulation workers that occurred at least 20 years after initial occupational exposure showed relative risks of about 5 associated with asbestos exposure, of about 10 associated with cigarette smoking, and of about 50 following joint exposure (15). For this same cohort there was a gradient with amount smoked, with heavily-smoking asbestos workers experiencing nearly 90 times the risk of nonsmoking (any tobacco form), nonexposed individuals. Because the bulk of the excess of lung cancer results from the synergism between smoking and asbestos, breaking either causal pathway may result in a significant reduction in risk to asbestos workers.

The industry with the largest number of workers with potential for exposure to asbestos is shipbuilding (17). This industry in the United States was only of moderate size until World War II, when it underwent massive expansion and became the largest single manufacturing industry in the country. The number of persons employed in United States shipyards was around 200,000 during the period 1915–1965, except for an increase to about 475,000 during World War I and a striking increase to about 1.7 million persons in late 1943. Because turnover among shipyard workers was high during the wartime escalation, the total number of individuals employed during World War II may have been as high as 4.5 million. Only limited data are available on exposure to particular substances among individual shipyard workers, although an environmental survey in 1945 of pipecovering operations in two Navy and two private shipyards showed asbestos exposures could be high. This survey uncovered no increased prevalence of asbestos disease, which led to a false sense of security that persisted for almost two decades. Then in 1964 a British series of 17 patients with mesothelioma was reported in Liverpool; five had worked in the ship-repair industry. Other cases subsequently were identified among shipyard workers of Plymouth and then elsewhere in Europe and recently in the United States. The mesotheliomas signaled the presence of earlier exposures to asbestos, but the recognition that asbestos exposures were widespread throughout the shipyards came only in the late 1970s, when pleural and parenchymal x-ray changes characteristic of asbestos disease were observed among long-term shipyard workers of virtually all trades, not just those directly handling asbestos products (17).

Also in the late 1970s lung cancer began to be identified among World War II shipyard workers in the United States (17). Four case-control studies of lung cancer have been conducted by the National Cancer Institute in areas along the Atlantic coast where mortality rates are high. In all areas there were elevated risks associated with prior work in area shipyards, particularly during World War II. In two of the areas (Georgia and Florida) major shipyards operated only during the war and closed shortly thereafter. In coastal Virginia, where the shipbuilding industry is still the area's largest single employer, the risk of lung cancer was elevated among those who had worked in the shipyards during World War II, but not among those first employed after 1950. These studies enabled detailed evaluation of the role of cigarette smoking upon the occupational association. In the combined data from all four studies, the increased risk of lung cancer among shipyard workers was seen in nearly all cigarette smoking categories. The largest absolute excess, however, occurred among heavy smokers, consistent with the synergistic relation between smoking and asbestos. Asbestos was also thought to be primarily responsible for the lung cancer excess in a cohort study of workers employed in the early 1950s at the Pearl Harbor Naval Shipyard in Hawaii. There was a 70% increase in lung cancer deaths among men whose particular jobs suggested exposure to asbestos, but no excess risk for the remainder of the workforce. In all of these studies, however, it is not possible to exclude the influence of carcinogens other than asbestos in shipyards.

Bischloromethyl Ether

Workers in chemical manufacturing plants in the United States, Germany, and Japan exposed to bischloromethyl ether (BCME) have demonstrated increased risks of lung cancer, with excesses over tenfold in the most heavily exposed (2). One of the most interesting features is the specificity of association with a particular histologic type of tumor, namely small- (or oat-) cell carcinoma, with these tumors typically occurring at unusually young ages.

The number of individuals exposed to BCME is not large, so that opportunities for additional research, eg, to further assess dose-exposure relationships, are limited. Nevertheless, one research problem concerns the relative roles of smoking and BCME exposure and their implications for mechanisms of carcinogenesis, because one study indicated that the relative increases in risk was far greater for workers who were nonsmokers (and ex-smokers) than smokers and hypothesized that heavy smoking actually may inhibit BCME-induced lung cancer (19). In addition, it is not known whether the carcinogenic effect established for BCME holds as well for chloromethyl methyl ether, but epidemiologic studies may shed little light on this issue because technical grade chloromethyl methyl ether is usually contaminated with BCME.

Chromium Compounds

The first clear indication that chromium compounds could induce lung tumors in man came from a review in the 1940s of the proportionate mortality experience of workers at six United States chromate-producing plants (20). Thirty-two deaths were attributed to lung cancer, in contrast to an expected level of slightly over one among a comparison group of employees in an oil-refining company. By the late 1970s lung cancer had been noted in excess in other chromate production workers and in chromate pigment and chrome-plating workers in the United States, England, Japan, and Norway (21). Further confirmation of an excess among British sodium chromate production workers has since been published (22), and elevated lung cancer has been reported among zinc chromate spray painters (23). Although the role of cigarette smoking has not been fully evaluated, the consistency of the findings and the magnitude of the excesses (ranging from somewhat less than two- to 30-fold) leave little doubt as to the carcinogenic potential of the compounds. Recent data from Japan suggest that small-cell cancers of the lung predominate when exposures are heavy (24). The relative influences of the various types of chromium compounds are less clear. Some hexavalent forms, eg, calcium chromate, are strongly carcinogenic in rats after intrabronchial implantation, whereas evidence for others is inadequate, and there has been little support from animal or from short-term tests of carcinogenicity or mutagenic activity for trivalent forms (2).

Mustard Gas

A constellation of respiratory tract tumors, including those of the trachea and bronchus, has been reported among Japanese workers who manufactured mustard gas during the 1930s and into World War II (25). Over 30 respiratory cancer deaths occurred whereas less than one was expected at prevailing Japanese national rates. A twofold increase of lung cancer also has been observed among workers heavily exposed to mustard gas in a German factory, and a still smaller excess in an updated followup among American soldiers occasionally exposed during World War I (2).

Nickel-Refining Processes

A tenfold excess of lung cancer (and an even greater relative increase of nasal cancer) was reported in the 1950s among men in a Welsh nickel refinery, consistent with the report of excess respiratory cancer among nickel refiners in the 1932 British Annual Report of the Chief Inspector of Factories and Workshops (26). Later followup confirmed that the increase was confined to those who had begun work before changes in operations took place in the early 1930s and so most likely was related to exposures to dusts during preliminary nickel ore smelting rather than to exposure to nickel carbonyl, a gas released in the refining. Studies in Britain, Canada, and Norway also show substantial increased risks of lung cancer among nickel refinery workers (2). Three small surveys have not found increased lung cancer mortality in men exposed to lower levels of nickel dusts and aerosols in non-refining processes, suggesting that nickel per se may not be sufficient to induce lung cancer, but the exact processes or nickel compounds responsible for the sharply increased cancer risk in refinery workers is uncertain. Some nickel compounds (eg, nickel subsulfide) but not others are carcinogenic in laboratory animals (2).

Polycyclic Aromatic Hydrocarbons

The suspicions of the first half of this century of increased risks of lung cancer among workers exposed to polycyclic aromatic hydrocarbons (PAH) in coal carbonization processes (gas retort houses, coke ovens, gas generators) were confirmed in the 1950s and 1960s. The largest investigation was the cohort study by Lloyd and co-workers of 59,000 men employed in Pittsburgh area steel mills in 1953 and followed for mortality thereafter (27). The most prominent finding was an increased death rate from lung cancer among those who worked at coke plants. The excess was concentrated among men who worked topside of the coke ovens, reaching ten times the mortality rate of other steel workers. Relative increases of about twofold have been reported among gas retort workers in Britain, and mortality was shown to increase with duration of employment among gas generator employees in Japan (2). A recent case-control study of lung cancer in eastern Pennsylvania found a significant increase among steel workers, with the excess (nearly twofold) primarily limited to long-term employees who began work in the 1930s (8). This study was the first to examine the role of cigarette smoking and found the greatest occupational excess among heavy smokers.

Soot, tar, and oils, substances associated with the first clearly recognized occupational cancers of the scrotum among London chimney sweeps in the 1700s, were also the first chemical substances for which carcinogenicity was demonstrated in laboratory animals in skin painting experiments in rabbits in Japan at the turn of this century. Their role in respiratory cancer is suggested by the increased lung cancer risks among roofers and aluminum reduction plant workers exposed to coal tar and pitch volatiles (28, 29).

Despite the observation of excess lung cancer risk in different countries and in different industrial settings, there has been some uncertainty as to the specific exposures responsible. Nevertheless a common denominator has been exposure to polycyclic aromatic hydrocarbons, a broad class of chemical compounds released in the carbonization processes and found in coal and petroleum, many of which (eg, benzo[a]pyrene) are carcinogenic in laboratory animals (2). Additional research is needed to determine which hydrocarbons may predominate and whether other exposures contribute to the excess risk in PAH-exposed groups. Ferric oxides had been considered as possibly influential in the excess risk among steel workers, because iron ore (hematite) miners in Britain experience increased lung cancer, but recent studies in Sweden and the United States Mesabi range suggest that the excess lung cancer among the miners is more likely caused by radon (30, 31).

Radiation (Radon)

Lung cancer has long been common among miners in certain areas of central Europe, accounting for as much as 30–50% of all deaths in the early 1900s. The cancers have also occurred in excess among uranium miners in the United States, Canada, and Czechoslovakia, fluorspar miners in Newfoundland, underground hematite miners in Cumberland, Cornish tin miners, and metal miners in Sweden and in the United States (32–34). A commonality among each of these occupational groups is exposure to ionizing radiation from α-rays emitted by inhaled radon dust particles. The likelihood that radiation is the cause of many of these lung tumors is suggested by the increased risk observed with increased radiation dose—the smoking-adjusted excess for white male uranium miners, eg, with highest exposure ($>$ 3700 working level months) reaching nearly 20-fold (32)—and by the specificity of the tumor type involved. Among United States uranium miners with higher levels of exposure, over three-fourths of the lung cancers were small-cell undifferentiated carcinomas, histologic types that usually account for less than one-fourth of lung cancers among American men (32). It had earlier been suggested that radon acts synergistically with cigarette smoking in enhancing lung cancer risk, but there has been some question during the 1970s as to the precise nature of the smoking-radiation relationship (35). The most recent analyses of the United States uranium miner data, however, show that the original proposition may be appropriate and that the effects of cumulative radon exposure and cumulative tobacco exposure tend to multiply each other (36). Further research may help unravel the potentially complex interrelationships between radiation (both high linear energy transfer α- and low linear energy transfer γ- and x-rays), smoking, and other factors and help provide clues to the mechanisms of radiation cancer and guidelines for inferring about risks associated with low level exposure. Low-dose exposures among radiologists and x-ray technicians have not resulted in increased lung cancer mortality, although a two-fold excess had been reported in British radiologists who entered the profession prior to 1920 when exposures were high (37, 38).

Suspected Occupational Lung Carcinogens

Substances for which there is experimental evidence of carcinogenicity and suggestive (but not conclusive) evidence from epidemiologic studies are included here.

Acrylonitrile

Acrylonitrile, used in the production of plastics, fibers, and synthetic rubber, has been associated with increases, on the order of about twofold or less, of lung cancer among workers in plants in the United States, Germany, and Great Britain (2, 39). In the American studies, even though the total number of cases was small (8 respiratory cancers observed, 4.4 expected in one; 9 vs 5.9 in the other), there was some suggestion of a trend of increased risk with increased exposure.

Beryllium

Much of the epidemiologic data to evaluate the carcinogenic potential of beryllium comes from studies of workers in plants in Pennsylvania and Ohio involved in the extraction of beryllium oxides from ores and the production of beryllium-copper alloys (40). In the largest compilation, 47 lung cancer deaths were observed during 1942–1975, whereas 34 were expected based on national rates. The excess reached nearly twofold among those followed 25 or more years since onset of exposure. Some controversy has surrounded this study (41), but ongoing extended followup should help clarify the risk among this population.

Vinyl Chloride

Vinyl chloride, a well-known liver carcinogen, also may affect the lung. An increased risk of lung cancer of less than twofold has been found among groups of workers in polymerization plants and among employees exposed to vinyl chloride dusts in a synthetic chemicals plants in the United States, although not among a group of heavily exposed Canadian workers (2, 42, 43). A 17% proportionate mortality increase was reported for polyvinyl chloride fabricators, where exposures were thought to be low.

Industrial Processes Suspected of Increasing Lung Cancer Risk

Three industrial processes have been associated with elevated lung cancer risk, but the evidence is not yet sufficient to consider the relationship one of cause and effect or to incriminate clearly any single exposure as responsible for the association.

Foundry Work

Although reviews of occupational mortality statistics in Great Britain had noted increased frequencies of lung cancer among molders, casters, and other foundry workers as early as the 1930s, it was not until the late 1970s that the association began to be clarified (44). In cohort studies of foundry workers in Finland, Canada, and the United States, increased lung cancer risks were reported. The increases in each study were on the order of two- to threefold among those employed at least 5 years. The excess was primarily among molders and casters in iron foundries in Finland, but extended to steel foundry workers in Canada. In addition, a proportionate mortality study among members of a molders union in the United States found 208 deaths caused by lung cancer, whereas 142 were expected. A recent case-control study also has found excess lung cancer among long-term foundry workers in the steel industry, particularly those beginning work prior to 1935, that was not caused by smoking, although the numbers of men involved were small (8). Therefore, the pattern of increased respiratory cancer seems consistent across different study methods in different countries and suggests that an occupational hazard exists. The exposures responsible for the increased lung cancer are not known. The PAHs, including benzo[a]pyrene, have been detected in the foundry atmosphere, particularly following shakeout procedures when castings are removed from molds, as have benzene, aromatic amines, chromium, nickel and various silica sands. Ongoing animal studies of the carcinogenicity of mold emissions, together with additional industrial hygiene characterization of the foundry environment and epidemiologic followup of exposed populations may help clarify the role of on the job exposures in the increased lung cancer rates among foundry workers.

Rubber Manufacturing

Observations of bladder tumors among workers in the rubber industry in Great Britain in the early 1950s helped lead to the establishment of ongoing cohort studies of four large groups of workers in Great Britain and the United States (45). In one, a 10-year followup of 41,000 workers at British rubber factories, 822 lung cancer deaths were observed during 1967–1976 compared to 717 expected based on prevailing rates in England and Wales. Lung cancer death rates were also elevated (638 observed, 517 expected) during 1946–1975 among 34,000 employees in one of 13 British factories. The overall lung cancer Standardized Mortality Ratios (SMRs) for groups of 29,000 and 19,000 men working in rubber plants in Akron, Ohio were not elevated, however, although about a twofold excess lung cancer morbidity was found among workers in tire casting and molding and fuel cell/deicer manufacture in the first group, whereas a case-control study within the other cohort noted small increases for several job categories, including compounding and mixing and shipping and receiving. Lung cancer mortality rates among females in both American cohorts was increased by two- to threefold, but the numbers of cancers observed were not large. In summary, the combined evidence suggests that lung cancer may occur somewhat more often among rubber workers, but the specific exposures (occupational or nonoccupational) responsible for the association have not been identified and a causal connection cannot be made.

Welding

In a recent review of epidemiologic studies providing information on lung cancer among welders, Beaumont and Weiss (46) list five with significantly elevated risk ratios and then present data showing a 30% excess of lung cancer among 3200 welders who were members of a local boilermakers' union. The excess reached 74% when only those followed at least 20 years since first employment were considered. In another cohort of 1000 welders, including those exposed to nickel oxides, lung cancer was increased by 50% (47). In addition, increased risks of lung cancer of this same order of magnitude (96 observed, 67 expected) have since been reported for welders and gas cutters in Sweden (48). The Swedish data on 26,000 welders also identified several cases of mesothelioma, suggesting that asbestos may be involved. In addition, a fourfold excess of lung cancer incidence was seen among the subgroup of Swedish stainless steel welders, suggesting a potential role for hexavalent chromium compounds. Additional investigation of cancer among welders is warranted to clarify the contribution of various occupational exposures among this large group of workers, and to evaluate confounding or interactive effects of smoking.

Possible Occupational Lung Carcinogens

For the eight substances described here carcinogenic activity has been demonstrated in animal experiments and there have been some reports of lung cancer among exposed workers. The epidemiologic observations for each substance are quite limited, however, so that these agents must be considered as possible human carcinogens essentially based only on evidence from laboratory animals.

Cadmium

In a cohort study of cadmium smelter workers in the eastern United States, 12 deaths due to respiratory cancer were observed where 5.1 were expected. Follow-up of other small groups of cadmium-nickel battery workers and cadmium-copper alloy factory workers in Sweden also showed somewhat more lung cancer than expected, but preliminary results from a cohort of 3026 battery workers in Great Britain are reported to show no significant excess of lung cancer (2).

Chlorinated Toluenes

Six cases of respiratory cancer, three in nonsmokers, have been reported among a small group of workers in Japan producing benzoyl chloride and other chlorinated toluenes (benzal chloride, benzotrichloride, and benzyl chloride), substances used in pharmaceutical products, certain dyes, and perfumes, and as chemical intermediates in the production of other chemicals (13).

Dimethyl Sulfate

The epidemiologic evidence linking lung cancer to dimethyl sulfate, an alkylating agent used in producing methyl derivatives that has caused cancer in rats following inhalation, is limited to case reports of lung cancer in exposed chemical factory workers (2).

Epichlorohydrin

This chemical, an alkylating agent used in the production of synthetic glycerin and epoxy resins, produced respiratory cancer in rats following inhalation (2). In a cohort mortality study (49) of 863 United States chemical factory workers exposed to epichlorohydrin, a small excess of lung cancer was found (6 observed, 4.2 expected). The relative increase was greater (4 observed, 1.6 expected) when comparison was restricted to men who had preceded work in the epichlorohydrin unit with work in the production of isopropanol, raising the possibility of an enhanced risk following sequential exposures to animal carcinogens.

Fiber Glass and Other Man-Made Fibers

Glass fibers of similar size and shape to those of asbestos have induced mesotheliomas following intratracheal implantation in rats (50). Several epidemiologic investigations of groups, typically small, of exposed workers have not shown increased respiratory cancer mortality, but recent data from a mortality study of mineral fiber production workers in 13 factories in several European countries show a nearly twofold excess of lung cancer among those with 30 or more years since initial employment (51). The findings suggest that the latent period for cancer induction may be long and signal the need for long-term followup among exposed cohorts.

Lead Compounds

An excess of lung cancers was reported among workers in lead smelters (22 observed, 15.8 expected) and battery plants (61 observed, 49.5 expected) in the United States (52). The role of lead, however, if any, in respiratory carcinogenesis is not understood and awaits further clarification.

Silica

Silica is a ubiquitous material that until recently had not been considered as a potential lung carcinogen. The induction of lymphomas in rats following silica exposures and the enhancement of benzopyrene-induced tumors by silica in hamsters (53, 54), however, and the observation of increased lung cancer among foundry workers (see previous section) suggest the need for further study. In addition, increased rates of lung cancer have been observed among patients with silicosis in Sweden (55) and in Canada (56). In the Canadian study 38 lung cancer deaths were recorded during 1940–1978, where only 15.3 were expected in the Ontario male population among men who were given workmen's compensation for silicosis prior to 1959, but no excess was found among more recent silicosis cases. Although exposures to other carcinogens could not be ruled out, the findings underscored the need for a reevaluation of silica as a potential human lung carcinogen.

Talc

Elevated respiratory cancer mortality has been reported among workers engaged in the mining and milling of nonasbestiform talc in the United States, although not in a cohort study in Italy (57, 58). In addition, increased lung cancer has been reported in workers exposed to fibrous talc that may have been contaminated with asbestos (58, 59). Further suggestion that nonfibrous talc may be involved in lung cancer risk comes from a recent proportionate mortality study of pottery workers, where an 80% excess of lung cancer (62 observed deaths, 34 expected) was associated with sanitary wares production, particularly with casting where use of talc dusts is heavy (60). Limited experimental data show that nonasbestiform talc can produce lung fibroses after inhalation by rats: the talc exposure in this experiment also yielded two lung tumors in 24 rats exposed for 1 year, compared to 1 lung tumor in 71 unexposed controls and 8 in 22 rats similarly exposed to chrysotile asbestos (58).

Industrial Processes Possibly Associated with Increased Lung Cancer

A review of all available reports mentioning occupation and cancer, including routinely or specially compiled national or local statistics linking the two (such as decennial occupational mortality supplements or other reviews of statements on occupation on death certificates or other records) would reveal a fairly long list of industries or subgroups of industries for which lung cancer rates over some period of time have been reported to be higher than in a reference population. This is to be expected, of course, when a large number of comparisons are made and when smoking prevalences vary, as they are known to do, by occupational category. Therefore it is difficult to cull from these reports the industrial processes that may be labeled as "possibly associated with increased lung cancer risk" and so warrant additional research. Nevertheless such a list of industries is presented below. For nearly all the industries chosen, mention of elevated lung cancer has been made in more than one report.

Construction

A recent case-control study of lung cancer in Jacksonville, Florida, where mortality rates are higher than in any other urban sector of the United States, revealed several significant occupational associations, including a 30% smoking-adjusted increased risk of this tumor associated with employment in construction jobs (61). The excess was primarily among those with reported exposures to asbestos. The results are consistent with previous reports of elevated lung cancer among construction workers in a case-control death certificate survey in neighboring Georgia (62) and in some (63, 64) but not all (65) occupational mortality surveys elsewhere in the United States and Great Britain.

Fishing

Two case-control studies in the United States have associated work in the fishing industry with two- to threefold increased rates of lung cancer (61, 64). A doubled rate of lung cancer was also seen in British occupational mortality statistics (63) but not among fishermen in Canada (66).

Painting

The suspicion that painters may experience increased lung cancer arises primarily from surveys of routinely collected mortality statistics (63, 65). In addition, an increased lung cancer death rate has been reported among spray painters of aircraft, with zinc chromate primer paints a suspected agent (23). In a cohort mortality study of 16,000 paint manufacturing workers, only a slight excess of lung cancer was found, but this was noteworthy because there were marked reductions of nonmalignant respiratory disease, suggesting that smoking may be less common among these workers (67). On the other hand, one survey of smoking patterns showed a higher prevalence of current smokers among painters than among a number of other blue collar occupations (68).

Pesticide Applications

Four cohorts of men likely to be heavily exposed to organic pesticides (16,000 pesticide applicators, 1400 workers engaged in the production of heptachlor and chlordane, 3800 licensed structural pest control workers in Florida, and 1700 exposed agricultural workers in East Germany) recently have been found to have 15–90% increased mortality from lung cancer (69, 71). In the latter two groups the SMRs increased to nearly threefold among those with 20 or more years exposure. The German workers also showed a predisposition for undifferentiated and small-cell lung tumors and were reported to have smoking habits comparable to the general male population of Germany. Another cohort study of 2000 organochlorine manufacturing plant workers showed fewer total respiratory cancer deaths than expected, but small increases were seen in some plants surveyed (69). Finally, a group of 2600 individuals recently exposed to pesticides has been assembled: only 13 cancer deaths were observed during 1971–1977, not an excessive number, but five were caused by lung cancer (69). Taken together the studies raise the possibility of a slightly increased lung cancer risk, but none was able to quantify exposure to specific chemicals because the groups handled a variety of substances, or to evaluate the influence of smoking. There is current interest in the carcinogenic potential of phenoxyacetic herbicides and dioxin, which have been implicated in an increase in soft-tissue sarcomas and histiocytic lymphomas among exposed individuals in Sweden (71). Cohort studies of Swedish railroad and forestry workers, and of workers in German and American chemical plants manufacturing the herbicide 2,4,5-T, have not indicated an excess of lung cancer, but the number of expected cases in all groups combined was small (2). Further research to evaluate cancer among pesticide workers seems clearly warranted in view of the widespread use of chemical insecticides, fungicides, and other pesticides in the past three decades.

Petroleum Refining

Although early interest of cancer in the petroleum industry focused on skin tumors following contact exposure to oils, and current interest focuses on the excesses of brain tumors observed among refinery and petrochemical workers in Texas and elsewhere, increased lung cancer also has been reported, although not consistently, among workers in the industry. In a cohort study of 20,000 employees in 17 United States refineries, no overall excess of lung cancer during 1962–1971 was found compared to national rates, but internal comparisons showed increasing mortality rates with increasing exposure to hydrocarbons (72). Among 35,000 men who had worked during 1951–1975 in eight British oil refineries, 416 lung cancer deaths were observed during 1951–1975, whereas 533 were expected, a decrease the study authors speculate may be related to proscriptions against smoking for certain jobs (73). Similarly, no increase in lung cancer mortality rates was observed among Quebec oil refinery workers (3 observed, 8.5 expected), among refinery workers in an Exxon plant in Louisiana (78 observed, 86 expected), or among workers in a Texas City petrochemical manufacturing plant (50 observed, 64 expected) (72, 74, 75). There also were deficits of death from nonmalignant respiratory disease in each of these studies, suggesting that workers adhered to strict antismoking rules. A cohort investigation of 22,000 Imperial Oil employees in Canada, however, revealed a nearly twofold excess of lung cancer among men with daily occupational contact with petroleum or its products, with the death rates increasing in proportion to duration of employment in the refineries (72). In addition, proportional mortality analyses of deaths among members of the Oil, Chemical, and Atomic Workers International Union in Texas showed excesses of respiratory cancer of 10–45%, although there was no evidence of increasing trends with duration of employment (76). A review of occupational statements on lung cancer death certificates in Louisiana also showed a higher frequency of petroleum employees, especially at older ages (64). Examination of death certificates in Los Angeles likewise showed a higher percentage of coal and petroleum products workers among men who died of lung cancer (65). In summary, the available studies present a mixed picture, and further study, particularly ones in which detailed histories of occupation, smoking, and other factors can be obtained on lung cancer patients, is needed to clarify whether groups of workers within this large industry are at increased risk of lung cancer, and if so, to identify the responsible carcinogens.

Sugar Cane Farming

Some of the highest rates of lung cancer in the United States are found in Louisiana's southern parishes along the lower reaches of the Mississippi river (see chapter 6). Reasons for the excess are not clear, but a recent case-control study, showing that 38% of those who died of the cancer had worked for at least 6 months as sugarcane workers, indicates that exposure within the industry may be relevant (77). Two cases of mesothelioma were detected, similar to the observation of mesothelioma in sugarcane workers in India, suggesting that the fibrous cane dust exposures may be involved. Independent evaluation of the association between lung cancer and sugarcane farming by an ongoing large case-control study in Louisiana should help determine the extent, if any, of risks related to the industry.

In concluding this review of occupational lung cancer, the paramount role of cigarette smoking should once again be acknowledged. There is no doubt that smoking is the major cause of lung tumors; but if there are many substances such as asbestos and radon that multiply the effects of cigarettes, the role of occupation assumes added importance. Continued studies of occupational groups may help better quantify such potential interactions and provide clues useful in formulating measures aimed at the reduction of cancer, not only among worker populations where exposures are high, but in the general population as well.

References

1. Decoufle P. Occupation. In: Schottenfeld D, Fraumeni J, eds, Cancer epidemiology and prevention. Philadelphia: W.B. Saunders, 1982:318–35.
2. International Agency for Research in Cancer. IARC monographs on the evaluation of the carcinogenic risk of chemicals to humans. Supplement 4. Lyon:IARC, 1982.
3. National Academy of Sciences. Medical and biologic effects of environmental pollutants. Arsenic. Washington, DC: NAS, 1977:195–215.
4. Lee AM, Fraumeni JF Jr. Arsenic and respiratory cancer in man: An occupational study. JNCI 1969;42:1045–52.
5. Lubin JH, Pottern LM, Blot WJ, Tokudome S, Stone BJ, Fraumeni JF Jr. Respiratory cancer among copper smelter workers: recent mortality statistics. JOM 1981;23:779–84.
6. Welch K, Higgins I, Oh M, Burchfiel C. Arsenic exposure, smoking and respiratory cancer in copper smelter workers. Arch Environ Health 1982; 37:325–35.
7. Logue JN, Koontz MD, Hattwick MA. A historical prospective mortality study of workers in copper and zinc refineries. JOM 1982;24:398–408.
8. Blot WJ, Brown LM, Pottern LM, Stone BJ, Fraumeni JF Jr. Lung cancer among long-term steel workers. Am J Epidemiol 1983; 117:706–16.
9. Pershagen G, Wall S, Taube A, Linnman L. On the interaction between occupational arsenic exposure and smoking and its relationship to lung cancer. Scand J Work Environ Health 1981;7:302–9.
10. Pinto SS, Henderson V, Enterline PE. Mortality experience of arsenic exposed workers. Arch Environ Health 1978; 33:325–31.
11. Brown CC, Chu KC. Implications of the multistage theory of carcinogenesis applied to occupational arsenic exposure. JNCI 1983; 70:455–63.
12. Enterline PE, Marsh GM. Cancer among workers exposed to arsenic and other substances in a copper smelter. Am J Epidemiol 1982;116:895–911.
13. International Agency for Research in Cancer. IARC monographs on the evaluation of the carcinogenic risk of chemicals to humans. Some industrial chemicals and dyestuff. Vol 29: 49–92, 1982.
14. Doll R. Mortality from lung cancer among asbestos workers. Br J Ind Med 1955;12:81–6.
15. Selikoff IJ, Hammond EC (eds). Health hazards of asbestos exposure. Ann NY Acad Sci 1979;330:53–126, 473–90.
16. Wignall BK, Fox AJ. Mortality of female gas mask assemblers. Br J Ind Med 1982;39:34–8.
17. Blot WJ, Fraumeni JF Jr. Cancer among shipyard workers. Banbury Rep 1981;9:37–49.
18. Whitwell F, Newhouse M, Bennett D. A study of the histological cell types of lung cancer in workers suffering from asbestosis in the United Kingdom. Br J Ind Med 1974;31:298–303.
19. Weiss W. The cigarette factor in lung cancer due to chloromethyl ether. JOM 1980;22:527–9.
20. Machle W, Gregorius F. Cancer of the respiratory system in the United States chromate-producing industry. Public Health Rep 1948;63:1114–27.
21. Hayes RB. Occupational exposure to chromium and cancer: a review. In: Reviews of cancer epidemiology, Vol 1. New York: Elsevier-North Holland, 1979.
22. Alderson MR, Rattan NS, Bidstrup L. Health of workmen in the chromate-producing industry in Britain. Br J Ind Med 1981;38:117–24.
23. Dalager NA, Mason TJ, Fraumeni JF Jr. Cancer mortality among workers exposed to zinc chromate paints. JOM 1980;22:25–9.
24. Abe S, Ohsaki Y, Kimura K, Tsuneta Y, Mikami H, Murao M. Chromate lung cancer with special reference to its cell type and relation to the manufacturing process. Cancer 1982;49:783–7.

25. Wada S, Nishimoto Y, Miyanishi M, Kambe S, Miller RW. Mustard gas as a cause of respiratory neoplasia in man. Lancet 1968;1:1161-3.
26. Doll R. Cancer of the lung and nose in nickel workers. Br J Ind Med 1958;15:217-23.
27. Lloyd JW. Long-term mortality study of steel workers. V. Respiratory cancer in coke plant workers. JOM 1971;13:53-68.
28. Hammond EC, Selikoff IJ, Lawler PL, Seidman H. Inhalation of benzpyrene and cancer in man. Ann NY Acad Sci 1976;271:116-24.
29. Gibbs GW, Horowitz I. Lung cancer mortality in aluminum reduction plant workers. JOM 1979;21:347-53.
30. Axelson O, Sjoberg A. Cancer incidence and exposure to iron oxide dust. JOM 1979;21:419-22.
31. Lawler AB, Mandel JS, Schuman LM, Lubin JH. Mortality study of iron-ore miners: preliminary results. In: Proceedings of 4th annual Rocky Mountain Center for Occupational and Environmental Health conference. Park City: Ann Arbor Science Press, 1982.
32. Lundin FE, Wagoner JR, Archer VE. Radon daughter exposure and respiratory cancer: quantitative and temporal aspects. NIOSH-NIEHS Joint Memo 1. Springfield, NTIS, 1971.
33. National Academy of Sciences. The effects on populations of exposure to low levels of ionizing radiation: 1980. Washington, DC: National Academy Press, 1980:308-30.
34. Fox AJ, Goldblatt P, Kinlen LJ. A study of the mortality of Cornish tin miners. Br J Ind Med 1981;38:378-80.
35. Lundin FE, Archer VE, Wagoner JR. An exposure-time-response model for lung cancer mortality in uranium miners: effects of radiation exposure, age, and cigarette smoking. In Breslow N, Whittmore A, eds, Energy and health. Philadelphia: Society for Industrial and Applied Mathematics (SIAM), 1979:243-64.
36. Whittemore AS, McMillan A. Lung cancer mortality among U.S. uranium miners: a reappraisal. JNCI 1983; 71:489-500.
37. Matanoski GM, Sartwell P, Elliot E, Tonascia J, Sternberg A. Cancer risks in radiologists and radiation workers. In: Boice J, Fraumeni J, eds, Relation carcinogenesis: epidemiology and biological significance. In press.
38. Smith PG, Doll R. Mortality from cancers and all causes among British radiologists. Br J Radiol 1981;54:187-94.
39. Delzell E, Monson RR. Mortality among rubber workers. VI. Men with potential exposure to acrylonitrile. JOM 1982;24:767-9.
40. Wagoner JK, Infante P, Bayliss DL. Beryllium: an etiologic agent in the induction of lung cancer, nonneoplastic respiratory disease, and heart disease among industrially exposed workers. Environ Res 1980;21:15-34.
41. Smith J. Beryllium report disputed by listed author. Science 1981;211:556-7.
42. Waxweiller RJ, Smith AH, Falk H, Tyroler HA. Excess lung cancer risk in a synthetic chemicals plant. Environ Health Perspect 1981;41:159-65.
43. Theriault G, Allard P. Cancer mortality of a group of Canadian workers exposed to vinyl chloride monomers. JOM 1982;23:671-6.
44. Palmer WG, Scott WD. Lung cancer in ferrous foundry workers: a review. Am Ind Hyg J 1981;42:329-40.
45. International Agency for Research on Cancer. IARC monographs on the evaluation of the carcinogenic risk of chemicals to humans. The rubber industry. Vol 28:183-226, 1982.
46. Beaumont JJ, Weiss N. Lung cancer among welders. JOM 1981;23:839-44.
47. Polednak AP. Mortality among welders, including a group exposed to nickel oxides. Arch Environ Health 1981;36:235-42.
48. Sjogren B, Hogstedt C, Malker H. Chromium and asbestos as two probable risk factors in lung cancer among welders. JOM 1982;24:874-5.
49. Enterline PE. Importance of sequential exposure in the production of epichlorohydrin and isopropanol. Am NY Acad Sci 1982;381:344-9.
50. Stanton MF, Wrench C. Mechanisms of mesothelioma induction with asbestos and fibrous glass. JNCI 1972;48:797-821.
51. Saracci R, Simonato L. Man-made vitreous fibers and workers' health: an overview of the epidemiologic evidence. Scand J Work Environ Health 1982;8:234-42.
52. Cooper WC, Gaffey WR. Mortality of lead workers. JOM 1975;17:100-7.
53. Wagner MM, Wagner JC. Lymphomas in the Wistar rat after intrapleural inoculation of silica. JNCI 1976;57:509-78.

54. Stenback F. Rowland J. Experimental respiratory carcinogensis in hamsters: environmental, physiochemical and biologic aspects. Oncology 1979;26:63–71.
55. Westerholm P. Silicosis observations in a case register. Scand J Work Environ Health 1980;6:1–86.
56. Finkelstein M, Kuziak R, Suranyi G. Mortality among miners receiving workmens compensation for silicosis in Ontario: 1940–1975. JOM 1982;24:663-6
57. Katsnelson BA, Mokronsova KA. Non-fibrous mineral dusts and malignant tumors. JOM 1979;21:15–20.
58. Lemen R, Dement J, eds. Dusts and disease. Park Forest South, IL: Pathotox, 1979:357–63,379–92.
59. Stille WT, Tabershaw IR. The mortality experience of upstate New York talc workers. JOM 1982;24:480–4.
60. Thomas TL. A preliminary investigation of mortality among workers in the pottery industry. Int J Epidemiol 1982;11:175–80.
61. Blot WJ, Davies JE, Brown LM, et al. Occupation and the high risk of lung cancer in northeast Florida. Cancer 1982;50:364–371.
62. Harrington JM, Blot WJ, Hoover RN, Housworth JW, Heath CW Jr, Fraumeni JF Jr: Lung cancer in coastal Georgia: a death certificate analysis of occupation. JNCI 1978;60:295–8.
63. Office of Population Censuses and Surveys. Occupational mortality 1970–72. London: Her Majesty's Stationary Office, 1978.
64. Gottieb MS, Pickle LW, Blot WJ, Fraumeni JF Jr. Lung cancer in Louisiana: death certificate analysis. JNCI 1979;63:1131–7.
65. Menck HR, Henderson BE. Occupational differences in rates of lung cancer. JOM 1976;18:797–801.
66. Howe GR, Lindsay JP. A follow-up study of a ten-percent sample of the Canadian labor force. Cancer mortality in males 1965–73. JNCI 1983;70:37–44.
67. Morgan RW, Kaplan SD, Gaffey WR. A general mortality study of production workers in the paint and coatings manufacturing industry. JOM 1981;23:13–21.
68. Sterling TD, Weinkan JJ. Smoking patterns by occupation, industry, sex, and race. Arch Environ Health 1978;33:313–7.
69. Blair A, Grauman DJ, Lubin JH, Fraumeni JF Jr. Lung cancer and other causes of death among licensed pesticide applicators. JNCI 1983; 71:31–38.
70. Barthel E. Increased risk of lung cancer in pesticide-exposed male agricultural workers. J Toxicol Environ Health 1981;8:1027–40.
71. Hardell L. Epidemiological studies on soft-tissue sarcoma and malignant lymphoma and their relation to phenoxy acid or chlorophenol exposure. Umex, Umex University Med Dissertations No. 65, 1981.
72. Bingham E, Trosset RP, Warshawsky D. Carcinogenic potential of petroleum hydrocarbon: a critical review of the literature. J Environ Pathol Toxicol 1980;3:483–563.
73. Rushton L, Alderson MR. An epidemiological survey of eight oil refineries in Britain. Br J Ind Med 1981;38:225–34.
74. Hanis NM, Holmes TM, Shallenberger LG, Jones KE. Epidemiologic study of refining and chemical plant workers. JOM 1982;24:203–12.
75. Waxweiler RJ, Alexander V, Leffingwell SS, Haring M, Lloyd JW. Mortality from brain tumor and other causes in a cohort of petrochemical workers. JNCI 1983;70:75–81.
76. Thomas TL, Waxweiler RJ, Mouie-Eraso R, Itaya S, Fraumeni JF Jr. Mortality patterns among workers in three Texas oil refineries. JOM 1982;24:135–41.
77. Rothschild H, Mulvey JJ. An increased risk for lung cancer mortality associated with sugarcane farming. JNCI 1982;68:755–60.

CHAPTER **5**

Air Pollution and Lung Cancer

CARL M. SHY

Department of Epidemiology, School of Public Health, University of North Carolina at Chapel Hill, Chapel Hill, North Carolina 27514

ABSTRACT

Evidence for a potential causal relationship between air pollution and lung cancer is derived from three lines of epidemiologic studies: an urban factor for lung cancer not entirely explained by the distribution of smoking habits; excess lung cancer in occupational cohorts exposed to tar, soot, and combustion of fossil fuels found in ambient air; and quantitative dose–response models based on population studies. The weakest link in these lines of evidence is the absence of an acceptable index of population exposure to ambient air carcinogens. Much of the urban excess can be explained by lifestyle factors, such as exposure to side stream tobacco smoke or intensity of smoking, or to differences in occupational exposures between urban and rural residents. Elucidation of the role of air pollution requires the study of cohorts exposed to specific classes of suspected atmospheric carcinogens and less reliance on crude indices of air carcinogens, such as benzo[*a*]pyrene.
Key Words: **Air pollution, lung cancer, epidemiology**

The possibility of a causal association between air pollution and lung cancer is based on three lines of epidemiologic evidence.

1. There is an urban factor for lung cancer risk; this factor is not explained by an urban excess of tobacco smoking habits.
2. Carcinogens are found in ambient air; examples are soot, tars, benzo[*a*]pyrene, and other combustion products of fossil fuels. Some of these substances are associated causally with lung cancer excess in exposed occupational cohorts.
3. Some cross-sectional geographic studies suggest a quantitative relationship between indices of atmospheric pollution and lung cancer.

In spite of these lines of evidence, I argue that we cannot draw firm conclusions about the contribution of ambient air pollution to the risk of lung cancer in human populations. None of the epidemiologic studies allows us to make a direct link between populations exposed to ambient air pollution and lung cancer incidence. In

Lung Cancer: Causes and Prevention.

this paper I address deficiencies in the above lines of evidence and suggest some epidemiologic approaches to the study of air pollution and lung cancer.

The Urban Factor

The simple ratio of age-adjusted lung cancer mortality rates in urban to rates in rural residents of the United States reveals a relative risk for urban residence of approximately 1.8, with a range of 1.2–2.8 in different studies (1-6). The findings of an urban excess are so consistent that the validity of the urban factor in lung cancer is not a serious issue.

Age- and smoking-standardized rates of lung cancer among urban and rural inhabitants are available from two prospective cohort studies. In his study of American Legion members who had resided in the same area of California for 10 or more years, Buell (7) compared members from Los Angeles and the San Francisco Bay area with members from other California counties and found an age- and smoking-adjusted lung cancer mortality ratio of 1.3, with a larger ratio among nonsmokers (3.3) and lower ratios among smokers (1.3, 1.1, and 1.6, for less than 1 pack, 1 pack, and more than 1 pack per day smokers, respectively). In the American Cancer Society's prospective study of 1 million men and women, Hammond and Horn (8) reported an age- and smoking-adjusted lung cancer mortality ratio of 1.3 for white males, age 50–69 years residing in cities of 50,000 or larger vs those residing in rural areas. Similar to the Buell study, a larger urban–rural ratio was found for nonsmokers than for smokers.

Because occupational exposures of urban and rural residents are likely to be different and to relate to lung cancer risks, the contribution of occupational exposures to the urban factor needs to be addressed. Based on the American Cancer Society's prospective study, Hammond and Garfinkel (9) obtained age- and smoking-adjusted standardized mortality ratios (SMR) for males who, at the time of enrollment in the prospective study, said that they had lived in their present neighborhood for at least 10 years. The SMRs were stratified by place of residence, and each stratum was subdivided by the presence or absence of occupational exposure to dust, fumes, vapors, gases or x-rays. To further evaluate the contribution of place of residence and occupational exposures to the lung cancer mortality experience of this population, each residence- and occupational exposure-specific SMR was divided by the SMR of the nonmetropolitan rural, nonoccupationally exposed study population. These results, shown as relative risks in Table 1, reveal increased lung cancer associated with occupational exposures within each place of residence category. Within metropolitan areas, the excess relative risk associated with occupational exposures ranges from 20% (1.34–1.14) to 30% (1.45–1.15). Within occupational exposure categories, the place of residence effect on excess relative risk varies from 15% among nonoccupationally exposed to 20–30% among occupationally exposed. However, it is likely that the 20–30% excess relative risk associated with place of residence among occupationally exposed persons does not fully control for occupational exposure effects, because occupational exposures in metropolitan areas are qualitatively different and probably have a

Table 1. Relative risk[a] of male lung cancer mortality standardized for smoking and age by place of residence and occupational exposure category[b]

Place of residence	Occupationally exposed to dust, fumes, gases	Not occupationally exposed to dust, fumes, gases
Metropolitan areas population 1 million +	1.45	1.15
Metropolitan areas population less than 1 million	1.34	1.14
Nonmetropolitan areas		
Towns	1.14	1.18
Rural areas	1.15	1.00

[a]Relative risk expressed as the ratio of the SMR for each residence/occupational exposure category to the SMR of the nonmetropolitan rural, nonoccupationally exposed population. Each SMR was standardized for age and smoking habits of the entire study population.
[b]Adapted from Hammond and Garfinkel (9).

greater lung cancer risk than occupational exposures in rural areas, where the work day is less likely to be spent in a closed industrial plant environment. Hence it seems reasonable to infer, from these data, that the urban factor is best represented by the 15% excess relative risk among persons not occupationally exposed, whereas the occupational factor is represented by the 20–30% excess relative risk among metropolitan residents. "Occupational exposure" is too heterogeneous a category to allow firm conclusions to be drawn about the relative magnitude of the occupational and urban effects from these data. The findings, however, implicate both an occupational exposure and urban residence contribution to the urban excess in lung cancer and suggest that occupational exposures are at least as important as, and probably more important than, the urban residence factor.

The nonoccupational urban residence effect on lung cancer risk may itself be a composite of several different risk factors such as personal air pollution, diet, stress, and ambient air pollution. The role of diet and stress in the urban component has not been assessed as yet. A few studies (10, 11) suggest a small but detectable increased risk associated with passive smoking. Differences in exposures of urban and rural residents to passive smoke have not been quantified. Hence, the contribution, if any, of passive cigarette smoke to the urban excess is unknown.

Carcinogens in Ambient Air

A variety of particulate and vapor-phase organics in ambient air manifest carcinogenic activity in experimental systems (12–14). Incomplete combustion of fossil fuels and of other organic hydrocarbons is the major source of organic particulates in ambient air, whereas vapor-phase organics are emitted as aerosols from various industrial activities, from combustion of fossil fuels and from natural sources. Particulate organics in urban air are initially separated from other constituents as a crude benzene extract and subdivided by stepwise extractions with ether, sodium hydroxide, and hydrochloric acid into acidic, basic, and neutral portions

(15). Chromatography of the neutral portion yields aliphatic, aromatic, and oxygenated fractions.

The aliphatic fractions, in the form of polycyclic aromatic hydrocarbons, has been more thoroughly investigated as carcinogens than other components of particulate organic air pollution. The relative carcinogenic activity of various polycyclic aromatics identified in urban air is listed in Table 2; potency is based on laboratory assays of compounds tested for carcinogenic activity. Formation of these compounds is greatly enhanced by incomplete, or oxygen-deficient, combustion of any material containing carbon and hydrogen. Lee et al (16) compiled a list of more than 100 aromatic hydrocarbons detected in particulate air samples. The large array of particulate organic matter compounds and the complexity of analyzing these compounds chemically creates a major barrier in assessing the carcinogenic potential of air pollution. There is a great need to define a few index compounds that represent the carcinogenic activity of atmospheric particulates from different source categories.

To date, benzo[*a*]pyrene (BaP) has been the most common air pollutant monitored as the carcinogenic indicator for urban air, a selection that is increasingly unsatisfactory. The BaP emissions are largely a product of inefficient combustion of fossil fuels; the major sources of atmospheric BaP in the United States (17) are coke production plants, burning coal refuse banks, forest fires, home fireplaces, and home coal-burning furnaces. With the shift in home heating from coal to oil,natural gas, and electricity, a major source of BaP has been nearly removed from the United States. For example, in 1966 (when the disappearance of coal-burning home furnaces was nearly complete), the annual median BaP for urban sites in the U.S. National Air Surveillance Network was 3.2 ng/m^3, whereas in

Table 2. Carcinogenic polycyclic organic matter identified in urban air[a]

Compound	Formula	Carcinogenicity
Polycyclic Aromatic Hydrocarbons		
Chrysene	$C_{18}H_{12}$	+
Benz[*a*]anthracene	$C_{18}H_{12}$	+
Dibenzo[*a,g*]fluorine	$C_{21}H_{14}$	+
Dibenz[*a,c*]anthracene	$C_{22}H_{14}$	+
Indeno[1,2,3,-*cd*]pyrene	$C_{22}H_{12}$	+
Benzo[*b*]fluoranthene	$C_{20}H_{12}$	+ +
Benzo[*j*]fluoranthene	$C_{20}H_{12}$	+ +
Benzo[*j*]aceanthrylene	$C_{20}H_{14}$	+ +
Dibenzo[*a,e*]pyrene	$C_{22}H_{14}$	+ +
Benzo[*c*]phenanthrene	$C_{18}H_{12}$	+ + +
Dibenzo[*a,h*]pyrene	$C_{22}H_{14}$	+ + +
Dibenzo[*a,i*]pyrene	$C_{22}H_{14}$	+ + +
Dibenz[*a,h*]anthracene	$C_{22}H_{14}$	+ + +
Benzo[*a*]pyrene	$C_{20}H_{12}$	+ + + +
Aza- and Iminoarenes		
Quinoline	C_9H_8N	+
Dibenz[*a,h*]acridine	$C_{21}H_{13}N$	+ +
Dibenz[*a,j*]acridine	$C_{21}H_{13}N$	+ +
Dibenzo[*c,g*]carbazole	$C_{20}H_{13}N$	+ + +

[a]From U.S. Environmental Protection Agency (18).

1975 this value was nearly tenfold lower, 0.5 ng/m^3 (18). Although measurements are unavailable, it is highly probable that BaP levels in urban air were 10–20 times greater in the 1930s and 1940s, prior to the conversion from home burning coal furnaces, compared with the 1960s and 1970s. Therefore, the time trend for BaP levels in the United States has been directly opposite to the lung cancer mortality trend, even considering a lag of 20–30 years.

There is no evidence that trends for atmospheric levels of other polycyclic aromatics have followed the decrease in BaP concentrations. Polycyclic aromatics emitted by automobiles, eg, coronene, are unrelated to BaP levels. Diesel exhaust contains insignificant amounts of BaP. Nitrogen analogs of polycyclic aromatic hydrocarbons, such as aza- and iminoarenes, also have carcinogenic potency in bioassay systems. These substances are found in urban air but their distribution, sources, and variations in air concentrations between cities are unknown.

The other major chromatographic fractions of the neutral portion (derived from crude benzene extracts of particulate air samples) are aliphatic and oxygenated hydrocarbons. Twenty to 65% of organic particulates in urban air consists of aliphatic hydrocarbons in the 16–36 carbon atom range. Although these compounds generally test negative as carcinogens, some of their photodecomposition products are epoxides and peroxides (12) and several chemicals in this category are known carcinogens in experimental animals. Among the oxygenated hydrocarbons found in particulate air samples are *o*-heterocyclic hydrocarbons, epoxides, peroxides, aldehydes, ketones, sugars, quinones, esters, and lactones. Environmental sources of these compounds are combustion of plant products including wood, volatilization and combustion of petroleum products, and industrial plasticizers (12). The concentration and distribution of these substances in urban air has not been studied.

The biologic activity and atmospheric distribution of compounds in the acidic and basic groups of the crude benzene extract from particulate air samples has received little attention. Some compounds in the basic group, namely dibenz[*a*,*b*] acridine and 2-naphthylamine, are known animal and/or human carcinogens.

Vapor-phase organics in ambient air include benzene, chloroform, formaldehyde, vinyl chloride, carbon tetrachloride, and a host of other compounds, such as aliphatic and olefinic hydrocarbons, aldehydes, ketones, fatty acids, and esters. An inherent problem in measuring these compounds in air samples is their high chemical reactivity and volatility. Sources of vapor-phase organics in ambient air include motor vehicle exhausts, industrial processes involving solvents, petroleum refining, solid waste incineration, open-dump burning, and forest fires. There are natural sources of volatile emissions, such as plants; methane and terpenes are major vapor-phase hydrocarbons from plants and decay products of plants.

Geographic Studies

Very few investigators have had available to them direct measurements of carcinogenic pollutants in air samples. More importantly, even when some index of carcinogenic pollution was derived and related to geographic variations in lung cancer mortality, the mortality rates could not be adjusted for variations in cigarette smoking habits, occupational exposures of individuals, or indoor sources of pollution. For example, Stocks (19) computed correlation coefficients between lung cancer mortality and atmospheric deposited matter (a crude and unreliable index of organic pollutants) in 58 county boroughs and 79 administrative areas of England. Although significant correlations were found in the 58 county boroughs, but not the administrative areas, smoking and occupation could not be factored in, and the latency issue was not addressed. Similarly, Carnow and Meier (20) performed a linear regression analysis of lung cancer mortality in the 48 contiguous states of the United States as a function of per capita state cigarette sales and a weighted average of BaP measurements from a few urban and rural locations in each state. The resulting regression coefficients were used to predict an increase of 5% in the lung cancer rate for each nanogram per cubic meter increment in BaP concentrations. Aside from the crude adjustment for cigarette smoking based on state sales, the derivation of a single BaP air concentration value for each state is inappropriate and implausible as a determinant of lung cancer mortality rates for an entire state. In addition, the 1967–1969 BaP levels used in the analysis do not represent concentrations, or geographic differences in concentrations that must have existed 20–30 years prior to the 1954–1961 time period selected by the authors for their mortality data.

Hammond and Garfinkel (9) used the American Cancer Society's prospective study of lung cancer in males (previously mentioned) to evaluate a possible ambient air pollution effect. Subjects were stratified according to three levels of atmospheric particulate matter (low, 35–99 $\mu g/m^3$; moderate, 100–129 $\mu g/m^3$; high, 130–180 $\mu g/m^3$) as measured in each city and three levels of benzene-soluble organics (low, 3.4–6.3 $\mu g/m^3$; moderate, 6.5–7.9 $\mu g/m^3$; high, 8.5–15.0 $\mu g/m^3$). Age-and smoking-standardized lung cancer mortality ratios failed to show any consistent pattern of association with these indices of air pollution among men either occupationally exposed or not occupationally exposed to dust, fumes, and gases.

Overall, the quantitative geographic studies of lung cancer and carcinogenic air pollution are highly unsatisfactory. No specific or encompassing index of population exposure to carcinogenic air pollution is available. Lack of data at the aggregate level on smoking, occupational exposure, or indoor exposure to air carcinogens makes it impossible to control for important potential confounding factors. Even feasible adjustments for industrial location have not been attempted. The geographic studies of lung cancer mortality are inevitably plagued by the uncontrolled confounders, which can be controlled plausibly only in individual risk studies.

Epidemiologic Evaluation of Atmospheric Carcinogens

If ambient air pollution, independent of cigarette smoking and occupation, accounts for some of the excess lung cancer risk found in urban areas, available indirect evidence suggests that this contribution is quite small. Greater precision of this estimate requires individual risk studies (as opposed to geographic or aggregate risk studies) that are difficult to design. The greatest obstacle remains the absence of an identifiable index of ambient carcinogenic air pollution. Specifically, benzo[*a*]pyrene, the most commonly measured organic hydrocarbon in air, is not a satisfactory index pollutant. No one compound or class of compounds seems appropriate to represent the diverse array of substances that can be found in the acidic, neutral, and basic fractions of benzene-soluble extracts from particulate air samples, and vapor-phase organics are not even present in these extracts. Direct measurements of an array of representative compounds from these different categories is analytically complex, expensive, and infeasible at the present time. To characterize human exposure to atmospheric carcinogens requires a meeting of minds of the analytical chemist and environmental epidemiologist. One approach would be to identify cohorts exposed to specific classes of suspected air carcinogens. Examples of these substances are formaldehyde, indoor cigarette smoke, classes of solvents in closed environments, and diesel exhaust. Exposed groups may best be studied in an occupational setting, although chemical measurements of exposure will be a difficult issue. General population studies in different urban environments are unlikely ever to provide satisfactory data, owing to the heterogeneity of exposure and our inability to characterize this exposure with any degree of chemical specificity.

References

1. Hoffman EF, Gilliam AG. Lung cancer mortality. Geographic Distribution in the United States for 1948-1949. Public Health Rep 1954;69:1033-42.
2. Griswold MH, Wilder CS, Culter SJ, et al. Cancer in Connecticut, 1935-1951. Hartford: Connecticut State Dept of Health 1955.
3. Mancuso TF, MacFarlane EM, Porterfield JD. Distribution of cancer mortality in Ohio. Am J Public Health 1955;45:58-70.
4. Zimmer EG, Haenszel W. Cancer in Iowa. U.S. Public Health Service Publ 466. Washington, DC: U.S. Government Printing Office, 1956.
5. Prindle RA. Some considerations in the interpretation of air pollution health effects data. J Air Poll Control 1959;9:12-9.
6. Levin ML, Haenszel W, Carroll BE, et al. Cancer incidence in urban and rural areas of New York State. JNCI 1960;24:1243-57.
7. Buell P. Relative impact of smoking and air pollution on lung cancer. Arch Environ Health 1967;15:291-7.
8. Hammond EC, Horn D. Smoking and death rates—report on 44 months of follow-up of 187,783 men. I. Total mortality. II. Death rates by cause. JAMA 1958;166:1159-72, 1294-1308.
9. Hammond EC, Garfinkel L. General air pollution and cancer in the United States. Prevent Med 1980;9:206-11.
10. Hirayama T. Non-smoking wives of heavy smokers have a higher risk of lung cancer. A study from Japan. Br Med J 1981;282:183-5.
11. Trichopoulos D, Kalandidi A, Sparros L, MacMahon B. Lung cancer and passive smoking. Int J Cancer 1981;27:1-4.
12. Hoffman D, Wynder EL. Organic particulate pollutants. In: Stern AC, ed, Air pollution , Vol II, 3rd ed. New York: Academic Press, 1977:361-455.
13. Committee on Medical and Biological Effects of Environmental Pollutants, National Research Council, National Academy of Sciences. Particulate polycyclic organic matter. Washington, DC: National Academy of Sciences, 1972.
14. Committee on Medical and Biological Effects of Environmental Pollutants, National Research Council, National Academy of Sciences. Vapor-Phase Organic Pollutants. Washington, DC: National Academy of Sciences, 1976.

15. Hueper WC, Koten P, Tabor EC, et al. Carcinogenic bioassays on air pollutants. Arch pathol 1962;74:89–116.
16. Lee ML, Novotny M, Bartle KD. Gas chromatography/mass spectrometric and nuclear magnetic resonance determination of polynuclear aromatic hydrocarbons in airborne particulates. Anal Chem 1976;48:1566–72.
17. U.S. Environmental Protection Agency. Preliminary assessment of the sources, control and population exposure to airborne polycyclic organic matter (POM) as indicated by benzo[*a*]pyrene (BaP). Office of Air Quality Planning and Standards, U.S. Environmental Protection Agency, Research Triangle Park, NC, 1978.
18. U.S. Environmental Protection Agency. Health assessment document for polycyclic organic matter. Washington, DC: Office of Research and Development, U.S. Environmental Protection Agency, May 1978.
19. Stocks P. Cancer and bronchitis mortality in relation to atmospheric deposits and smoke. Br Med J 1959;1:74–9.
20. Carnow BW, Meier P. Air pollution and pulmonary cancer. Arch Environ Health 1973;27:207–8.

CHAPTER 6

The Causes of Lung Cancer in Louisiana

PELAYO CORREA*, LINDA WILLIAMS PICKLE**, ELIZABETH FONTHAM*, NANCY DALAGER**, YOUPING LIN*, WILLIAM HAENSZEL,*** and WILLIAM D. JOHNSON*

*Departments of Pathology and Biometry, Louisiana State University Medical Center, New Orleans, Louisiana 70112

**Environmental Epidemiology Branch, National Cancer Institute, Landow 3C15, Bethesda, Maryland 20205

***Illinois Cancer Council, Chicago, Illinois 60603

ABSTRACT

Lung cancer accounts for most of the excessive cancer mortality reported for Louisiana residents. A case-control study involving interviews with 1338 lung cancer patients and 1393 comparison subjects recently has been conducted. All newly diagnosed cases from all southern Louisiana hospitals as well as those from Alexandria and Shreveport hospitals were identified. Questions were asked about residential history, occupation, diet, smoking and drinking habits, source of drinking water, ancestry, income, education, and previous medical history. Preliminary results, including attributable risks for the main causative factors, are presented.

Key Words: **Forestry, oil/gas extraction, sugar cane, chemical manufacture, petrochemical manufacture, metal processing, shipbuilding, motor freight handling, wood dust, mineral oil, smoking, drinking water, fruit intake, vegetable intake, fishing, transportation industry**

South Louisiana has the dubious distinction of displaying some of the highest lung cancer rates in the country. Higher than average rates have been reported for approximately 50 years. Table 1 shows data for three time periods. In 1930–1932 Louisiana lung cancer death rates in males were higher than those for the United States. More recent data show that the excess has persisted. Rates in black males have surpassed those of white males. (1, 2).

Lung Cancer: Causes and Prevention.

Table 1. Lung cancer death rates in three time periods[a]

Period/Population[b]	Louisiana	United States
1930–1932		
(adjusted to 1930 United States population)		
WM	4.0	3.1
WF	1.6	1.8
BM	1.9	1.4
BF	0.5	0.8
1950–1967		
(adjusted to 1960 United States population)		
WM	19.3	16.3
WF	1.8	2.2
BM	14.4	16.3
BF	1.5	2.2
1975–1977		
(adjusted to 1970 United States population)		
WM	81.8	66.2
WF	18.9	16.6
BM	82.1	77.2
BF	16.6	15.8

[a] Because of differences in population adjustment, rates can be compared only to each other within each time period.
[b] Abbreviations: WM, white males; WF, white females; BM, black males; BF, black females.

This type of clustering of cancer in the deltas of big rivers has been observed before, and hypotheses to explain its causes have abounded, mostly based on anecdotal thinking. A good example is provided by the conclusion reached by Alfred Haviland in 1875 after studying the geographic distribution of cancer in England (3):

> So, in cancer, the maps teach us that the high, dry sites on the older rocks are the places where cancer does not thrive, and that it does thrive in the vales by the sides of large rivers which overflow their banks, and in the neighbourhood of which are to be found the drifts of ages of washings from the inhabited country above. Where there is a tendency to cancer, let the patient be removed to the high, dry sites; and perchance if whole families were thus to emigrate, we should not hear so much of the hereditary character of this or of many other diseases.

Today, more than a century later, we still do not know whether the high frequency of cancer in the valleys near big rivers is due to river pollution as suggested by Haviland, to industrial occupational hazards, or to the lifestyle adopted by the inhabitants of those lands.

In an attempt to apply scientific methodology to study this problem, the National Cancer Institute and Louisiana State University have conducted a collaborative case-control study of lung cancer in South Louisiana. The same methodology has been applied in a smaller study in the north of the state, where cancer rates are lower, under the sponsorship of the Louisiana Chapter of the American Cancer Society. Preliminary results of these studies are reported here.

Materials and Methods

Current primary lung cancer cases were identified from admission diagnosis and pathology records of all participating hospitals in 29 Louisiana parishes (counties) including all southern parishes plus one central (Rapides) and two northern parishes (Caddo and Bossier). All major hospitals in the study area participated except in the city of New Orleans where, for logistic reasons, interviewing was limited to two large hospitals serving the medically uninsured population and two large private hospitals. A control was randomly selected from patients attending the same hospital and matched to the case by race, sex, and age (within 5 years). Patients whose main diagnosis was emphysema, chronic bronchitis, chronic obstructive pulmonary disease, or cancer of the larynx, oral cavity, esophagus, or bladder were excluded from the control selection procedures. The admission diagnoses of the controls were distributed in the following categories: cardiovascular, 15.3%; gastrointestinal, 13%; musculoskeletal, 10%; genitourinary, 7.3%; ophthalmology and otorhinolaryngology, 6.6%; other tumors, 5%; diabetes, 5%; trauma 3.7%; peripheral vascular, 3.7%; pulmonary, 2.7%; cerebrovascular, 2.5%; infections, 2%.

Local professional interviewers, trained for this study and thoroughly familiar with the local culture, carried out personal interviews with the subjects (76% of the cases and 89% of the controls) or their next of kin. The questions covered occupation, residency, diet, smoking and drinking habits, health, water supply, and other related items. Histologic confirmation was obtained for 97% of the cases. Table 2 shows the number of acceptable completed interviews by sex, race, and location. An additional 34 cases of bronchioalveolar carcinoma were interviewed but are not included in the analysis.

Odds ratios were based on the products of the diagonals in 2 × 2 tables. Adjustments for smoking characteristics made by the direct method.

Table 2. Number of interviews[a]

	Cases	Controls
South Louisiana[a]		
WM	641	665
WF	201	217
BM	304	317
BF	73	75
Subtotal	1219	1274
North Louisiana[a]		
WM	62	62
WF	19	19
BM	29	29
BF	9	9
Subtotal	119	119
Total	1338	1393

[a]Abbreviations as in Table 1.

Results

Smoking

Tables 3 and 4 show the odds ratio for each smoking category. The increase in risk with increasing amounts of cigarette use is evident in all sex–race groups. The results show the same general pattern observed in other studies, but the excess risk for each category of smoking when compared to that for nonsmokers is greater in Louisiana than in most other studies. The number of black females is admittedly small, and the results for them are unreliable.

Of the white male lung cancer patients, 97.7% were smokers. The corresponding figures for other race–sex groups were: black males, 97.6%; white females, 88%; and black females, 94%. Overall, fewer than 3% of males and about 10% of female lung cancer patients were nonsmokers.

Table 3. Odds ratios for lung cancer in Louisiana by pack-years of cigarettes smoked

	Odds ratio[a]			
Pack-years	**WM**	**WF**	**BM**	**BF**
0	1.0	1.0	1.0	1.0
1-20	3.6	1.5	4.0	13.3
21-40	9.5	7.7	14.6	19.5
41+	24.5	26.2	18.2	52.8
Total	17.2	8.6	13.1	22.0

[a]Abbreviations as in Table 1.

Table 4. Odds ratios for lung cancer in Louisiana by smoking characterististics[a]

	Odds ratio
Nonsmokers	1.0
Filter[a]	8.4
Nonfilter[a]	15.2
Age started[a]	
<16	24.2
16-20	17.4
21+	8.3
Current smoker	12.6
Quit	
3-5 years	7.7
6-20	7.0
20+	3.9
Inhale	
None	4.6
Mouth	6.3
Chest	11.3

[a]Adjusted for sex and age.

Table 5. Lung cancer risk by social class (SC) and smoking categories

	Odds ratio	
Category (pack-years)	**High SC**	**Low SC**
Nonsmokers	1.0	0.90
≤20	2.79	4.28
21–50	9.44	11.84
51+	19.52	17.68

Increasing risks are seen for nonfilter versus filter cigarettes; earlier versus later starting age; nonquitters versus quitters, and deep versus light inhalation. The data for socioeconomic class suggest higher risks in the lower socioeconomic classes for light and moderate smokers but not for heavy smokers (Table 5). These results leave no doubt that smoking is the undisputed, overwhelming major cause of lung cancer in Louisiana.

Occupation

Odds ratios were calculated for all "ever employed" in occupation categories represented in our sample. Table 6 lists the results for occupations with elevated risks or occupations for which previous studies have suggested a positive association with lung cancer. Results are given for white males only because of small numbers and absence of positive associations for white females and blacks of both sexes. Only workers in the "forestry" category exhibited a significantly elevated risk; most of them were sawmill workers. After adjusting for smoking history, our study failed to detect any positive association with some Louisiana occupations previously suspected as playing a role in lung cancer causation, such as sugarcane farming, oil and gas extraction, construction, chemical manufacturing and processing, petrochemical manufacturing and processing, metal processing, and shipbuilding.

To enhance the possibility of detecting occupational effects that might not be uncovered by the summary classification of unusual occupations, we identified cases and controls who had worked in suspect occupations for 10 or more years and compared them with a selected group of cases and controls whose occupations suggested low exposure to carcinogens in the workplace (hunting and trapping,

Table 6. Odds ratio[a] for pertinent occupations, white males

	Odds ratio	
Occupation	**Unadjusted**	**Adjusted for smoking**
Forestry	1.56	1.67[b]
Petroleum refining	1.15	1.02
Printing	1.49	1.64
Fishing	1.72	1.20

[a]Never employed in the occupation = unit risk.
[b]Significant at 0.05 level.

transportation and public utilities, wholesale and retail trade, finance, services, public administration). Included in this category were: professionals, technical, managerial, clerical, sales, amusement, recreation, and motion pictures. This group also excluded subjects who reported suspect exposures while employed in gasoline service stations, laundry and dry cleaning businesses, electrical and electronic engineering, chemistry, and agricultural sciences, or as farm advisers, commercial artists, and painters. Even after this effort to maximize the case-control contrasts of occupations, only forestry and lumber manufacturing gave positive significant associations after adjustments were made for smoking. Suggestive, but not statistically significant associations were noted for construction, petroleum processing, transportation, and motor freight handling.

Occupational Exposures to Suspect Materials

A list of 46 suspect materials was covered by specific questions in the interview. Table 7 shows the exposures with positive or borderline findings. After adjustments are made for smoking, only wood dust and mineral oil mist carry a significant excess risk. Known lung carcinogens such as asbestos, nickel, and chromium, display elevated but not statistically significant risks in our series.

Living Near Industrial Plants

Table 8 reports the results of our inquiry concerning proximity of residence to an industrial plant. Of the many types of plants mentioned, lumber mills and petroleum refineries showed a significantly elevated relative risk.

Drinking Water Source

Table 9 shows odds ratios for lung cancer by source of drinking water. Risks for persons born and currently living in locations served by surface water (S-S) did not deviate significantly from those born and currently living in locations served by ground water (G-G) (17).

Table 7. Odds ratio[a] for occupational exposures, white males

	Odds Ratio	
Material	**Unadjusted**	**Adjusted for smoking**
Wood dust	1.44[b]	1.40[b]
Mineral oil mist	2.10[b]	2.13[b]
Asbestos	1.39	1.32
Mustard gas	1.44	2.38
Nickel	1.44	1.89
Chromium	2.28	2.40
Cotton	1.42	1.70
Coal dust	2.02[b]	1.47
Lead	1.53	1.50

[a]Never exposed to the material = unit risk.
[b]Significant at 0.05 level.

Table 8. Odds ratio[a] of lung cancer for subjects less than 2 miles from industrial plants

Plant	Odds ratio	
	Unadjusted	Adjusted for sex, race, and smoking history
Any plant	1.17	1.28[b]
Lumber	4.25[b]	3.60[b]
Petroleum refining	1.21	1.47[b]
Chemical plant	0.86	0.90

[a]Resided two or more miles away = unit risk.
[b]Significant at 0.05 level.

Table 9. Odds ratios of lung cancer by drinking water source (S-S vs G-G)[a]

	Odds ratio
White males	0.99
White females	1.25
Black males	0.89
Black females	2.13
All subjects	1.02

[a]Persons born and residing in areas served by ground water supplies (G-G) = unit risk.

Nutrition

Detailed information was collected for 74 diet items. The intake of fresh fruits and vegetables was negatively associated with lung cancer risk. The foods that discriminated best between cases and controls were broccoli, lettuce, carrots, bananas, oranges, and fruit juice. To assess possible dose-response effects we created a composite index of fruit and vegetable consumption. For the 18 items in this category, intake was rated as low (<25 percentile), medium (25-74 percentile), or high (75 + percentile) based on the frequency distribution of consumption for individual foods. Values for 2, 5, and 9 were assigned for low, medium, and high exposure for each item.

Some results of this analysis are shown in Table 10. A clear enhancement of risk by low intake of fresh fruits and vegetables is seen, independent of cigarette smoking. The numbers of cases for some of the exposure combinations in the table are small and yield confidence limits that include unity. Inspection of this table, however, suggests that insufficient intake of fruits and vegetables increases lung cancer risk in light and moderate smokers. When the same kind of tabulation is restricted to the six items that seem to have a more pronounced effect as shown in Table 11 (lettuce, broccoli, carrots, bananas, oranges, and fruit juices) the effect is seen in all smoking categories. This suggests that the protective effect of fresh fruits and vegetables may be restricted to specific items. Further research is needed to clarify this point.

Table 10. Odds ratios for lung cancer in white males of Louisiana by pack-years of cigarettes smoked and levels of consumption of fresh fruits and vegetables (18 items)

	Pack-years of cigarettes					
All fresh fruits and vegetables	0	1–20	21–40	41+	Crude	Adjusted for smoking
High	1.0	2.3	7.4	28.0	1.0	1.0
Medium	0.8	4.0	12.0	27.3	1.2	1.1
Low	1.9	6.5	11.4	31.9	1.6	1.3
Crude	1.0	3.8	9.9	26.8		
Adjusted for vegetables	1.0	3.6	9.7	26.6		

Table 11. Odds ratios for lung cancer in white males of Louisiana by pack-years of cigarettes smoked and levels of consumption of lettuce, broccoli, carrots, bananas, oranges, and fruit juices

	Pack-years of cigarettes					
Fruits and vegetables	0	1–20	21–40	41+	Crude	Adjusted for pack-years
High	1.0	3.1	12.2	28.5	1.0	1.0
Medium	1.5	5.8	15.6	36.6	1.5	1.3
Low	2.6	9.4	17.2	52.0	2.3	1.8
Crude	1.0	3.7	9.4	27.5		
Adjusted for vegetables	1.0	3.5	9.7	24.2		

Discussion

Alton Ochsner, to whom this volume is dedicated, correctly identified the beginning of the epidemic of lung cancer in Louisiana (4). His abundant clinical practice convinced him that cigarette smoking was the main reason for the epidemic. The high mortality rate for Louisiana was pinpointed by the National Cancer Institute (5) and specifically localized to the southern part of the state by the county maps (6). In 1975 Blot and Fraumeni (7) studied the correlation between industry and clusters of high lung cancer risk counties in Louisiana and other states and reported excessive rates for males in counties where paper, chemical, petroleum, and transportation industries were located. In 1977 DeRouen and Diem correlated parish-specific lung cancer rates with drinking water source information and reported a positive association between surface water and lung cancer rates limited to nonwhite males (8). After studying similar correlations for tumors of other organs, the authors dismissed the observation as nonspecific. Voors and co-workers did multiple regression analysis of lung cancer and environmental parameters and, in 1978 reported an association between lung cancer and residency in the wetlands, especially marked for South Louisiana (9). The relationship between lung cancer and nutrition has been explored by Lopez and his associates who, in 1979 and 1980, reported a negative correlation between lung cancer and β-carotene intake (10,11). Death certificates have been used extensively by Gottlieb and her colleagues (12–16). These studies have revealed an excess risk associated with shipbuilding, fishing, and oil-related industries. Acadian ancestry was associated with higher rates in older patients. These studies also revealed an association between surface water and lung cancer in nonwhite males only, as previously reported by DeRouen and Diem. This was again interpreted as artifactual, especially because the confounding effects of smoking and other environmental factors cannot be controlled in death certificate-based studies. Death certificate studies have been combined with next of kin interviews by Rothschild (17–19) and co-workers, who reported increased risks of lung cancer and mesothelioma in workers in the sugarcane industry. The same team described a continued rise in lung cancer rates in South Louisiana after the first report by Mason and McKay, later confirmed by Blot and Fraumeni (20). A study of histologic types by Rothschild and co-workers concluded that the distribution of histologic types was similar in low- and high-risk areas of Louisiana (19). Their findings are consistent with recent trends of decline in the proportion of squamous cell carcinoma and increase in the relative frequency of adenocarcinoma and small-cell carcinoma.

In terms of the magnitude of risks and the proportion of the population exposed to the risk factors cigarette smoking overshadows all other factors—occupation, air pollution, nutrition—considered in this report. The data in hand suggest that as much as 90% of all lung cancer cases in Louisiana are attributable to cigarette smoking. The second most important factor appears to be nutrition, which may be responsible for approximately 30% increase in the relative risk.

Our data in no way exonerate other factors as agents responsible for lung cancer deaths. One limitation of our study, shared by most studies available today, is that our controls are patients attending the hospital for other diseases. Both cases and controls are therefore "sick people" and no comparison to normal "healthy" subjects is made; this may obscure some of the etiologic associations. Some of the occupations and exposures listed in Tables 6 and 7, although not statistically significant, probably represent etiologic factors in lung cancer. Because some of them are avoidable by sound industrial hygiene practices, possible preventive programs should be designed and implemented. What our study indicates is that they are not responsible for a sizable proportion of the risk.

If prevention of the disease is contemplated, the strongest effort should be directed toward prevention of smoking. The second most important factor is nutrition, and more research is needed to evaluate the possible effects of improving the dietary intake of fresh fruits and vegetables.

Acknowledgments

Work in South Louisiana was supported by contract No N01-CP-91023 of the National Cancer Institute, U.S. Public Health Service. Work in North Louisiana was supported by a grant from the Louisiana Division of the American Cancer Society.

References

1. Gover M. Cancer Mortality in the U.S. III Geographic variation in recorded cancer mortality for detailed sites for an average of the years 1930–32. U.S. Public Health Service, U.S.Government Printing Office, Washington, DC. Bulletin No. 257. 1940.
2. Ballinger T. Personal communication. 1983
3. Haviland A. The geographic distribution of heart disease and dropsy, cancer in females and phtisis in females. London: Smith, Elder and Co., 1875.
4. Ochsner A, DeBakey M. Symposium on Cancer. Primary pulmonary malignancy treated by total pneumonectomy; analysis of 79 collected cases and presentation of 7 personal cases. Surg Gynec Obstet 1939;68:435–451.
5. Burbank F. Patterns in cancer mortality in the U.S. National Cancer Institute Monogr 33, Washington, DC: NCI, 1971.
6. Mason TJ, McKay FW, Hoover R, et al. Atlas of cancer mortality for U.S. counties 1950–1969. Washington, DC: U.S. Government Printing Office, 1975.
7. Blot WJ, Fraumeni JF. Geographic patterns of lung cancer: industrial correlations. Am J Epidemiol 1976;103:539–50.
8. DeRouen TA, Diem JE. Relationships between cancer mortality in Louisiana and drinking water source and other possible causative agents. In: Origins of human cancer. Editors: H.H. Hiatt, J.D. Watson, J.A. Winsten. Cold Spring Harbor, New York. Cold Spring Harbor Laboratory, 1977:331–45.
9. Voors AW, Johnson WD, Steele SH, Rothschild H. Relationship between respiratory cancer and wetland residency in Louisiana. Arch Environ Health 1978;33:124–9.
10. Lopez A, Yates B, Johnson WD, Nze R. The role of vitamin A and ascorbic acid in relation to respiratory system cancer. Am Soc Clin Nutr Abstracts 1979;553A.
11. Lopez A, LeGardeur BY, Johnson WD. Relationship between vitamin A and respiratory cancer. Am Fed Clin Res 1980; (abstract)
12. Gottlieb MS, Pickle LW, Blot WJ, Fraumeni JF. Lung cancer in Louisiana: death certificate analysis. JNCI 1979;63:1133–1137.
13. Gottlieb MS, Stedman RB. Lung cancer in shipbuilding and related industries in Louisiana. Southern Med J 1979;72:1099–1101.
14. Gottlieb MS. Lung cancer and petroleum industry in Louisiana. JOM 1980;22:384–388.
15. Gottlieb MS, Carr JK. Mortality studies on lung, pancreas, esophageal and other cancers in Louisiana. In: Quantification of occupational risk. Banbury Rep 9. Editors: M. Sneiderman, R. Peto. Cold Spring Harbor, New York. Cold Spring Harbor Laboratory, 1981:195–204.
16. Gottlieb MS, Carr JK, Clarkson JR. Drinking water and cancer in Louisiana. Am J Epidemiol 1982;116:652–67.
17. Rothschild H, Voors AW, Weed S, et al. Trends in respiratory system cancer mortality in Louisiana: Geographic distribution in 1950–69 and 1967–76 compared. Am J Publ Health 1979; 69:380–1.
18. Rothschild H, Mulvey JJ. An increased risk for lung cancer mortality associated with sugar cane farming. JNCI 1982;68:755–60.
19. Rothschild H, Buechner H, Welsh R, et al. Histologic typing of lung cancer in Louisiana. Cancer 1982;49:1874–7.
20. Blot WJ, Fraumeni JF. Changing patterns of lung cancer in the U.S. Am J Epidemiol 1982; 115:664–73.

CHAPTER 7

The Causes of Lung Cancer in Texas

PATRICIA A. BUFFLER,* LINDA WILLIAMS PICKLE,**
THOMAS J. MASON,** and CHARLES CONTANT**

* Epidemiology Research Unit, The University of Texas Health Science Center at Houston, School of Public Health, Houston, Texas 77025
**Environmental Epidemiology Branch, National Cancer Institute, Landow 3C15, Bethesda, Maryland 20205

ABSTRACT

A population-based case-comparison interview study of lung cancer was conducted from 1979 to 1982 in six Texas coastal counties—Orange, Jefferson, Chambers, Harris, Galveston, and Brazoria—to evaluate the association of lung cancer with occupational and other environmental exposures. Lung cancer mortality rates in these counties consistently have exceeded lung cancer mortality rates observed for Texas and the United States from 1950–1969 to 1970–1975 for both sexes and races (white and nonwhites).

Histologically and cytologically confirmed incident cases diagnosed during the interval July 1976 to June 1980 among white male and female residents aged 30–79 years were ascertained from participating hospitals in the six-county area. Both population-based and decedent comparisons were selected and matched on age, race, sex, region of residence, and vital status at time of ascertainment.

The exposures of primary interest in the study of lung cancer are those associated with occupation (employment in specific industries and occupations) in conjunction with tobacco, alcohol, diet, and residential exposures.
Key Words: **Smoking history, petrochemical industry, histologic types, construction workers, chemical manufacturing, transportation**

Introduction and Background

Data presented by Doll and Peto (1) and related reports (2) indicate that respiratory cancer sites, dominated by lung cancer, show the most dramatic increases of all cancer sites over the past 30 years. The role of smoking in the etiology of respiratory cancer has been well documented. In addition, lung cancer is

Lung Cancer: Causes and Prevention.

recognized as possibly the most important work-related cancer. However, the interaction between smoking and occupational exposures and the increased risk that may be attributed to an occupational exposure has not been very well characterized for a large number of workplace exposures.

A population-based case-comparison interview study of lung cancer, obtaining detailed occupational histories, was conducted in six Texas coastal counties where lung cancer mortality rates were elevated (3). Figure 1 shows the location of the counties of Orange, Jefferson, Chambers, Brazoria, Galveston, and Harris, a highly industrialized area where Houston is located. Approximately 25% (3.5 million) of the total state population in 1980 resided in this southeastern coastal area, the majority (77.5%) in Harris County.

Newly diagnosed, histologically confirmed cases of lung cancer in white females (including Hispanic) were ascertained from July 1977 through June 1980 in Harris County (3 years) and from July 1976 through June 1980 for the surrounding five counties. Similarly, cases among white males (including Hispanic) were ascertained for four years (July 1976 through June 1980) for the five less urban but industrialized counties, excluding Harris County. Background lung cancer mortality rates for white males and females were examined by Texas State Economic Area

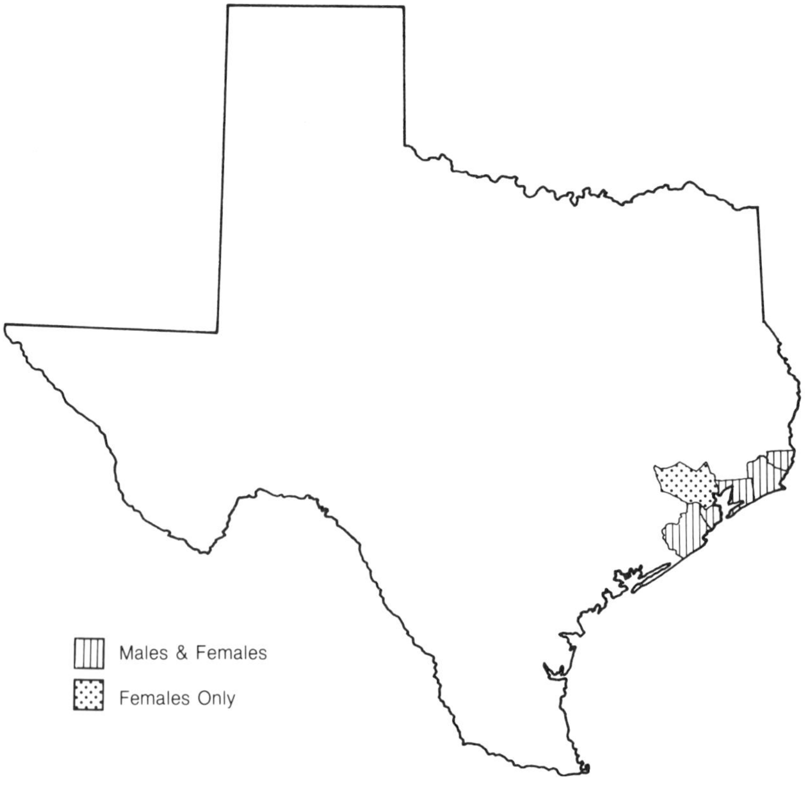

Figure 1. Texas lung cancer study area.

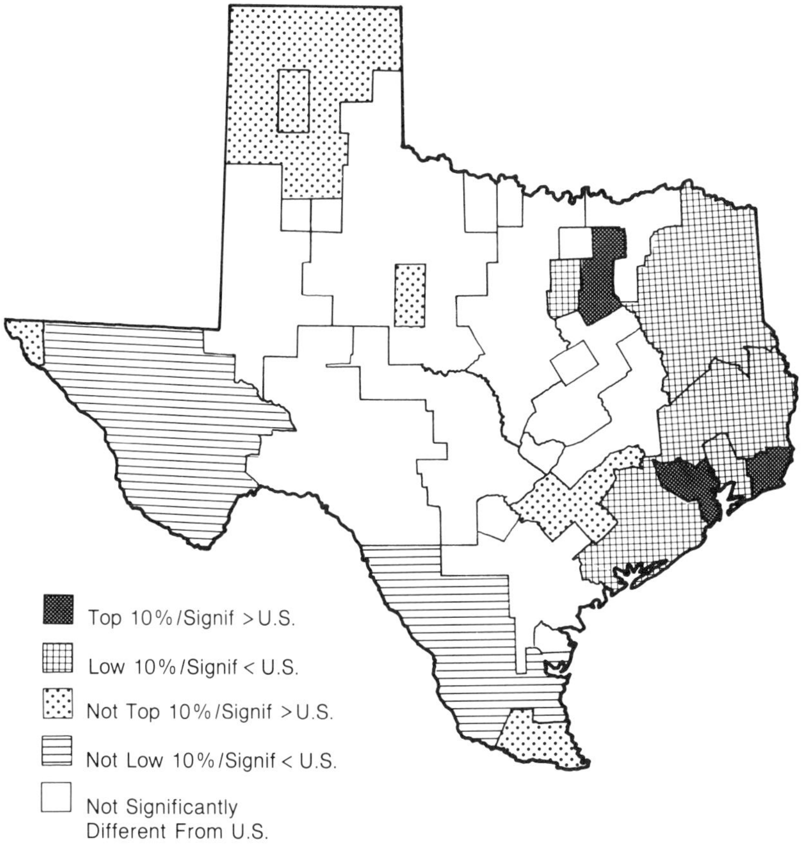

Figure 2. Lung cancer mortality 1970–1975 for white males.

(SEA) for the time period (1970 to 1975[1]) immediately preceeding the case-comparison study. As shown in Figures 2 and 3, these maps consistently document the significantly higher lung cancer mortality rates observed earlier for both white males and white females in these Texas coastal counties. The dark areas along the upper Texas coast are the Beaumont SEA (Orange and Jefferson counties), the Houston SEA (Harris County), and the Galveston SEA (Galveston County). Age-adjusted mortality rates (adjusted to the 1960 United States population) in these areas are in the top 10% of rates for SEAs in the United States and are significantly higher than the white male or white female lung cancer mortality rate for the total United States population. For white females in Harris County, this excess was notable for both the rate and the trend in the rate from 1950 to 1975 (4). For all ages, combined, the overall excess in lung cancer mortality in the Texas study area is approximately 30–40%, but this is considerably greater for some age groups.

Occupational and industrial exposures of importance for residents of the Texas coastal area include those associated with shipbuilding and repair, chemical and

[1]Excluding deaths for 1972.

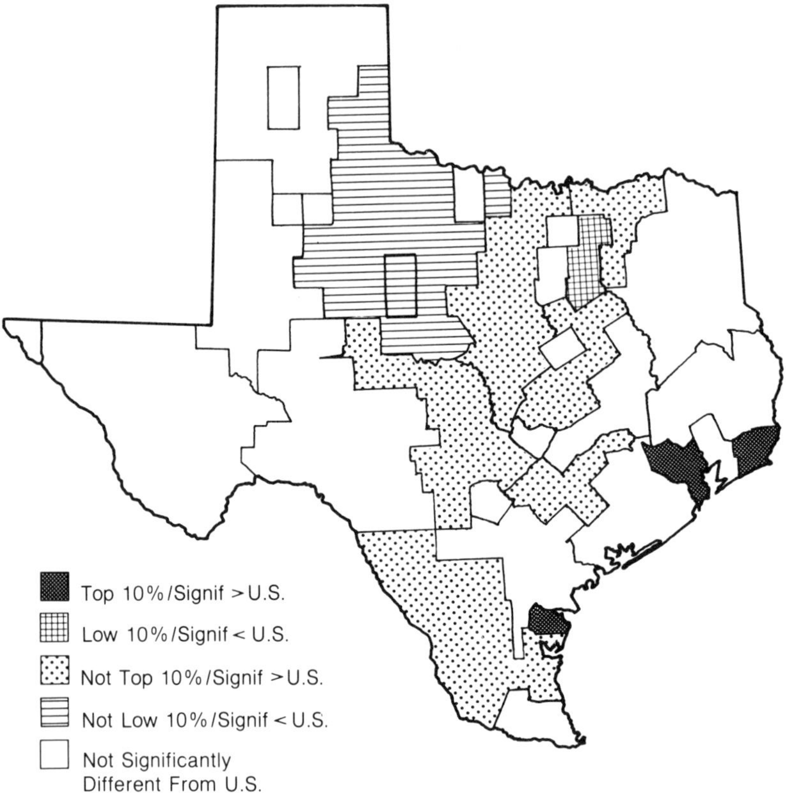

Figure 3. Lung cancer mortality 1970–1975 for white females.

petrochemical manufacturing, petroleum refining, construction, and metal industries. The largest United States based chemical and synthetic rubber production facilities are located in the study area, so a high proportion of the working population currently is employed or has been employed in these industries. For some of the smaller counties, such as Orange and Jefferson, where a single industry is dominant, as high as 27% of the working population reported being currently employed in chemical and allied products manufacturing compared with 2% for Harris County (5).

Methods

Histologically confirmed incident cases of lung cancer diagnosed among white male and female residents (including Hispanic) of the study counties for the designated time intervals (July 1977 through June 1980 for females in Harris County and July 1976 through June 1980 for males and females in other counties) were ascertained by review of hospital and state records. Hospitals in the study area that were not already participating in the Statewide Cancer Reporting Program were contacted and asked to participate in the study. Population-based and decedent comparison subjects were selected from state and federal records and matched to cases on age, race, sex, vital status at time of ascertainment, and county of residence (Harris County or other five counties). Hispanic study subjects were identified systematically by use of an algorithm to identify Spanish surname. Medical records were abstracted by state-trained abstractors to obtain relevant disease and demographic data. Following contact with the family physician (for cases only), personal interviews were conducted with study subjects or with the next of kin of decedent cases and comparison subjects, using established criteria for selecting the most appropriate next of kin respondents. Interviews were conducted by trained interviewers in the home using a standardized interview protocol. Detailed information regarding the primary exposures of interest was collected, specifically smoking history, work history, residential history, and drinking history.

Industries of employment were coded to the Standard Industrial Classification (SIC) (6) and occupations were coded using the *Dictionary of Occupational Titles* (7). The Mantel-Haenszel summary chi-square and odds ratio statistics were calculated (8). Confidence intervals (95%) were calculated using the method of Miettinem (9).

Results

A total of 56 of the 67 hospitals in the six-county Texas study participated in the study, including all of the seven large hospitals (500 or more beds). Ten of the 11 smaller hospitals that did not participate were located in Harris County. Therefore we were able to ascertain 92.2% (1520 cases) of the total 1649 incident white male and female lung cancer cases (including Hispanic) estimated for the 3- to 4-year interval (mid-1976 or 1977 to mid-1980). The number of incident cases was estimated by adjusting age–race–sex–county mortality rates by population growth and an incidence: mortality ratio of 1.35:1.0. Case ascertainment was higher for residents of counties other than Harris County, 97.2% vs 82.1% (Table 1). A total of 766 female and 754 male cases were ascertained representing, respectively, 88.7 and 96.1% of the total estimated incident cases ascertained. Hispanic females appear to be poorly ascertained (38.1%), but this may be related to the classification based on Spanish surname which may not be an effective technique for ascertaining married Hispanic females.

All ascertained cases will be used for determining age–race–sex and county lung cancer incidence rates for the study area. A total of 88.9% of the ascertained cases were included in the interview study. Some cases (110, or 7.2%) lacked histologic or cytologic confirmation of lung cancer and were ineligible for the case-comparison study. For the majority of these cases (79, or 71.8%) the basis of the lung cancer diagnosis was radiologic or clinical evidence. There was insufficient diagnostic information available on the remaining 31 cases. Additional losses of study subjects in the case-comparison study were related to race and residential eligibility criteria; unable to locate; moved out of interview area; physician,

Table 1. Lung cancer case ascertainment in Texas study by sex, ethnic group, and area, 1976–1980

	Number estimated	Number ascertained[a] (%)	Number cases interviewed[b]
White Females			
Anglo	822	750 (91.2)	449
Spanish surname	42	16 (38.1)	11
Total	864	766 (88.7)	460
White Males			
Anglo	767	730 (95.2)	460
Spanish surname	18	24 (133.3)	15
Total	785	754 (96.1)	475
Area			
Harris County (females only, 1977–1980)	567	468 (82.1)	275
Other counties	1082	1052 (97.2)	660
Total	1649	1520 (92.2)	935

[a]Includes 110 cases without histologic confirmation and an additional 15 cases estimated to be ineligible, in terms of race and residence criteria.
[b]Excludes cases ineligible; not located; refusals by physician, hospital, or study subject; and cases interviewed and subsequently identified as ineligible, or data to be of poor quality.

Table 2. Texas lung cancer study population by sex, study group, and ethnicity

	Study group		
	Cases	Controls	Totals
Total			
Female	460	482	942
Male	475	466	941
Total	935	948	1883
Spanish surname			
Female	11	20	31
Male	15	19	34
Total	26	39	65

hospital, and subject refusals; and poor quality interview data. Overall study subject refusal rates were 7.7% and 10.7% for decedent cases and controls respectively, and 13.5% and 20.6% for living cases and controls, respectively. A total of 935 interviews was completed with eligible cases (460 females and 475 males) and 948 interviews with frequency matched comparison subjects (Table 2). Included in these totals are 26 Spanish surname cases and 39 comparison subjects. Separate analyses are not presented at this time for these study subjects.

The average duration of time study subjects resided in the county of diagnosis or in the six-county study area is over 25 years for all study groups. The majority of both male (86%) and female (82%) cases were decedent cases and were slightly older at time of diagnosis than the living cases (Tables 3 and 4). The distribution of age at diagnosis is compared for male and female study groups in Figure 4. A higher proportion of the female cases was diagnosed before age 60 (45.4%) than male cases diagnosed before age 60 (34%).

Table 3. Number and percentage of male lung cancer cases by age at diagnosis and type of respondent, Texas, 1976 to 1980

Age at diagnosis (years)	Type of respondent								Total			
	Self				Next of kin							
	Cases		Controls		Cases		Controls		Cases		Controls	
	No	%	No	%	No	%	No	%	No	%	No	%
30–39	1	1.5	1	1.6	3	0.7	2	0.5	4	0.8	3	0.6
40–49	5	7.5	7	10.9	28	6.9	34	8.5	33	7.0	41	8.8
50–59	23	34.3	22	34.4	102	25.0	98	24.4	125	26.2	120	25.7
60–69	31	47.0	23	35.9	165	40.4	164	40.8	196	41.3	18.7	40.2
70–79 +	7	10.6	11	17.2	110	27.0	104	25.9	117	24.7	11.5	24.7
		100.0		100.0		100.0		100.0		100.0		100.0
Totals	67		64		408		402		475		466	

Table 4. Number and percentage of female lung cancer cases by age at diagnosis and type of respondent, Texas, 1976 to 1980

Age at diagnosis (years)	Type of respondent								Total			
	Self				Next of kin							
	Cases		Controls		Cases		Controls		Cases		Controls	
	No	%	No	%	No	%	No	%	No	%	No	%
30–39	0	0.0	3	2.6	6	1.6	5	1.4	6	1.3	8	1.7
40–49	9	11.1	12	10.3	40	10.6	50	13.7	49	10.6	62	12.9
50–59	36	44.4	55	47.4	118	31.1	104	28.4	154	33.5	159	33.0
60–69	24	29.6	34	29.3	153	40.4	135	36.9	177	38.5	169	35.1
70–79 +	12	14.8	12	10.3	62	16.4	72	19.7	74	16.1	84	17.4
		100.0		100.0		100.0		100.0		100.0		100.0
Totals	81		116		379		366		460		482	

Proportions of male and female cases and comparison subjects using tobacco, cigarettes, alcohol, or who "ever lived with household member who smoked regularly" are compared in Table 5. Ninety-seven percent of the male cases and 91% of the female cases reported ever smoking cigarettes but a higher proportion of the female than male cases reported smoking cigarettes currently, 68% vs 54%. Proportions of heavy smokers and use of alcohol (ever) were higher for cases than comparison subjects and for males than females. An extremely high proportion of both female cases and comparison subjects report having lived with a household member who smoked regularly, 93% vs 88%.

Although the patterns of risk differed for males and females (Table 6), the odds ratios for all smoking variables were statistically significant at the $p = .05$ level. Among males, ex-smokers had a risk higher than current smokers, whereas in females the risk was lower in ex-smokers. The highest odds ratio for females was observed for current smokers, 7.9 vs 5.0 for ex-smokers. Odds ratios for the ac-

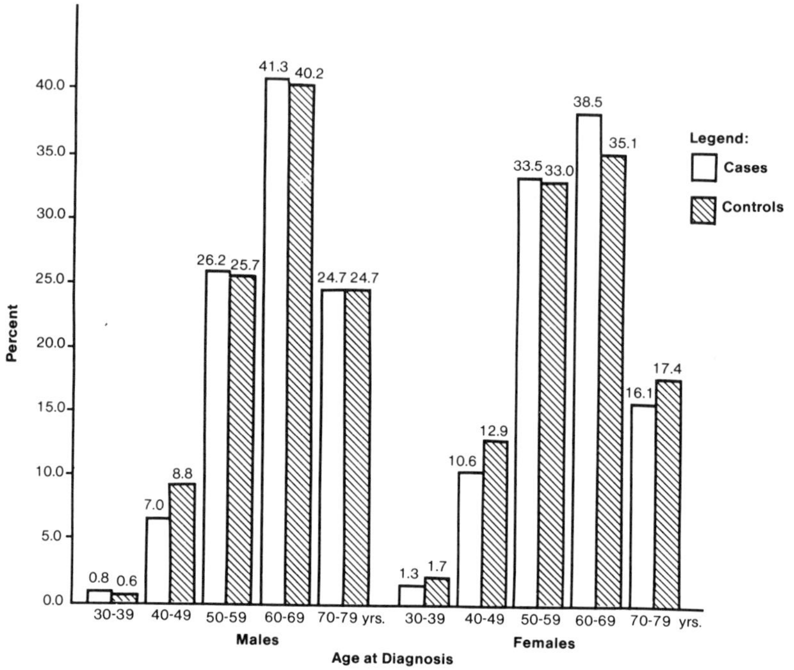

Figure 4. Age distribution (age at diagnosis) for male and female study subjects, Texas lung cancer study, 1976–1980. Clear columns, cases; shaded columns, controls.

cumulated lifetime cigarette dose, expressed as pack-years, were higher for males in the low and moderate categories but associated with a similar gradient in both males and females. No difference in risk was associated with the use of filtered cigarettes for either males or females.

The role of "passive smoking" in contributing to risk of lung cancer was examined (Table 7). In this analysis the crude (or unadjusted) odds ratio are increased and significant for both males and females, 1.4 and 2.1, respectively. However, when the confounding effect of individual subject smoking was controlled by stratifying the

Table 5. Proportion of cases and controls reporting use of tobacco, cigarettes and alcohol by sex, Texas lung cancer study, 1976–1980

	Males		Females	
	Cases	Controls	Cases	Controls
Tobacco (ever)	0.99	0.90	0.91	0.59
Cigarettes (ever)	0.97	0.80	0.91	0.59
Cigarettes (current)	0.54	0.47	0.68	0.38
Cigarettes (light)	0.08	0.10	0.08	0.17
Cigarettes (heavy)	0.45	0.29	0.34	0.13
Alcohol (ever)	0.86	0.81	0.78	0.63
Lived with a smoker	0.76	0.70	0.93	0.88

Table 6. Odds ratios[a] associated with smoking variables for males and females, Texas lung cancer study, 1976–1980

	Males	Females
Ever smoked	10.12	6.89
Current smoker	9.59	7.89
Ex-smoker	10.85	5.00
Pack-years		
Low (0–35)	6.24	3.21
Moderate (36–63)	9.39	7.98
High (64 +)	13.05	13.35
Filtered cigarettes		
Yes	9.39	7.11
No	10.25	6.06
Both	12.27	7.09

[a]All odds ratios significant at $p < .05$.

male and female study groups into smokers (ever) and nonsmokers (never) and examining the adjusted odds ratios, there was no significant increase in risk associated with passive smoking. In fact, the odds ratios for nonsmokers living with a regular smoker were not increased for either males or females, 0.52 and 0.78, respectively. However, odds ratios for smokers living with a regular smoker were increased, although not significantly, 1.28 and 1.80 for males and females. The overall odds ratios (adjusted) associated with passive smoking were only slightly increased and not significant for either males or females, 1.2 and 1.3, respectively. When the possibility of a ''passive smoking'' effect was examined among nonsmokers by number of years lived with a regular smoker, there was very little difference in risk for females who lived with a regular smoker for 0-32 years (Table 8). The odds ratios for males suggest an increase by are based on smaller numbers than the analysis in females.

Table 7. Odds ratios for passive smoking (household member smoked regularly) in Texas male and female lung cancer studies, 1976–1980

	Yes		No		Odds	95%	
	Case	Control	Case	Control	ratio	Confidence interval	χ^2
Males							
Crude	363	329	93	119	1.41[a]	1.04, 1.92	4.8
Self ever smoked							
No	5	56	6	34	0.52	0.15, 1.74	1.2
Yes	357	273	87	85	1.28	0.91, 1.79	2.0
Overall (MOR)					1.20	0.87, 1.65	1.18
Females							
Crude	429	425	24	51	2.12[a]	1.29, 3.50	9.05
Self ever smoked							
No	33	164	8	32	0.78	0.34, 1.81	0.3
Yes	396	260	16	19	1.80	0.92, 3.58	3.0
Overall (MOR)					1.30	0.78, 2.18	1.0

[a]$p < .05$.

Table 8. Odds ratios associated with passive smoking

Ever live with household member who smoked	Number	Odds ratio	Confidence interval	χ^2
Males				
Total nonsmokers	61	0.52	0.15, 1.74	1.2
0–32 years	49	0.40	0.10, 1.58	1.8
33+ years	10	1.56	0.30, 8.05	0.3
Females				
Total nonsmokers	201	0.78	0.34, 1.81	0.3
0–32 years	97	0.62	0.24, 1.63	0.9
33+ years	99	0.93	0.38, 2.28	0.0

Histologic types of lung cancer were classified according to the World Health Organization (WHO) classification (10). The four major cell types account for 75–85% of the cases in both the male and female series and the cell type distribution by age group is shown for males and females in Table 9. Adenocarcinoma is the predominant lung cancer cell type in both young (30–49 years) males and females, comprising 37.8% (males) and 38.9% (females) of all lung cancers among persons aged 30–49 years at diagnosis. There is a marked shift with age in this pattern such that for both males and females aged 70 or older at diagnosis the predominant cell type is squamous or epidermoid (accounting for 40.5% of all cases among males and 31.0% among females). Overall, squamous was the predominant cell type among males (42.2%) and adenocarcinoma among females (35.5%). These patterns held for both smokers and nonsmokers except for nonsmoking males, in whom 6 of 11 (54.5%) cases were adenocarcinoma.

The risk associated with smoking was examined by cell type, specifically odds ratios for smoking categories within the adenocarcinoma series compared with nonadenocarcinoma cases (Tables 10 and 11). The odds ratios for smoking categories based on pack-years were all significant, emphasizing the increased risk of lung cancer (all types) associated with smoking. However, the gradient of risk, in both males and females, was markedly different for adenocarcinoma compared with nonadenocarcinoma (all other lung cancer) cell types. There were 104 cases of

Table 9. Male and female lung cancer cases by histologic type and age, Texas, 1976–1980

	Males						Females					
	30–49 years		50–69 years		70+ years		30–49 years		50–69 years		70+ years	
Cell type	No	%	No	%	No	%	No	%	No	%	No	%
Squamous	8	21.6	112	34.8	47	40.5	11	20.4	74	22.6	22	31.0
Small cell	4	10.8	64	20.1	16	13.8	10	18.5	92	28.1	11	15.5
Adenocarcinoma	14	37.8	73	22.9	17	14.7	21	38.9	99	30.3	19	26.8
Large cell	2	5.4	19	6.0	9	7.8	4	7.4	11	3.4	3	4.2
Other		24.4		16.2		23.2		14.8		15.7		12.5
Total		100.0		100.0		100.0		100.0		100.0		100.0

Table 10. Odds ratios associated with smoking for lung cancer cell types in males, Texas lung cancer study, 1976–1980

Cell type	Smoking category (pack-years)	Odds ratio	Confidence intervals	χ^2
Adenocarcinoma	Low	3.85	1.44, 10.31	8.04
	Moderate	4.45	1.72, 11.48	10.93
	High	5.38	2.14, 13.56	15.21
Nonadenocarcinoma	Low	6.60	2.75, 15.84	21.57
	Moderate	11.30	4.87, 26.19	43.75
	High	15.41	6.73, 35.25	63.34

Table 11. Odds ratios associated with smoking for lung cancer cell types in females, Texas lung cancer study, 1976–1980

Cell type	Smoking category (pack-years)	Odds ratio	Confidence intervals	χ^2
Adenocarcinoma	Low	2.16	1.18, 3.98	6.37
	Moderate	4.32	2.40, 7.79	26.11
	High	7.80	4.28, 14.20	52.93
Nonadenocarcinoma	Low	4.17	2.34, 7.43	25.80
	Moderate	10.97	6.27, 19.20	86.87
	High	18.90	10.61, 33.67	128.13

adenocarcinoma in the male series and 139 in the female series. A much steeper increase in risk associated with lifetime cigarette dose (pack-years) is observed for all other lung cancer cell types compared to adenocarcinoma. These patterns are summarized in Figure 5.

Preliminary analyses of the detailed work histories is based on the usual occupation and usual industry of employment as reported or as summarized from the work history for self and spouse. Examination of the work histories indicates that approximately 78% of the study subjects spent more than half of their reported working time employed in the occupation reported as their usual occupation. Usual industry of employment was determined by selecting the industry in which a subject was reported to have been employed for the longest duration of time. Odds ratios, adjusted for smoking (ever/never) were determined to identify whether an increased risk was associated with employment in a given occupation or industry for both males and females. Using the Professional/Technical category as a referent for males (odds ratio = 1), none of the odds ratios for the other occupational categories was significantly increased (Table 12). Odds ratios (OR) for usual industry of employment were similarly calculated using the sales category (SIC 50–59) as the referent (OR = 1.0) (Table 13). Significantly elevated odds ratios were observed for several industrial categories, specifically construction (SIC 15–17), chemical manufacturing (SIC 28), metal manufacturing (SIC 33–34), and transportation (SIC 40–49). In addition, an elevated odds ratio (OR = 2.44) of borderline statistical significance (at the .05 level) is observed for oil and gas extraction (SIC 13).

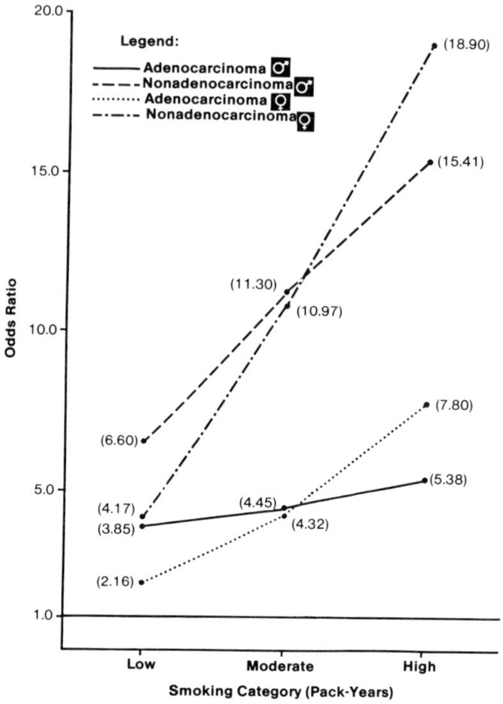

Figure 5. Odds ratios associated with smoking by lung cancer cell type.

The majority (approximately 60%) of the females reported their usual occupation as housewife. Using this category as the referent (OR = 1.0), smoking-adjusted odds ratios (ever/never) were calculated for the remaining categories (Table 14). Although there are several categories with elevated odds ratios, only the odds ratio for the clerical category (1.57) is significant. The odds ratio for the service category (1.57) is similarly increased, and of borderline statistical significance.

Table 12. Adjusted[a] odds ratios for usual occupation in Texas male lung cancer study, 1976–1980

Occupation category	Total number in category (cases and controls)	Odds ratio	Confidence interval	χ^2
Clerical/Sales	94	0.61	0.36, 1.04	3.33
Service	50	1.12	0.60, 2.09	0.13
Agriculture	39	0.89	0.44, 1.84	0.09
Processing	77	0.80	0.47, 1.38	0.63
Machine trades	77	1.37	0.78, 2.39	1.19
Bench work	14	1.04	0.34, 3.19	0.01
Structural work	275	1.46	0.96, 2.20	3.15
Miscellaneous	140	0.89	0.55, 1.44	0.22
Professional/Technical	157	1.00	— —	—

[a]Adjusted for smoking (ever/never).

Table 13. Adjusted[a] odds ratios for usual industry of employment in Texas male lung cancer study, 1976–1980

Industry category (SIC number)	Total number in category	Odds ratio	Confidence interval	χ^2
Agriculture (01–09)	30	1.64	0.70, 3.83	1.31
Oil/gas extract (13)	28	2.44	1.00, 5.97	3.82
Other mining (10–12, 14)	8	0.72	0.19, 2.80	0.22
Construction (15–17)	150	2.56[b]	1.49, 4.41	11.50
Chemical (28)	60	2.16[b]	1.10, 4.24	5.04
Petroleum (29)	178	1.54	0.91, 2.60	2.63
Metals (33–34)	25	3.38[b]	1.36, 8.39	6.90
Shipbuilding (373)	27	1.91	0.83, 4.42	2.29
Other manufacturing (20–39 minus above)	52	1.55	0.77, 3.12	1.51
Transportation (40–49)	120	2.57[b]	1.47, 4.52	10.88
Personal services (60–69, 80, 91–97)	65	1.73	0.91, 3.29	2.76
Professional/Governmental (70–79, 81–87)	85	1.34	0.73, 2.44	0.91
Sales (50–59)	97	1.00	— —	—

[a]Adjusted for smoking (ever/never).
[b]$p < .05$

Table 14. Adjusted[a] odds ratios for usual occupation in Texas female lung cancer study, 1976–1980

Occupation category	Total number in category	Odds ratio	Confidence interval	χ^2
Clerical	161	1.57[b]	1.07, 2.31	5.27
Service	88	1.57	0.96, 2.57	3.22
Agriculture	3	0.74	0.14, 3.92	0.12
Processing	2	4.22	0.43, 41.33	1.53
Machine trades	2	2.66	0.45, 15.93	1.15
Bench work	11	1.67	0.47, 5.97	0.62
Structural	2	5.22	0.79, 34.59	2.93
Miscellaneous	8	2.27	0.52, 9.98	1.18
Professional/Technical	110	1.15	0.75, 1.76	0.40
Housewife	551	1.00	— —	—

[a]Adjusted for smoking (ever/never).
[b]$p < .05$

There were too few observations in the remaining categories for a meaningful analysis. A similar analysis of usual industry of employment for females indicated no categories of concern except for the possible exception of the increase noted for the category of other manufacturing (Table 15).

Smoking-adjusted odds ratios were also examined for the usual occupation and industry of employment for the spouses of both males and females. The only significantly increased odds ratio observed was for the usual industry of employment for spouses of female lung cancer cases. The Construction industry, with 146 cases and controls reporting this as the usual industry for their spouse, was associated with an increased odds ratio of 1.74 (1.04, 2.92; $\chi^2 = 4.40$).

Table 15. Adjusted[a] odds ratios for usual industry of employment in Texas female lung cancer study, 1976–1980

Industry category	Total number in category	Odds ratio	Confidence interval	χ^2
Agriculture	6	0.91	0.24, 3.53	0.02
Oil/gas extract	4	2.01	0.37, 10.84	0.66
Other mining	0	—	— —	—
Construction	2	4.95	0.75, 32.69	2.76
Chemical	2	3.93	0.40, 39.06	1.37
Petroleum	6	0.43	0.91, 2.00	1.16
Metals	2	3.93	0.40, 39.06	1.37
Shipbuilding	2	3.93	0.40, 39.06	1.37
Other manufacturing	23	2.70	0.95, 7.67	3.50
Transportation	12	0.78	0.22, 2.76	0.15
Services	74	1.26	0.75, 2.13	0.75
Professional/Governmental	93	1.08	0.69, 1.69	0.12
Sales	113	1.23	0.80, 1.90	0.92
Housewife	592	1.00	— —	—

[a]Adjusted for smoking (ever/never).

Table 16. Odds ratios for household member regularly employed in specific industry for Texas lung cancer study, 1976–1980: Males

Industry	Yes: Case	Yes: Control	Odds ratio	95% Confidence interval	χ^2
Asbestos manufacturing	6	2	2.60	0.60, 11.25	1.76
Cement manufacturing	5	5	0.99	0.30, 3.25	0.00
Insulation manufacturing	4	1	2.99	0.47, 19.04	1.48
Coal mining	11	4	2.57	0.86, 7.71	3.06
Shipyard/shipbuilding	58	52	1.11	0.75, 1.65	2.27
Demolition	5	3	1.54	0.40, 5.93	0.41
High-rise construction	11	9	1.19	0.50, 2.84	0.16

Table 17. Odds ratios for household member regularly employed in specific industry for Texas lung cancer study, 1976–1980: Females

Industry	Yes: Case	Yes: Control	Odds ratio	95% Confidence interval	χ^2
Asbestos manufacturing	5	10	0.55	0.20, 1.50	1.29
Cement manufacturing	20	18	1.17	0.02, 2.23	0.24
Insulation manufacturing	9	4	2.24	0.73, 6.94	2.07
Coal mining	7	12	0.63	0.25, 1.57	1.00
Shipyard/shipbuilding	99	102	1.02	0.75, 1.39	0.02
Demolition	5	7	0.77	0.25, 2.33	0.02
High-rise construction	37	26	1.52	0.91, 2.55	2.60

In addition to these analyses specific questions were asked regarding whether anyone in the household ever worked in the following industries: asbestos, cement, or insulation manufacturing; coal mining; shipyards and shipbuilding; demolition;

high-rise construction. For both males and females a large number of cases and controls reported having a household member employed in a shipyard or in shipbuilding, but this was not associated with an increased odds ratio (1.11 for males and 1.02 for females) (Tables 16 and 17). Among males there were no statistically significant increases; however, the odds ratios for asbestos manufacturing, insulation manufacturing, and coal mining are increased. Similarly, for females the odds ratio is increased for insulation manufacturing and high-rise construction but not significantly.

Discussion

The availability of fairly large numbers of male and female incident lung cancer cases and comparison subjects in an interview study with detailed occupational histories provides an important basis for examining the contribution of occupational exposures to lung cancer in males and females. Recognizing the strong increase in lung cancer risk associated with cigarette smoking, such analyses need to control for smoking differences. Our preliminary analysis of usual occupation and industry of employment with a broad smoking adjustment (ever/never) indicates several occupational and industrial associations that need to be pursued in future analyses. Specifically, odds ratios are significantly increased for usual employment in several industries (construction, chemical, metal, and transportation) for males and the clerical occupations for females. In addition, there are several associations suggested by increased odds ratios, which are not statistically significant. For males, an increased risk is suggested for occupations in the structural category and employment in industries related to oil and gas extraction (SIC 13), petroleum refining (SIC 60–69), and shipbuilding (SIC 373). For females, occupations in the service category and industries in the other manufacturing group are associated with fairly stable increased odds ratios.

Future analysis of these data will examine the possible interaction of smoking with occupational and industrial groups and a possible need to employ more specific smoking strata. Examination of odds ratios for smoking strata within occupational and industrial categories suggested that an ever/never smoking classification would be sufficient to control for the confounding effect of smoking in the examination of overall risks associated with usual employment in specific occupational and industrial categories as presented here. However, this broad classification may not be sufficiently specific for an examination of interaction of smoking with workplace exposures. In these analyses the classification of "exposed" within a specific category is based upon the "usual" occupation or industry of employment rather than "ever employed" in a given work environment. The use of the usual pattern may be more conservative in the detection of occupational and industrial associations and is perhaps the more appropriate designation to use for a preliminary examination of the data. As noted, the use of the usual occupation and industry of employment did introduce some special constraints on the analysis of the female patterns in that the usual occupation and industry for over

60% of the cases and controls was "Housewife." We will employ a number of more specific designations of occupational and industrial variables in future analyses.

Even with these recognized limitations, the suggestion which clearly emerges from our data is that there may be a wider variety of workplace exposures associated with substantial increments in the risk of lung cancer than currently recognized. In addition, use of the full work history, including dates will surely aid in refining the preliminary associations reported here.

The relationship of lung cancer cell type with age at time of diagnosis warrants further scrutiny in that the highest odds ratios for the smoking variables were observed for the youngest age group (< 57 years at time of diagnosis). The lack of a "passive smoking" effect when the confounding effect of smoking of individual study subjects is considered, is not consistent with early reports. Although subsequent reports are also not consistent with regard to this association, it may be that the study population available was not sufficiently large to detect a fairly low level effect and that this association needs to be assessed in a considerably larger study population.

These preliminary analyses demonstrate a strong and consistent smoking effect in males and females for all types of lung cancer. The risk differentials associated with cigarette smoking observed for adenocarcinoma and other lung cancer cell types are striking and consistent with findings of others (11). In addition, they reemphasize earlier suggestions that perhaps specific environmental exposures are more strongly associated with specific types of lung cancer. In addition, these data suggest that perhaps lung cancer is more similar in males and females than previously regarded and that the observed differentials in risk by sex are principally due to exposure differentials.

Acknowledgments

The authors thank Drs. Irene Easling and Keith Burau and their capable and dedicated staff for their invaluable assistance with the data collection and data management for this study. We also wish to acknowledge the valuable consultation and assistance of Dr. Robert Hardy (UTSPH), Dr. Reuel A. Stallones (UTSPH), Dr. David T. Carr (M.D. Anderson Hospital and Tumor Institute), Dr. S. Donald Greenberg (Baylor College of Medicine), the staff of the Texas State Health Department Statewide Cancer Reporting Program and Bureau of Vital Statistics, and the American Lung Association, San Jacinto Chapter. And lastly, we wish to acknowledge the assistance of the many hospitals, physicians, agencies, and individuals without whom it would not have been possible for us to successfully complete this study.

References

1. Doll R, Peto R. The causes of cancer: quantitative estimates of avoidable risks of cancer in the United States today. Oxford: Oxford University Press, 1981.

2. U.S. Congress Office of Technology Assessment. Assessment of technologies for determining cancer risks from the environment. OTA-H-138. Washington, DC: U.S. Government Printing Office, June 1981.
3. Mason TJ, McKay FW, Hoover R, Blot WJ, Fraumeni JF. Atlas of cancer mortality for U.S. Counties: 1950–69. U.S. Department of Health, Education and Welfare Publ (NIH) 75-780. Washington, DC: U.S. Government Printing Office, 1974.
4. National Cancer Institute, Environmental Epidemiology Branch. Cancer mortality maps by State Economic Area, 1970–75. Unpublished report, 1983.
5. U.S. Bureau of the Census, U.S. Census of Population: 1970. General Social and Economic Characteristics Texas PC (1)-C45. Washington, DC: U.S. Government Printing Office, 1972.
6. Office of Management and the Budget. Standard industrial classification manual. Washington DC: U.S. Government Printing Office, 1972.
7. U.S. Department of Labor. Dictionary of occupational titles, 4th ed. Washington, DC: U.S. Government Printing Office, 1977.
8. Mantel N, Haenszel W. Statistical aspects of the analysis of data from retrospective studies of disease. JNCI 1959;22:719–48.
9. Miettinen O. Simple internal estimation of risk ratio. Am J Epidemiol 1974;100:515–16.
10. World Health Organization. International classification of disease for oncology (ICD-0), 1st ed. Geneva: WHO, 1976.
11. Rosenow EC, Carr DT. Bronchogenic carcinoma. CA 1979;29(4):233–45.

CHAPTER 8

Recent Case–Control Studies of Lung Cancer in the United States

LINDA WILLIAMS PICKLE,* PELAYO CORREA** and ELIZABETH FONTHAM**

*Population Studies Section, Environmental Epidemiology Branch, National Cancer Institute, Landow Building 3C15, Bethesda, Maryland 20205
**Department of Pathology, Louisiana State University Medical Center, New Orleans, Louisiana 70112

ABSTRACT

United States county lung cancer mortality rates were elevated among whites along the Gulf and Atlantic Coasts during 1950–1969. Rates in these areas have continued to rise faster than the overall United States rate, making geographic differences even more pronounced. Although cigarette smoking is accepted as the predominant cause of lung cancer in the United States, these geographic differences, as well as results of correlation studies, suggest the presence of other environmental determinants.

Case-control interview studies first initiated in these high-rate areas concentrated on the collection of smoking and occupational information. Recent studies, however, have suggested other possible risk factors for lung cancer: various occupational exposures, some of which may act synergistically with cigarette smoking; air pollution; genetic resistance or susceptibility; "passive" exposures in the home, including cigarette smoking and dusts on workers clothing; and nutritional deficiencies. Results from case-control studies published since 1978 are reviewed, concentrating on studies conducted along the Gulf and Atlantic Coasts. Preliminary results of an ongoing analysis of "Cajun lifestyle" and lung cancer in Louisiana are presented to illustrate the complex issues now under investigation for this cancer site.

Key Words: **Epidemiology, ethnic groups, lung neoplasms, nutrition, occupations, questionnaires, smoking**

Both incidence and mortality rates for cancer of the lung are highest of all cancer sites among men in this country (1) and, if current trends continue, will soon be the leading site of cancer among women (2). Cigarette smoking is now accepted as the

1984 Verlag Chemie International, Inc.
Lung Cancer: Causes and Prevention.

predominant cause of lung cancer, but this association was a controversial one when first proposed 30 years ago. Early studies of lung cancer therefore concentrated on assessing smoking habits to confirm this finding. Later, correlation studies and differing geographic patterns suggested that other factors were operating. As the hypothesized etiology of lung cancer has grown more complex, so have the studies designed to test these associations. We trace here the development of case-control studies of lung cancer during recent years, compare their results, and describe data currently being analyzed. As an example of the increasing complexity of these etiologic studies, preliminary results of an analysis of lifestyle and lung cancer in southern Louisiana are presented (also see chapter 6).

Maps of cancer mortality rates by county published for the years 1950–1969 (3) identified clusters of counties with high white male rates in urban centers in the northeast and Great Lakes regions, and along the Gulf and southern Atlantic coasts. Patterns for white females and for nonwhites (4) were less remarkable, with high rates seen primarily in urban areas. An ecologic study relating these mortality rates to demographic and industrial patterns at the county level showed significant correlations in areas that had concentrations of petrochemical, paper, and shipbuilding industries (5). Other studies have suggested additional causal factors, such as immunologic and nutritional deficiencies, as well as air pollution and specific occupational carcinogens in the workplace (6).

The geographic differences in lung cancer mortality have become even more pronounced over time. A map of the 1970–1975 mortality rates for white males (Figure 1) shows that the clustering of high-rate areas is even more concentrated in the southeast; the cluster in Louisiana now extends northward along the Mississippi River to Tennessee; this pattern is not seen for white females (Figure 2). If we look at areas that have high mortality rates and a significantly increasing rate of change over the past 25 years, we see even more striking geographic differences by sex (Figure 3 and 4). These differential patterns of mortality suggest that factors unique to males, eg, smoking habits and occupational exposures, are operating. This evidence combined with the accumulating evidence that exposures found in the workplace could cause cancer experimentally led the first large field studies of lung cancer in the 1970s to concentrate on tobacco and occupational exposures. As the number of suspected lung cancer carcinogens has increased, field studies have been designed to gather additional information.

To briefly review terminology, case-control studies in epidemiology are observational studies of humans who are selected either because they have the disease of interest (the cases) or because they do not (the controls). The exposure rates to suspected carcinogens in the case and control groups are compared to identify potential causal factors of the disease. However, there are different types of case-control studies, determined by the methods by which cases are identified and controls selected. For example, cases may be identified from the total population of the study area by means of a tumor registry, or may be identified only at certain representative hospitals in the area. Controls may be general population controls, chosen at random from the community, or may be hospitalized patients. Cases and controls also may be selected through death certificates or from personnel records at a particular manufacturing plant.

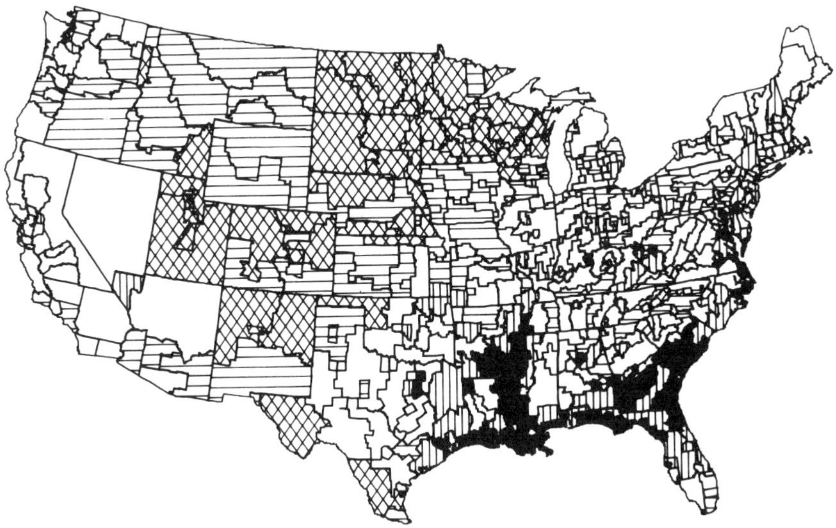

Figure 1. Lung cancer mortality rates for white males, 1970-1975, by State Economic Area; age standardized to 1960 United States population. Solid black, in highest decile, significantly greater than United States rate; vertical hatching, not in highest decile, significantly greater than United States rate; cross hatching, in lowest decile, significantly less than United States rate; horizontal hatching, not in lowest decile, significantly less than United States rate; clear, not significantly different from United States rate.

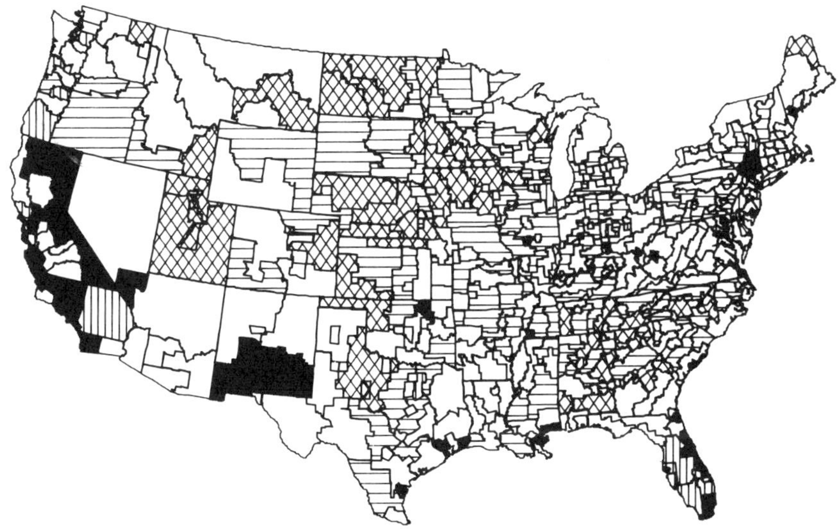

Figure 2. Lung cancer mortaility rates for white females, 1970-1975, by State Economic Area; age standardized to 1960 United States population. Solid black, in highest decile, significantly greater than United States rate; vertical hatching, not in highest decile, significantly greater than United States rate; cross hatching, in lowest decile, significantly less than United States rate; horizontal hatching, not in lowest decile, significantly less than United States rate; clear, not significantly different from United States rate.

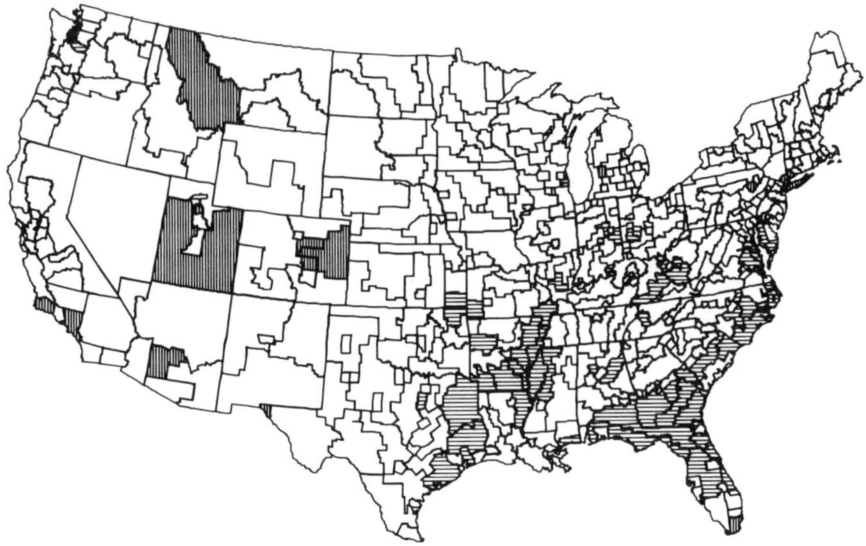

Figure 3. Lung cancer mortality rates for 1970–1975 and time trends for 1950–1975, for white males by State Economic Area; age standardized to 1960 United States population. Horizontal hatching, mortality rate and time trend significantly greater than United States rate and trend; vertical hatching mortality rate and time trend significantly less than United States rate and trend.

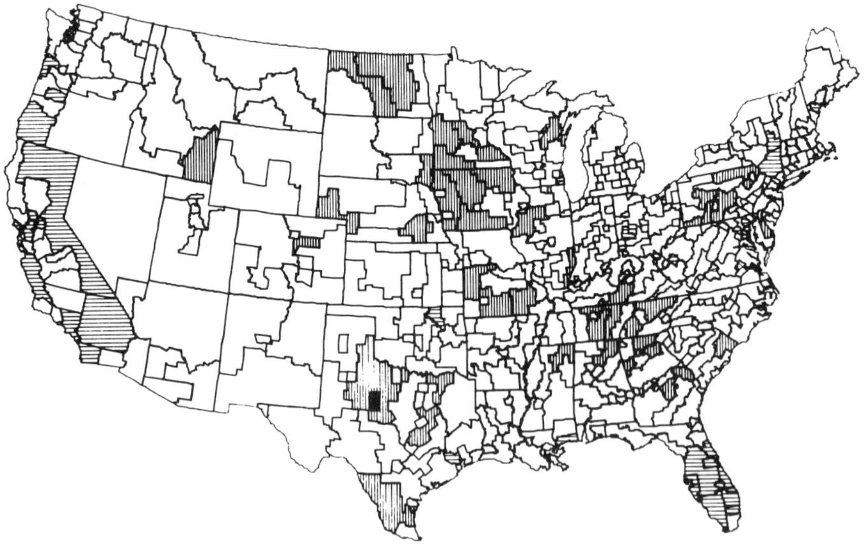

Figure 4. Lung cancer mortality rates for 1970–1975 and time trends for 1950–1975, for white females by State Economic Area; age standardized to 1960 United States population. Horizontal hatching, mortality rate and time trend significantly greater than United States rate and trend; vertical hatching, mortality rate and time trend significantly less than United States rate and trend.

Company records, death certificates, and tumor registry data can provide only limited information. More often than not, smoking information is not available. Most of the recent studies have used in-person interviews of the cases and controls or their next of kin to elicit more information than is usually available from these other sources. Of course, an interview study is time consuming and costly, and its success depends on the ability of patients to recall information about themselves or their relatives many years prior to interview, but it often is the only means of obtaining some kinds of information.

Figure 5 shows the location of recently reported case-control interview studies; these have been conducted primarily in coastal areas where white male mortality rates were elevated. Table 1 lists the reports of case-control studies in the United States published in the last four years (7–22). These include studies in the workplace, death certificate studies, studies from tumor registry data and interview studies that are either hospital or population based. The data for the last three shown are being analyzed now; preliminary data from Texas and Louisiana are presented here (Chapters 6 and 7, this volume). If we compare the information collected by these studies over time, a trend toward increasing complexity is seen (Table 2). Studies conducted in the early 1970s focused on occupation and smoking; recently completed studies included questions concerning diet, residential exposures, and "passive" exposures, such as smoking or occupational exposures by the spouse. As the complexity of study design and questionnaires has increased, so have the length of time required to interview the subject, the cost to conduct the study, the required sample size, and the complexity of statistical techniques necessary to process the massive amount of information available for each person. What once could be analyzed quickly with pencil and paper now takes months with sophisticated computer programs.

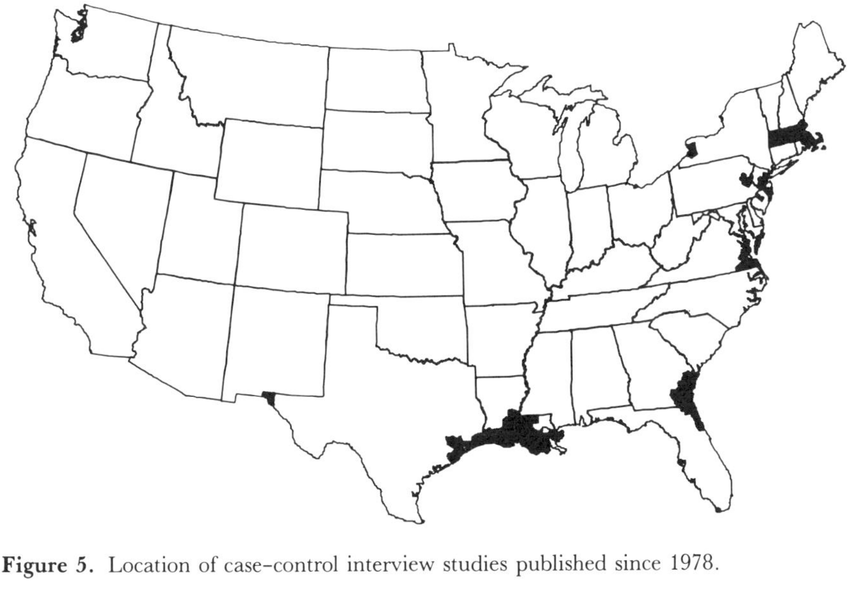

Figure 5. Location of case-control interview studies published since 1978.

Table 1. Recent case-control studies of lung cancer in the United States

First author	Year published	Location	Source of cases	Source of controls
Work records				
Egan-Baum	1981	United States	Workers	Death certificate
Silverstein	1981	Midwest	Workers	Death certificate
Death certificate				
Harrington	1978	Georgia	Death certificate	Death certificate
Gottlieb	1979	Louisiana	Death certificate	Death certificate
Gottlieb	1980	Louisiana	Death certificate	Death certificate
Tumor registry				
Rom	1982	Texas	Tumor registry	Tumor registry
Combination				
Wegman	1978	Massachusetts	Tumor registry Interviews	Tumor registry Interviews
Hinds	1981	Hawaii	Tumor registry Hospital	Population Interviews
Hinds	1982	Hawaii	Tumor registry Tuberculosis registry	Population Interviews
In-person interview				
Blot	1978	Georgia	Hospital Death certificate	Hospital Death certificate
Mettlin	1979	New York	Hospital	Hospital
Blot	1980	Virginia	Death certificate	Death certificate
Blot	1982	Florida	Hospital Death certificate	Hospital Death certificate
Vena	1982	New York	Hospital	Hospital
Rothschild	1982	Louisiana	Death certificate	Death certificate
Blot	1983	Pennsylvania	Death certificate	Death certificate
Correa	a,b	Louisiana	Hospital	Hospital
Buffler	a,c	Texas	Hospital, registry	Population
Altman	a	New Jersey	Hospital, registry	Population

[a]work in progress
[b]see Chapter 6
[c]see Chapter 7

Table 2. Questions included in recent interview studies

First author	Year published	State	Smoking	Occupation	Residence	Medical	Alcohol	Diet	Spouse's exposures
Blot	1978	GA	X	X	X	X			
Mettlin	1979	NY	X					X	
Blot	1980	VA	X	X	X	X			X
Blot	1982	FL	X	X	X	X			
Vena	1982	NY	X	X	X				
Rothschild	1982	LA	X	X	X				
Blot	1983	PA	X	X	X	X		X	
Correa	a,b	LA	X	X	X	X	X	X	X
Buffler	a,c	TX	X	X	X	X	X	X	X
Altman	a	NJ	X	X	X	X	X	X	X

[a]work in progress
[b]see Chapter 6
[c]see Chapter 7

A comparison of results for these studies does show certain consistencies, despite the variation of study design and information sources. Table 3 summarizes the industries reportedly linked to an elevated lung cancer risk by the general studies, either death certificate or interview studies. The results of studies conducted in a particular industry or plant (7, 8) are too specific for this kind of comparison. Relative risks for the shipbuilding industry were elevated in all four coastal areas studied (10, 12, 14, 15), although the excess risk in Virginia was limited to those men employed prior to 1950 (14). The fishing, construction, and wood or forestry industries had high estimated risks in several of these studies; the preliminary analysis of the Louisiana data supports these findings (see Chapter 6). The correlation seen between county lung cancer mortality rates and the paper industry has not been confirmed by these studies; this may be because of the close proximity of the lumber/sawmill industry to the paper plants, rather than a factor directly related to paper manufacturing. Equivocal results have been seen for employment in the petrochemical industry, which was also shown to be correlated with high mortality rates; nonsignificant risks of approximately 1.4 were seen in several areas, including coastal Texas. Other industries reported to be associated with high lung cancer risk are the sugarcane farming (17) and steel manufacturing (18) industries. Except for asbestos, the agents that may be responsible for these increases have not been isolated. It is important to note that some of these analyses have not controlled for smoking and so may not be comparable to the others.

Table 3. Industries with >25% excess lung cancer risk reported by recent case-control studies

Industry	Study	Odds ratio[a]	Controlled for smoking?
Shipbuilding	LA, 1979	2.0	
	GA, 1978	1.6	Yes
	VA, 1980	1.7 (prior to 1950)	Yes
	LA, 1982	1.5 NS	
	FL, 1982	1.4 NS	Yes
Construction	GA, 1978	2.0	
	LA, 1979	1.3 NS	
	FL, 1982	1.4	Yes
	PA, 1983	1.4 NS	
Fishing	LA, 1979	1.8	
	FL, 1982	3.2	
Wood/paper	GA, 1978	1.3 NS (coastal = 3.3.)	
	FL, 1982	1.7 (lumber/wood)	Yes
		2.3 (forestry)	
Chemical	GA, 1978	1.5 NS (includes painters)	
	LA, 1979	1.4 NS (age < 63)	
	PA, 1983	1.4 NS	
Petroleum	LA, 1979	1.3 NS (refining)	
		1.6 (crude, age > 62)	
Metal manufacturing	LA, 1979	1.3 NS	
	PA, 1983	1.8 (steel)	Yes
		1.6 (zinc)	Yes
Sugarcane farming	LA, 1982	2.4	Yes

[a]NS denotes not significantly different from 1.0, $\alpha = 0.05$.

Examination of nearness of residences to manufacturing plants has so far proved unproductive (Table 4); the positive association with residence near an oil refinery in Louisiana (10) was not significant and was based on the address given on the death certificate, possibly irrelevant to actual lifetime exposure. The positive association reported for a general measure of air pollution (16) was seen only among persons who had lived in the areas with heavy pollution for over 50 years. No elevation in risk was seen for residents near a nonferrous smelter in El Paso, Texas (20). Several methodologic problems have hampered the analysis of residential exposures to date: (1) uncertainty as to the latent period for lung cancer development (eg, which of the residences over a lifetime should be examined for nearness to a potential carcinogen source?); (2) variation in measurement techniques for potential pollutants; (3) inability to adequately model weather effects on the dispersion of these pollutants; and (4) a lag in the development of suitable statistical tests for comparing residential exposures of lung cancer cases and controls. Until at least some of these problems are resolved, evaluation of residential factors and lung cancer will lag behind other investigations.

Other factors have been examined as potential risk factors for lung cancer. As shown in Table 5, ethnic factors (10, 22), prior medical conditions (23), and nutritional deficiencies (13) have been suggested as causing an increased risk. Reports have been published from studies outside the United States on the relationship between "passive" smoking (24, 25), or exposure to someone else's smoke, and subsequent lung cancer; a review of worldwide literature is beyond the scope of this chapter, but this hypothesis is provocative and certainly will be tested during the ongoing analysis of the Texas, New Jersey, and Louisiana data.

Table 4. Reported associations of lung cancer risk and residential exposures

First author	Year published	State	Association[a]	Industry
Gottlieb	1979	LA	+ (NS)	Oil refineries
Rom	1982	TX	0	Nonferrous smelter
Vena	1982	NY	+ (>50 years)	General air pollution (Total suspended particulates)

[a]NS = not significant, + denotes a positive association, 0 denotes no association.

Table 5. Other results from recent case-control studies

First author	Year published	State	Association[a]	Exposure
Mettlin	1979	NY	–	Vitamin A intake
Gottlieb	1979	LA	+	Probable Acadian ancestry
Hinds	1981	HA	–	Ethnic group and smoking differences among women
Hinds	1972	HA	+	Prior tuberculosis infection in nonsmoking women

[a] + denotes positive association, – denotes negative association.

It should be evident at this point that as information has accumulated concerning the causes of lung cancer, studies have been refined to test more specific hypotheses. Information concerning specific exposures is easier to obtain for some factors than others; for example, whether a person ever smoked cigarettes usually can be ascertained by asking a spouse or relative, but the lifetime pattern of quitting and restarting, the number of cigarettes smoked per day, and type of cigarette smoked, all information required to estimate a lifetime dose of cigarettes, is much more difficult to obtain (26). Some information, such as exposure to a specific chemical, cannot be obtained at all because no long-term exposure records are kept at each workplace and the worker is often unaware of specific exposures. To illustrate the difficulties facing the epidemiologist in designing and analyzing such complex studies, preliminary data are presented from an ongoing study of Cajun lifestyle and lung cancer in southern Louisiana.

Louisiana Lung Cancer Study—Methods

Correa has described this study briefly in Chapter 6. Cases of lung cancer occurring from 1979 to 1981 among residents of 26 southern Louisiana parishes (Figure 6) were identified primarily from pathology records, supplemented by hospital records and death certificates; controls were selected from hospital records, matched on age (within 5 years), sex, race, parish of residence, and hospital if possible. All major hospitals were included in the study except in the New Orleans Tri-Parish area, where large hospitals were included so that approximately half of the incident cases were ascertained. Correa's study also includes interviews from several northern parishes, but only the data collected under contract with our branch at the National Cancer Institute (NCI) are presented here. A total of 1253 cases and 1274 controls were interviewed successfully, usually while still in the hospital; for the 19% of subjects who had died or were too disabled to respond, the spouse or next of kin was interviewed. Four interviews were dropped from this analysis because of poor quality data.

Results

Because the earlier Louisiana death certificate study (10) had found an increased risk of lung cancer among persons thought to be Cajuns, our questionnaire included an extensive series of questions about the subject's ancestry. Our first problem in trying to confirm the earlier finding was defining a Cajun. "Cajun" is thought to be a corruption of the term "Acadian," the settlers who migrated to southern Louisiana from Nova Scotia in the late 1700s (27). "Cajun" today is thought to refer more to a lifestyle than to a specific genetic trait, because of the length of time since the immigration of relatively few Acadians and the adoption of the Cajun lifestyle by other residents of the area. Three relevant questions were asked about Cajun ancestry: (1) Do you consider yourself a Cajun? (2) Was French

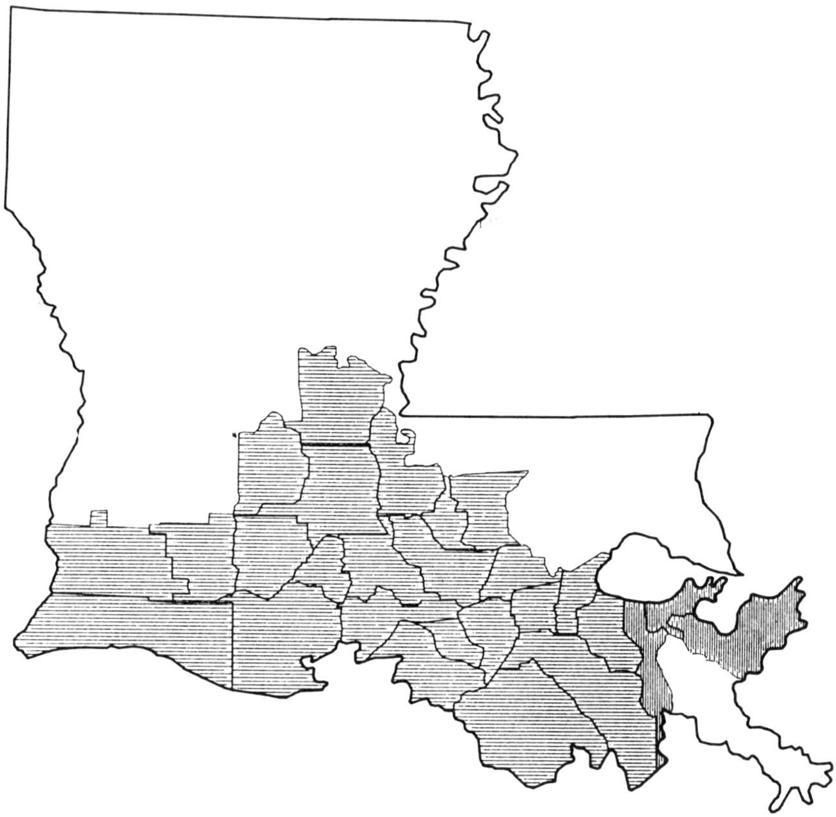

Figure 6. Louisiana lung cancer study area. Vertical hatching, Tri-Parish area; horizontal hatching, other parishes included.

spoken in your home when you were a child? and (3) Are you a descendant of the original Acadian settlers?

Table 6 shows the results of these questions by sex and race. Over 50% of the white respondents considered themselves Cajuns, and over half had spoken French in their homes; on the other hand, only 15% claimed Acadian ancestry, but over half could not answer this question. Fewer blacks answered affirmatively; in fact, one respondent stated that he could not be Cajun because he was black. Because of this possible bias in interpretation and response, and the small number of blacks who considered themselves Cajun, results from only the white subjects are presented here.

By combining answers to the three questions, we can form a gradient of probability of being a Cajun. As shown in Table 7, calculating crude odds ratios (ORs) for each of these Cajun categories versus the definite non-Cajun group (ie, those who answered negatively to all three questions) shows an elevation of lung cancer risk for the two most probable white male Cajun groups (OR = 1.2 and 1.4, respectively). For convenience, we will refer to these as Cajuns and Acadians,

Table 6. Proportion responding "yes" to LSU ethnic group questions, by sex and race

	White males (N = 1307) %	White females (N = 425) %	Black males (N = 620) %	Black females (N = 149) %
1. Do you consider yourself a Cajun?	56	51	19	18
2. Was French spoken in your home when you were a child?	51	50	36	40
3. Were any of your relatives among the original Acadian settlers?	16	14	5	10

respectively. Combining these two most likely Cajun groups, because of the number of missing answers to the Acadian question, yields an odds ratio of 1.25 [95% confidence interval (CI) of 0.99–1.57] for white males. We examined differences in certain exposures to try to explain this apparent risk. Our first thought was that this must result from differences in smoking patterns, but Table 8 shows only minimal differences in the percentage of smokers, mean amount, and number of years smoked for the two Cajun groups compared to the non-Cajuns. However, members of both Cajun groups were more likely to have rolled their own cigarettes and used brands of tobacco different from those used by the non-Cajuns.

Other a priori risk factors to be examined were employment in the shipbuilding or petrochemical industries. Table 9 shows the proportions ever employed in selected industries by Cajun class; fewer Cajuns than others had ever worked in the petrochemical industry and only a slightly higher percentage worked in the shipbuilding industry. Many more Cajuns worked in the fishing industry, which had an elevated odds ratio from the earlier death certificate study, and in agriculture, both sugarcane farming and other types.

Finally, because our overall analysis of the Louisiana data found a significant 30% reduction in risk for lung cancer among frequent consumers of fruits and vegetables (28), we compared the reported frequency of consumption of certain food items for Cajuns versus the non-Cajun group. Results are shown in Table 10. The Cajun/Acadian group reported significantly more servings of seafood, hot spices, organ meats, beans, and rice; the larger Cajun group reported more

Table 7. Odds ratios (OR) by degree of Cajun background

				White males		White females	
Cajun	French	Acadian		N	OR	N	OR
–	–	–	(Referent)	552	1.0	190	1.0
–	+	–		46	0.9	24	1.2
+	–	–		96	0.8	25	1.2
+	+	–		531	1.2	168	0.9
+	+	+		94	1.4	22	1.0

Table 8. Smoking patterns among Cajun groups, white males

	Cajun, French, Acadian	Cajun, French, not Acadian	Not Cajun
Ever smoked cigarettes (%)	85	81	83
Ever smoked nonfilter cigarettes (%)	82	72[a]	80
Ever smoked filter cigarettes (%)	60	53	55
Ever rolled own cigarettes (%)	63[a]	63[a]	45
Ever smoked home grown tobacco (%)	6	2	4
For smokers only:			
Mean No cigarettes/day			
Nonfilter	30	31	29
Filter	29	34	33
No years smoked			
Nonfilter	19	18	19
Filter	14	14	15

[a]Significantly different from non-Cajuns, $\alpha = .05$.

Table 9. Percentage employed in selected industries by Cajun group, white males

Industry	Cajun, French, Acadian	Cajun, French, not Acadian	Not Cajun
Shipbuilding	10	9	8
Chemical manufacturing	9	7[a]	16
Petroleum manufacturing	6[a]	6[a]	13
Fishing	8[a]	5[a]	2
Agriculture			
Sugarcane	4[a]	5[a]	0.5
Other	31[a]	38[a]	17

[a]Significantly different from non-Cajuns, $\alpha = .05$.

poultry, organ meat, beans, and rice consumption, and fewer servings of pork, fruits, and vegetables.

In an attempt to explain the elevated odds ratio seen for the two white male Cajun groups, we controlled for fruit and vegetable intake, as well as any cigarette smoking, beer consumption, and employment in the agriculture, sugarcane, or fishing industries. The crude estimated risk of 1.42 for the Cajun/Acadian group was reduced only to 1.30 (95% CI = 0.80 – 2.12); the combined odds ratio of 1.25 was nearly unchanged (OR = 1.23, 95% CI = 0.95 – 1.58). However, the addition of variables to the model indicating the consumption of hand-rolled cigarettes and the number of packages of tobacco used per week reduced these risk estimates to 1.16 and 1.12, respectively. Therefore, although there are measurably and significantly different patterns of occupation and diet for Cajuns, controlling for these exposures did not reduce the estimated lung cancer risk as much as controlling for smoking hand-rolled cigarettes. The risk associated with ever smoking

Table 10. Significant[a] differences in mean frequency of consumption by Cajun group vs. non-Cajuns—white males

Food Item	Cajun, French, Acadian	Cajun, French, not Acadian
Beef		
Poultry		+
Pork		−
Seafood	+	
Organ meat	+	+
Fruits		−
Vegetables		−
Beans	+	+
Hot spices	+	

[a] $\alpha = .05$ t test after normalizing square root transformation; + denotes greater frequency of consumption, − denotes lower frequency of consumption, compared to non-Cajuns.

hand-rolled cigarettes in the overall study group is 11.7, compared to 8.7 for persons who only smoked commercial cigarettes (both compared to never smokers). We plan further analyses to examine the effects of varying tar content of commercial cigarettes and of the brands of tobacco used for hand-rolled cigarettes. These preliminary analyses suggest that differences in type of tobacco used, rather than amount smoked, is responsible for the elevated risk seen among white male Cajuns.

Summary

In summary, etiologic studies of lung cancer have progressed from studies of usual occupation and smoking habits to studies of many complex, possibly interrelated factors. Questionnaires now elicit information about occupational and residential histories, specific chemical exposures, and lifetime usage of tobacco, alcohol, and food items, as well as family histories of other cancers and of chronic lung disease in an attempt to assess susceptibility. Cigarette smoking is by far the major risk factor for lung cancer, but risks may vary with the type of cigarette smoked. Recent studies have suggested smaller elevations for employment in several industries and a possible protective effect of vegetable intake. However, interactions that may exist among these factors have not been assessed adequately by studies to date. As the hypotheses have been refined, study design and consequently questionnaire design have become so complex that we may have reached the limit of the ability of respondents to provide useful information; the scope of studies has broadened recently to include even information on the occupation and smoking patterns of the spouse and close relatives of the patient—the patients themselves have a difficult time with these questions, but with a disease as rapidly fatal as lung cancer, this information is even more difficult to obtain from next of kin respondents (26). Epidemiologists planning future case–control studies of lung cancer should address this issue of availability and accuracy of information before undertaking their studies and should consider utilizing information from medical records, industrial hygienists, and laboratory tests, where possible, to supplement their questionnaire data.

Acknowledgments

The authors thank Neil Howard, Merry Rabb, Linda Smith, and Paul Gentile of ORI, Inc, for computer support, and James B. Pearson Jr, for editorial and technical assistance.

References

1. Young JL Jr, Percy CL, Asire AJ, eds. Surveillance, Epidemiology, and End Results: incidence and mortality data, 1973-77 NCI Monogr 51. Bethesda, MD: National Cancer Institute 1981.
2. Horm JW, Asire, AJ. Changes in lung cancer incidence and mortality rates among Americans: 1968-1978. JNCI 1982;69:833-837.
3. Mason TJ, McKay FW, Hoover R, Blot WJ, and Fraumeni JF Jr. Atlas of cancer mortality for U.S. counties: 1950-1969. U.S. Department of Health, Education and Welfare Publ (NIH) 75-780. Washington, DC: U.S. Government Printing Office, 1975.
4. Mason TJ, McKay FW, Hoover R, Blot WJ, and Fraumeni JF Jr. Atlas of cancer mortality among US nonwhites: 1950-1969. U.S. Department of Health, Education and Welfare Publ (NIH) 76-1204. Washington, DC: U.S. Government Printing Office, 1976.
5. Blot WJ, Fraumeni JF Jr. Geographic patterns of lung cancer: industrial correlations. Am J Epidemiol 1976;103:539-50.
6. Fraumeni JF Jr, Blot WJ. Lung and pleura. In: Schottenfeld D, Fraumeni JF Jr, eds, Cancer epidemiology and prevention. Philadelphia: WB Saunders, 1982, 564-82.
7. Egan-Baum E, Miller BA, Waxweiler RJ. Lung cancer and other mortality patterns among foundrymen. Scand J Work Environ Health 1981;7(suppl 4):147-55.
8. Silverstein M, Mirer F, Kotelchuck D, Silverstein B, Bennett M. Mortality among workers in a die-casting and electroplating plant. Scand J Work Environ Health 1981;7(Suppl 4):156-65.
9. Harrington JM, Blot WJ, Hoover RN, Housworth WJ, Heath CW, Fraumeni JF Jr. Lung cancer in coastal Georgia: a death certificate analysis of occupation. JNCI 1978;60:295-8.
10. Gottlieb MS, Pickle LW, Blot WJ, Fraumeni JF Jr. Lung cancer in Louisiana: death certificate analysis. JNCI 1979;63:1131-7.
11. Gottlieb MS. Lung cancer and the petroleum industry in Louisiana. JOM 1980;22:384-8.
12. Blot WJ, Harrington JM, Toledo A, Hoover R, Heath CW, Fraumeni JF Jr. Lung cancer after employment in shipyards during World War II. N Engl J Med 1978;299:620-4.
13. Mettlin C, Graham S, Swanson M. Vitamin A and lung cancer. JNCI 1979;62:1435-8.
14. Blot WJ, Morris LE, Stroube R, Tagnon I, Fraumeni JF Jr. Lung and laryngeal cancers in relation to shipyard employment in coastal Virginia. JNCI 1980;65:571-5.
15. Blot WJ, Davies JE, Brown LM, et al. Occupation and the high risk of lung cancer in northeast Florida. Cancer 1982;50:364-71.
16. Vena JE. Air pollution as a risk factor in lung cancer. Am J Epidemiol 1982;116:42-56.
17. Rothschild H, Mulvey JJ. An increased risk for lung cancer mortality associated with sugarcane farming. JNCI 1982;68:755-60.
18. Blot WJ, Brown LM, Pottern LM, Stone BJ, Fraumeni JF Jr. Lung cancer among long-term steel workers. Am J Epidemiol 1983;117:706-16.
19. Altman R, Mason TJ, Stemhagen A. Lung cancer in New Jersey. Personal communication 1983.
20. Rom WN, Varley G, Lyon JL, Shopkow S. Lung cancer mortality among residents living near the El Paso smelter. Br J Ind Med 1982;39:269-72.
21. Wegman DH, Peters JM. Oat cell lung cancer in selected occupations. JOM 1978;20:793-6.

22. Hinds MW, Stemmermann GN, Yang HY, Kolonel LN, Lee J, Wegner E. Differences in lung cancer risk from smoking among Japanese, Chinese, and Hawaiian women in Hawaii. Int J Cancer 1981;27:297-302.
23. Hinds MW, Cohen HI, Kolonel LN. Tuberculosis and lung cancer risk in nonsmoking women. Am Rev Respir Dis 1982;125:776-8.
24. Hirayama T. Non-smoking wives of heavy smokers have a higher risk of lung cancer: a study from Japan. Br Med J 1981;282:183-5.
25. Trichopoulos D, Kalandidi A, Sparros L, MacMahon B. Lung cancer and passive smoking. Int J Cancer 1981;27:1-4.
26. Pickle LW, Brown LM, Blot WJ. Information available from surrogate respondents in interview studies. Am J Epidemiol 1983;118:99-108.
27. Bertrand A. Louisiana and its Cajuns. Unpublished manuscript.
28. Falk R. Investigation of vitamin A and diet as etiologic factors in the development of lung cancer. Unpublished Masters thesis, Georgetown University, Washington, DC, 1982.

CHAPTER 9

The Epidemiologic Meaning of Histology in Lung Cancer

JOHN W. BERG

Department of Pathology, University of Colorado School of Medicine, 4200 East Ninth Avenue, Denver, Colorado 80262

ABSTRACT

Much has changed since Kreyberg described a simple relationship between cigarettes and lung cancer histology. First, histologic nomenclature has become more elaborate. Currently diagnoses for primary lung cancer fall into about 75 categories in the International Classification of Diseases for Oncology (ICD-O). Most of these diagnoses have not been evaluated epidemiologically. Second, not only do different causes produce different histologic, grade, and site distributions of lung cancer types, but also cigarettes apparently produce different histologic, grade, and site distributions in men and women and in blacks and whites. Therefore, the male–female ratio no longer serves as a simple indicator of whether a cancer type is linked to cigarettes or not. Third, indications for biopsy and incentives for classifications have changed, altering the composition of the large pool of unproved or unclassified cases. A broad concept of "demographic distances," derived from separating age, sex, race, and time influences on histology, appears to help organize and simplify classification.
Key Words: **Lung cancer, histologic classification, epidemiologic pathology**

As far as I am aware, epidemiologists rarely do case–control lung cancer studies anymore. Furthermore, whereas lung cancer is an almost unavoidable part of any cohort study of mortality, histologic types usually are not investigated separately. Descriptive epidemiology, of course, has been considered unworthy of grant support for quite a few years now. Despite these current fashions, I believe in the continued value of descriptive epidemiology as it applies to what pathologists consider different types of cancer. Such descriptions can help pathologists evaluate schemes of histologic classification by indicating whether two patterns have the same or different demographic distributions and so whether they are more or less likely to be mere facets of the same disease. Also, cancers with different causes can arise in the

Lung Cancer: Causes and Prevention.

same organ and the proper grouping by histologies can add a great deal of power to epidemiologic studies.

The classic example of epidemiologic help from histologic typing of cancers, of course, was Kreyberg's sharpening of the cigarette–lung cancer association by dividing lung cancer into two groups, one of which, containing squamous cell and oat cell types, was much more completely limited to smokers than were cancers in the other group, which contained adenocarcinomas, bronchial carcinoids, sarcomas, etc (1). It was not even necessary to do epidemiologic studies on less common types to see to which group they belonged; the sex ratio was about 10:1 in group 1 and much closer to unity in group 2 (see Table 1). The data from that time also suggested that the cancers of group 2 actually differed somewhat in their relation to smoking. Specifically, the male–female ratio for adenocarcinomas was high enough to suggest (correctly) that some, although not all, adenocarcinomas were caused by cigarettes.

Now, almost 30 years later, the situation has become more complex in several ways. First of all, the nomenclature for lung cancer has expanded greatly. In 1977, just after the general adoption of the enlarged histologic code of the International Classification of Diseases for Oncology (ICD-O),(2) Surveillance, Epidemiology, End Results (SEER) abstractors found diagnoses of primary lung cancer falling into 70 different rubrics, not including grade differences. Considering the 1977 diagnoses as a 10% sample of the total United States cases and projecting the SEER distribution of cases to the whole country, there were 22 diagnoses that were estimated to have been used more than 100 times that year (Table 2). The other 48 diagnoses were not negligible, however, in the sense that they could be grouped into another six categories, such as sarcomas or lymphomas, each of which also should contain more than 100 cases in a year's collection. We must expect the use of many of the new terms to increase so that the list of the commonly used terms in Table 2 will broaden.

On looking over the entire list of diagnoses it seems likely that many are synonyms. If all similar terms are grouped, however, we are defeating the purpose of ICD-O expansion, which was developed in the belief that these distinctions often would prove important. I shall return to this problem below. A second problem is that it is not clear which of the multitude of diagnoses are strongly associated with cigarette smoking. As I said, case–control studies on specific histologic types seem

Table 1. Relative frequencies and male/female ratios for several types of lung cancer from Connecticut for two time periods[a]

	Percentage of all lung cancers		M/F ratio	
	1950–1964	1973–1977	1950–1964	1973–1977
Squamous cell carcinoma	31.6	24.9	10.9/1	5.8/1
Oat cell carcinoma	4.5	11.9	8.4/1	2.3/1
Bronchiolar carcinomas	2.2	3.0	1.4/1	1.0/1
Other adenocarcinomas	10.8	21.3	2.5/1	1.8/1

[a]1950–1964: 7294 reviewed cases; 1973–1977: 7008 cases.

Table 2. Lung cancer diagnoses expected 100 times or more a year in the United States

ICD-O number	Diagnosis[a,b]
8000/3	Malignant neoplasm, NOS
8001/3	Malignant tumor cells
8010/3	Carcinoma, NOS
8012/3	Large-cell carcinoma
8020/3	Undifferentiated carcinoma
8021/3	Anaplastic carcinoma
8031/3	Giant-cell carcinoma
8041/3	Small-cell carcinoma
8042/3	Oat cell carcinoma
8070/3	Squamous cell carcinoma, NOS
8071/3	Keratinizing squamous-cell carcinoma
8072/3	Large-cell, nonkeratinizing squamous-cell carcinoma
8140/3	Adenocarcinoma, NOS
8200/3	Cylindroid adenocarcinoma
8240/3	Malignant carcinoid
8250/5	Bronchioloalveolar adenocarcinoma
8251/3	Alveolar adenocarcinoma
8260/3	Papillary adenocarcinoma
8310/3	Clear cell carcinoma
8480/3	Mucus adenocarcinoma
8481/3	Mucin-producing carcinoma
8560/3	Adenosquamous carcinoma
	Plus collective groups:
	Other squamous cell carcinoma variants (8)
	Other adenocarcinomas (12)
	Other carcinomas not in previous groups (9)
	Sarcomas (5)
	Lymphomas (7)
	Mixed and miscellaneous (7)

[a]NOS not otherwise specified.
[b]Numbers in parentheses are numbers of separate types in the "10%" sample. More types would be expected in a full series.

no longer to be done and, as Table 1 illustrates, the sex ratio no longer is as clear an indicator of cigarette association as it once was. Partly, of course, this is because more and more women smokers are reaching the cancer age. Beyond this, however, is another completely unanticipated finding. Cigarettes do not seem to be producing the same histologic distribution of cancers in women smokers as they produced in men. As can be deduced from Table 1, there has been a much greater increase in oat cell carcinomas in women than would have been predicted from the increase in squamous cell cancers, the archetype cigarette cancer in white males. We have estimated that more than a quarter of cigarette cancers in women are of the oat cell type (3). Perhaps a restudy of the pathogenesis of cigarette cancers in men and women would suggest reasons for the differences. The main reason for emphasizing the situation here is that this is just more evidence, on top of the well-known relationships of occupational causes to different types of lung cancer (4), that the different histologic types have different epidemiologies even within Kreyberg's two groups.

Still other evidence on the same point comes from looking at the histologic distributions in United States males from different ethnic and racial groups. In a report on differing relative frequencies of histologic types for each cancer site in blacks and whites, one of the more important differences is in types of lung cancer (Table 3). On average, registry-specific SEER data showed lung cancer to be 19% higher in black men than in white men (age-adjusted rates). One way of looking at this excess is to say that it is made up entirely of squamous cell cancers. The other cancer types actually had somewhat lower frequencies relative to all reported cancers as well as lower frequencies relative to typed lung cancers. Presumably the high rates in black men resulted principally from their smoking habits but why was only one cell type selectively increased?

In describing the above differences in histology that emerged in the 1970s, it would have been much easier and more straightforward to have been able to have presented findings in terms of incidence rates of cumulative probabilities of developing a specific type of lung cancer. This, however, would have been substantially misleading. The difficulty lies in the greater number of lung cancers that were not given a specific diagnosis but were called merely "cancer" or "carcinoma" if they were confirmed microscopically at all. Besides being frequent, the nonspecific diagnoses are not distributed evenly among all ages nor has their contribution to the total cancer rate stayed the same over time. Figures 1 and 2 illustrate these facts for unconfirmed and confirmed nonspecific diagnoses of lung cancer in white men. It is obvious that the calculation of age-adjusted rates would be distorted badly by the fact that less than half the men in the oldest age group had received specific diagnoses. (This is not the time to raise the question of what so many completely unconfirmed cases do to the total lung cancer rates.) The changes in proportion of confirmed cases and specific diagnoses with time also make comparisons over time misleading. Finally, in addition to the age and time differences shown in the figures, we found race and sex differences that would confuse the picture further, even when one specific age group was being examined. I am sure that better ways will be found to describe sex, race, and time differences than I have used. My intent here is only to indicate why care must be taken in any attempt to describe histologic differences or trends.

My own recent work has been on different, although related, problems. One goal has been to encourage more use of histologic information by cancer registries. To this end, I have developed an automated monitoring system designed to

Table 3. Type distribution of 2928 histologically proved and classified lung cancers in blacks compared with the distribution in whites from the same registries[a]

Type	Percentage of total	
	Black	White
Squamous cell	54	42
Oat cell	16	20
Bronchiolar	4	6
Other adenocarcinomas	23	29
Other and mixed types	3	3

[a]After age and sex adjustment to the population of black lung cancer patients. Data from Ref 5.

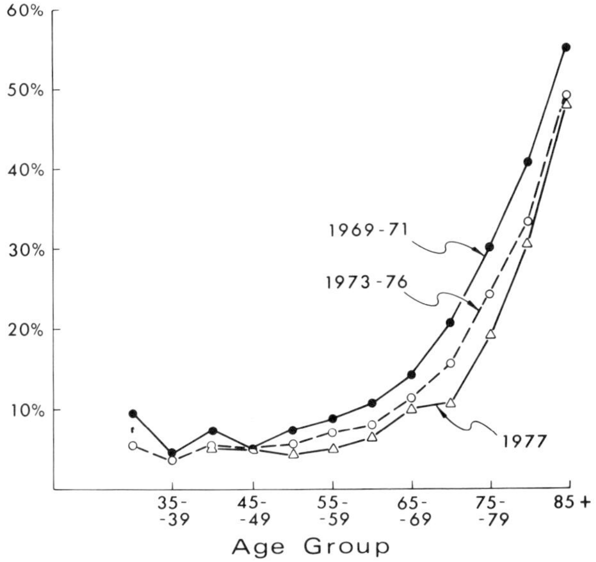

Figure 1. Percentage of all lung cancers in white males diagnosed as "cancer" or "carcinoma" without microscopic confirmation: 1969–1971 data from TNCS (Third National Cancer Survey); other data from SEER.

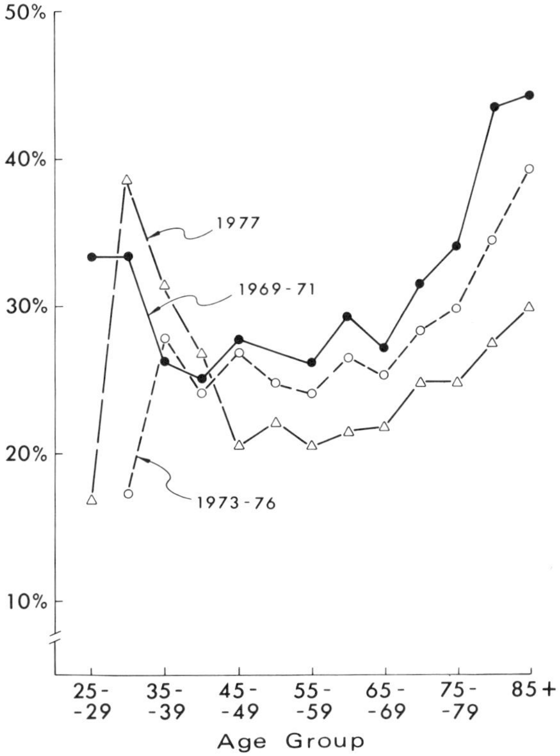

Figure 2. Percentage of microscopically confirmed lung cancer cases in white males diagnosed simply as "cancer" or "carcinoma" without further typing. Data sources as in Figure 1.

recognize and signal any sudden increases in special tumor types, such as the increase of mesotheliomas because of asbestos, hepatic angiosarcomas because of vinyl chloride, etc. The concept seemed a simple one, namely that in such instances relative frequency increases would be large and so true incidence rates, which take a long time to generate, would not be needed. Up to a point, system design was simple also. The difficulties emerged when I began to realize how many alternatives existed just for the coding of site and type. Lung cancers generate site problems only in one small but important area: should mesotheliomas arising from visceral pleura and growing into the lung be assigned to the lung rather than to the pleura? There were enough tumors so coded that it seemed best to leave them be and solve the problem of determining total mesothelioma frequency another way, namely by listing it as one of the histologies in which relative frequency was calculated for all sites of the body taken together as well as for each particular site.

As indicated earlier the real problem for handling lung data was the large number of possible histologic diagnoses. If what really was a single kind of lung cancer had the cases divided among several categories, a true increase might not result in a statistically significant rise in any one of the component groups. On the other hand, a difference in preference for particular diagnoses between the study and standard populations easily could give rise to false-positive results. If the other mistake was made and there was too much grouping, important changes easily could be missed, just as the sex and racial differences I have described for lung cancer would not be as apparent if one restricted one's attention to Kreyberg's groups I and II. I do not pretend to have built the final answers into the monitoring program but the substantial recoding of the data employed there to bring like things all together and keep unlike things apart has been based in large part upon a systematic examination of relationships between diagnoses. These relationships for lung cancers are the subject of the last part of this paper.

Originally, it appeared that the organization of histologic data would have to be based only on "common sense" and other unquantified judgments. However, the opportunity to work with National Cancer Institutes (NCI) staff on the SEER monograph (5) brought access to data on more than 325,000 cancers. Coupling this with 180,000 Third National Cancer Survey (TNCS) cases (Ref 6 and the public use tape) constituted a data set of over half a million cases, roughly representing the equivalent of 80% coverage of the entire United States for a year. Initially, only 58 histologies were studied because in all years except 1977 histologies had been coded by the simpler Manual of Tumor Nomenclature and Coding (MOTNAC) (7) code, not ICD-O.

The organization of these diagnoses was approached in stepwise fashion. If the data set contained less than 15 examples of a diagnosis there were considered to be too few cases for statistical analysis. Then cases usually were added to an appropriate, more general group. For example, the few patients with liposarcomas of the lung were grouped with the larger set diagnosed simply as "sarcoma." The few diagnoses, such as "melanoma of the lung", that did not easily fit into a broader grouping simply were not considered further in the analyses. In the second step, logically possible groupings of case sets with 15 or more patients in each were compared statistically by procedures described in Appendix A. For example, among the sarcomas only leiomyosarcomas were frequent enough to test separately. Comparing them with the remaining sarcomas as to age distribution, sex ratio, and black–white ratio yielded a combined probability of 0.40 that the two patient sets had been drawn from the same population. Hence, I added to the monitoring system a summary category of "all soft tissue sarcomas of the lung." By contrast, when pulmonary lymphomas were compared, although the non-Hodgkin lymphomas looked demographically homogeneous, the comparison of these with pulmonary Hodgkin disease patients yielded a P value of 0.0008 so a summary category for all lymphomas was not felt to be appropriate.

After the logical, commonsense relationships had been tested and "permissible" groupings accomplished, all possible comparisons of the resultant groups were done in the same way. Occasionally, it was possible to make additional groupings because a smaller group was found to fit with one possible parent group but not with any other. For lung cancers the most important finding was that patients with some kind of adenosquamous cancers (MOTNAC groups 8433, 8563, and 8573 seemed to be alike) were significantly different from patients with squamous cell carcinoma ($P \ll 0.001$) but not from patients with adenocarcinomas ($P = 0.17$). Hence the system, although also reporting each of the above mentioned MOTNAC groups separately, also included them in a summary category of "all adenocarcinomas" but did not use a summary category for "all adenosquamous carcinomas." (Bronchiolar carcinomas were significantly unlike other adenocarcinomas so they were not included in that summary tabulation.)

Table 4 represents the groupings as they looked at the end of this stage of data condensation. (It differs from Table 2 in that the simpler MOTNAC classification was used; data on the new separations of ICD-O only became available later and

Table 4. Classification of lung cancers after logical groupings that were not forbidden by probability tests[a]

I. Carcinomas
- A. Squamous cell carcinomas 807, 805, 812, (808)[b]
- B. Small-cell carcinomas 804
- C. Mucus-secreting carcinoma 848
- D. Bronchiolar alveolar carcinomas 825, 826
- E. Other adenocarcinomas 814, 820, (829), 843, 849, 855, 856, 857, (894)
- F. Giant and spindle cell carcinomas 803
- G. Malignant carcinoids 824
- H. Clear cell carcinomas 832, (832)
- I. Solid carcinomas (823), 851
- J. Carcinomas, unspecified 801

II. Other types
- A. Mixed carcinosarcomas (895), 898, (908)
- B. Mesotheliomas 905
- C. Soft-tissue sarcomas (869), 880, (881), (882), (833), (885), 889, (890), (891), (899), (912), (915), (954)
- D. Hodgkin disease 865
- E. Non-Hodgkin lymphomas 959, (960), (961), 962, (963), 964
- F. Other specific types (858), (872), (877), (896), (972) (not treated as a group)

III. Cancer, not further specified, 800, and cases without microscopic confirmation

[a]Titles and MOTNAC histology codes included.
[b]Numbers in parentheses are for less than 15 cases. Assigned arbitrarily.

are considered below.) One unexpected separation that was maintained was that "mucus-secreting" adenocarcinomas differed significantly from other adenocarcinomas because they occurred in younger patients. This separation is considered below. It may also surprise some that the patients with giant-spindle cell carcinomas were demographically different from adenocarcinoma patients, because the former tumor is considered a variant of the latter in many classifications. On the other hand, the small group of "solid" carcinomas was kept separate because it was not significantly different from any of the large categories and the statistical test therefore gave no suggestion for a grouping.

These results for lung cancer were fairly typical in that groups that were large tended to differ significantly from all other large groups and many of the small groups did not differ significantly from any of the larger groups unless the large group was very different indeed. An example of a very different group among lung cancers would be bronchial carcinoid patients. There were more women than men with this type of cancer and the average age was much lower than for any other group of patients. The main reason I emphasize these generalities is because statistical results depend on group sizes as well as on the magnitude of group differences. Hence they are not suitable for exhibiting degrees of resemblance of groups in any but a yes–no sense. They were used for my purposes in the monitoring program because I had nothing better and I thought some objective approach to grouping was preferable to a completely subjective scheme. To order histologic types into a truly objective classification and exhibit degrees of resemblance something more is needed.

The answer is simple when most of the differences among cancer types is expressed in terms of a single relationship, such as the sex ratio in the earlier data of Table 1. Ordering cancers by the sex ratio of the patient groups was essentially equivalent to ordering them by their degree of association with cigarettes. Today we have lost that simplicity and I suspect there is no indirect way to link lung cancer types with specific etiologies. Direct case–control or cohort studies will have to be done to answer basic questions.

Until these direct studies are available, is there a way of getting closer, at least to demographic resemblance, in case it has some relation to epidemiologic resemblance? There is a large literature on numerical taxonomy but it is not as immediately useful as may be first thought. It does address the problems of grouping and ordering biologic types on the basis of a set of characteristics; however, not only does there seem to be less than complete agreement as to how to go about the task, but the most successful methods rely on there being a great many characteristics measurable for each species or other group that is to be put in a hierarchy. For cancers we have few characteristics and it is not clear how to get optimal use of them. My probing in this area has been superficial, enough to convince me that it is a promising approach but not enough to be sure that I have a workable solution, much less an optimal one. The details of the methods used for the data presented here and associated technical problems are described in Appendix B. Here I outline the concept briefly and then show how it seems to put some of the newer nomenclatures in perspective and may offer more than the statistical tests.

Demographic distance as used here is a single number combining measures of the differences in mean age, the spread of ages around the means, the differences in sex ratios, and the differences in black-white ratios of the patient groups for the two cancers being compared. Each of the four differences is expressed on a scale that over the whole range of cancer comparisons gives it about equal weight with the others. Table 5 gives the distances between four major lung cancer types. To put the numbers on the table in perspective, values below 20 are quite close, values as high as 300 separate quite unlike groups, and scores between 20 and 50 suggest some but not great similarity. In the table the large distances between bronchial carcinoids and the other types reflect a large age difference as well as the fact that a majority of patients were women. Among the other types age differences are small so that differences in sex ratios dominate the picture with the excess of squamous cell cancers in black men also contributing to that cancer's distance from the others. The utility of the measure for me was not here where it tells what I already know, but in clarifying less clear situations. Table 6, for example, presents the relatively near neighbors for the histologic groupings of Table 4. The closest pair is mucus-secreting carcinoma and the major group of other adenocarcinomas. Hence, one would not be merging groups that really were unlike if the "statistically significant" age difference between the groups referred to above were ignored. The relative closeness of carcinosarcoma and giant-spindle cell carcinoma is interesting because some feel that the sarcomatous part of a carcinosarcoma usually is spindle-cell metaplasia of the carcinoma. On the other hand, carcinosarcomas also are close to other groups, suggesting a generally central location in the four-dimensional demographic space. Certainly, a similar central location makes sense for the group "carcinoma, NOS" (NOS = not otherwise specified) because it should be made up of a mixture of the specific types. "Cancer, NOS" stands off from the other groups because it, more than "carcinoma," was a diagnosis in older patients.

Table 7 uses demographic differences to help answer another question: is there any suggestion that the grade of a particular kind of lung cancer may have any epidemiologic relevance? There are 14 possible grade comparisons for the four cancer types with the largest number of cases (squamous cell and adenocarcinomas had enough cases in all four grade groups but oat cell cancers and "cancer, NOS" only had enough cases for grades 3 and 4). Seven, ie, half, of the comparisons indicated statistically significant demographic differences between patients with different grades of the same kind of cancers. The distances were not shown on the

Table 5. Demographic distances between principal types of lung cancer on an arbitrary scale

	Squamous cell	Oat cell	Adenocarcinoma	Bronchiolar carcinoma
Oat cell carcinoma	64	—	—	—
Adenocarcinoma	86	38	—	—
Bronchiolar carcinoma	110	55	36	—
Bronchial carcinoids	284	245	217	223

Table 6. Close demographic distances (less than 50 on an arbitrary scale) for the lung cancer groups of Table 4

I. Carcinomas
   A. Squamous cell carcinoma: carcinoma, NOS, 47
   B. Small-cell carcinoma: adenocarcinoma, 38; carcinoma, NOS, 33
   C. Mucus-secreting carcinoma: adenocarcinomas, 26; bronchiolar carcinoma, 38; clear cell carcinoma, 38; carcinosarcoma, 41
   D. Bronchiolar carcinoma: mucus-secreting carcinoma, adenocarcinomas, 36; solid carcinomas, 38
   E. Other adenocarcinomas small-cell carcinoma, 38; mucus-secreting carcinoma, 26; bronchiolar carcinoma, 36; carcinoma, NOS, 44; carcinosarcoma, 42
   F. Giant and spindle cell carcinoma: carcinosarcoma, 44
   G. Malignant carcinoids: none
   H. Clear cell carcinomas: mucus-secreting carcinoma, 38
   I. Solid carcinoma: bronchiolar carcinoma, 38
   J. Carcinomas, NOS: squamous cell carcinoma, 47; small-cell carcinoma, 33; adenocarcinoma, 44

II. Other types
   A. Carcinosarcomas: see C, E, F above. Also non-Hodgkin lymphomas, 44
   B. Mesotheliomas: none
   C. Soft-tissue sarcomas: none
   D. Hodgkin disease: none
   E. Non-Hodgkin lymphomas: carcinosarcomas, 44

III. Cancer, NOS: none

table because they were not statistically significant and usually were under 20 if there were adequate numbers of patients in both groups. What the table tells me is that because I feel the difference between bronchiolar carcinoma and other adenocarcinomas is important, I should feel the same way about some of the grade differences for squamous cell and adenocarcinomas and look for further differences in pathogenesis if not in etiology between the grade groups.

Finally, in Table 8 the distances and P values are given for the new distinctions ICD-O made within the simpler groups of MOTNAC, or at least for those distinctions with enough patients in each new group. The two separations that seem most

Table 7. Cancer grade and demographic distance[a]

1. Squamous cell carcinoma:
   Grades 1, 2, 3 compared with grade 4. Distances 36, 31, and 24.
   Grade 4 was relatively more common in women, less common in blacks.

2. Adenocarcinoma, NOS:
   Grade 2 compared with grades 3 and 4. Distances 36 and 41.
   Grade 2 was found more often in women.

3. Oat cell carcinoma:
   Grade 3 compared with grade 4. Distance 29.
   Grade 4 found more often in women.

4. Carcinoma, NOS:
   Grade 3 compared with grade 4. Distance 21.
   Grade 4 less often found in blacks.

[a]Patient groups with the same histologic type but different grades that were significantly different demographically.

Table 8. Significance tests and demographic distances of new separation of lung cancer introduced by ICD-O

	P	Distance
Squamous cell carcinoma		
8071 Keratinizing vs 8072 large cell, nonkeratinizing	<0.001	60
Oat cell carcinoma		
8041 Small cell vs 8042 oat cell	0.11	13
Bronchioloalveolar carcinoma		
8250 Bronchioloalveolar vs 8251 Alveolar	0.78	20
8480 Mucinous vs 8481 mucus-producing	0.11	40
8012 Large-cell carcinoma vs 8010 carcinoma, NOS	<0.05	44
8001 Malignant tumor cells vs 8000 cancer, NOS	<0.05	65
8021 Anaplastic cancer vs 8020 undifferentiated cancer	0.98	6
8021 Anaplastic cancer vs 8022 pleomorphic cancer	<0.05	84
8022 Pleomorphic cancer vs 8020 undifferentiated cancer	<0.05	81

important are the separation of pleomorphic carcinoma from undifferentiated and anaplastic carcinoma (actually all of these terms would have been coded to "carcinoma, NOS" in MOTNAC), and the separation of keratinizing and nonkeratinizing squamous cell carcinomas. The 8000/3–8001/3 difference presumably measures differences in cytology and biopsy use.

In conclusion, I believe that, although there is no substitute for direct epidemiologic evidence, demographic differences as measured by statistical tests and distances can be helpful in dealing with the plethora of apparently different cancer types of a given organ and possibly also in prioritizing distinctions that should be made between types in epidemiologic studies. I also believe that even for lung cancer there is important work to be done with regard to describing and understanding how different types of cancer are generated either because the causes are different or, as we seem to see now, because although the cause is the same, patients of different sexes and races respond differently.

Acknowledgments

This work was supported in part by grant CA-15823 from the National Institutes of Health and by a departmental gift from R.J. Reynolds Industries, Inc.

Appendix A. Testing the Statistical Significance of Demographic Differences Between Groups of Cancer Patients

Age, sex, and race were the variables examined. Fortuitously, most age distributions were nearly normal; at least, no transformation did anything but increase nonnormality. Mean ages thus were compared and as a weighted average of the differences of 12 possible subgroups: two sexes, two races (black and white) and three time periods (TNCS, 1969–1971; SEER originally with MOTNAC coding, 1973–1976; SEER with ICD-O coding, 1977). The individual differences were weighted by the inverse of their variances and a t test done on the weighted average distance to obtain the probability of the null hypothesis of no difference being true. Relatively frequently a problem arose because a very small group produced a comparison with such low variance that it completely dominated the weighted average. Hence, the computer program included a check to see whether either of the groups with the lowest variance for the difference had less than five patients; if so, that group was discarded and the weighted average recalculated. The variances of the groups also were tested and an appropriate modification of the t test was taken if the P value for the hypothesis of equal variance in the pairs of groups being compared was not met.

The sex ratios were compared by the Mantel-Haenszel procedure, dividing the cases into 108 possible strata: 18 age groups × 2 races × 3 time periods. Again, occasionally there were problems with small groups. Following Mantel and Fleiss (8), if any of the expected values of the totals was less than 5, the test was not used. Instead the corrected G test was used as recommended by Sokal and Rohlf (9) on the crude totals. Race differences were examined in the same way. The three resulting P values were combined as recommended by Fisher (10) into a summary P value. In generating the summary value, if the combined P value of the ratios of age variances was smaller than the P value of the weighted differences of the age means, the former value instead of the latter was used on the basis that it was stronger evidence that the two groups were different. This in turn was justified on the grounds that the use of statistical tests had a different emphasis than usual here: groups were to be combined unless it could be shown that they were unlikely at the 5% level to have been drawn from the same underlying population.

Appendix B. The Calculation of Demographic Distances

It should be emphasized that the procedure is in the process of development and analysis. Although it gives commonsense results here, its full use has not been studied. In particular, it has not been determined whether the distances can be used successfully for multidimensional scaling, our next step in generating a visualizable, consistent hierarchy and organization of cancer types.

The first step was to find a symmetrical measure, ie, one that gave the same value when we measured the distance from B to A as from A to B. The square of the weighted mean age difference fitted this definition as well. The "relative risk" value generated by the Mantel-Haenzel (M-H) procedure did not, because it was a ratio, but the square of the log of the relative risk did. The same ratio, of course, could be calculated from the four crude numbers of the G Test if there were not enough cases for the M-H test. Finally, it seemed that in this context, the within-group age variance was independent enough of the mean age that it too should be used in the distance calculations. Because variances are compared by ratios, again the square of the log of this ratio was utilized.

The next standard step is to normalize the variable so that each measure has equal weight. This was tried using the results of all comparisons at all sites. This clearly did not work well. Many of the age comparisons, perhaps half, had been large and statistically significantly different and the distribution of the differences was badly overweighted by extreme values. Perhaps this would not have mattered if the other measures had behaved the same but, by contrast, unusually few of the racial distributions had differed significantly and the differences in sex distribution fell somewhere in between. The current weights were arrived at by considering only a subset of test results that were forced into a more normal range. For the age differences, all with P values greater than 0.05 were included. An additional 4% were randomly selected from those differences with $0.05 < P < 0.01$ and 1% selected from those with $P < 0.01$. The same was done with the sex and age variance values, whereas for the race values enough with P values greater than 0.05 were discarded that the significant differences made up 5% of the totals. These subsets then were used to calculate scaling adjustments that came closer to giving each variable equal weight, but the results of this new weighting scheme still need to be evaluated.

After weighting, the four squared distances were added and in standard fashion (11) a summary distance was calculated $(\Sigma d^2/4)^{1/2}$ so that the results would be compatible with results from sites for which patients were either all men or all women.

References

1. Kreyberg L. Histological lung cancer types. Oslo: Norwegian Universities Press, 1962.
2. World Health Organization. (ICD-O) International classification of diseases for oncology. Geneva: WHO, 1976.
3. Berg JW, Percy C, Horm JW. Recent changes in the pattern of occurrence of oat cell carcinomas of the lung. In: Magnus K, ed, Trends in cancer incidence. Washington, DC: Hemisphere Publishing, 1982.
4. Berg JW. Epidemiology of the different histologic types of lung cancer. AEC Symp Ser 1970;21:93-104.
5. Young JL Jr, Percy CL, Asire AJ, eds. Surveillance, Epidemiology and End Results: Incidence and mortality data 1973-77. National Cancer Institute Monogr 57. Washington, DC: U.S. Department of Health and Human Services, 1981.
6. Cutler SJ, Young JL Jr, eds. Third national cancer survey: Incidence data. National Cancer Institute Monogr 41. Washington, DC: U.S. Department of Health, Education and Welfare, 1975.
7. American Cancer Society. Manual of tumor nomenclature and coding, 1968 ed. New York: ACS, 1968.
8. Mantel N, Fleiss JL. Minimum expected cell size requirements for the Mantel-Haenszel one-degree of freedom chi-square test and a related rapid procedure. Am J Epidemiol 1980;112:129-34.
9. Sokal RR, Rohlf FJ. Biometry. San Francisco: WH Freeman, 1969.
10. Fisher RA. Statistical methods for research workers, 13th ed. Edinburgh: Oliver and Boyd, 1958.
11. Sneath PHA, Sokal RR. Numerical toxonomy. San Francisco: Freeman WH, 1973.

CHAPTER **10**

Lung Cancer in Nonsmokers and Low-Risk Populations

JOSEPH L. LYON, ELECTRA D. AVLON, and JOHN W. GARDNER

Department of Family and Community Medicine, University of Utah, 50 North Medical Drive, Salt Lake City, Utah 84132

ABSTRACT

Lung cancer occurs independent of cigarette smoking, but at an incidence rate between 10 to 20% of that observed in smokers. The histologic pattern of tumors in nonsmokers is also different from smokers. Data are presented estimating lung cancer incidence in several nonsmoking populations, including Mormons and Seventh-Day Adventists, and discussing the causes of lung cancer in nonsmokers, including occupation and place of residence. Time trends in lung cancer incidence in nonsmokers are also presented in light of concern over the possible worsening of the urban environment. The interaction of cigarette smoking with other environmental carcinogens is discussed based on the evidence we can deduce from nonsmokers.
Key Words: **Lung cancer, smoking, nonsmokers, passive smoking, diet, occupational exposures, pollution, urban-rural**

Introduction

The airways leading to the lung and the lung itself are in continuous contact with the external environment because of their function of providing gaseous exchange between our internal environment and the external environment. The mucosal cells lining the respiratory tract come into contact with any respirable chemicals that are present in the external environment. Some of these chemicals are carcinogenic, and lung cancer occurs in a small proportion of people so exposed. The model of exposure is cigarette smoking and its association with cancer of the trachea, bronchi, and lung. Lung cancer, however, does occur at a much lower incidence rate in individuals who do not smoke tobacco products (1).

Lung Cancer: Causes and Prevention.

In this chapter we give a brief review of the epidemiologic literature on lung cancer, estimate the range of incidence of lung cancer in nonsmokers, and also discuss lung cancer incidence in some low-risk populations. We discuss potential confounding factors that influence lung cancer incidence or mortality in nonsmokers and point out the problems these confounding factors may cause when nonsmokers are used as a comparison group without adjustments being made for the confounding factors.

Results and Discussion

The published data for the United States for the year 1914 estimate a lung cancer mortality rate of 1.6 for men and 1.3 for women (2). Most critics agree that these mortality figures underestimate the true incidence of the disease and are severely biased by lack of diagnostic accuracy and underreporting (3). Only with the increased interest in the association between cigarette smoking and lung cancer, beginning in the late 1940s, do estimates of lung cancer in nonsmokers become more available.

Table 1 contains estimates derived from several cohort studies. Based on United States national samples, there appears to be an increase for men (mortality rates increasing from 13.3 to 22.8 per 100,000 between 1958 and 1966–1968) (2, 4). No increase was noted for women during the same interval; however, there are a number of problems with the classification of exposure for males that are discussed here. Other estimates of incidence rates in nonsmokers from both the United States Veterans' cohort and the American Cancer Society cohort yield remarkably similar age Standardized Mortality Rates (SMRs) (12.7 and 13.4 deaths per 100,000 person-years) (5, 6) and are cited by Enstrom (2).

Other studies have also calculated rates that are close to these, although using other age-standardization procedures. In their last published report on the follow-up study of British physicians, Doll and Peto (7) estimated a mortality rate for nonsmokers of 10 per 100,000 (Table 2). Enstrom (2), using Utah and California Mormon men who were known to be highly active in their church and thus assumed to be nonsmokers, estimated a rate of 24.5 deaths per 100,000. However, Gardner and Lyon (8) studying the Utah portion of the same group, arrived at a much lower mortality estimate, 9.2 deaths per 100,000 (Tables 3 and 4). The age-standardization procedure uses a different referent age in all three studies.

Table 1. Age-adjusted lung cancer mortality rates for United States nonsmokers in selected cohort studies by sex[a]

Sex	U.S. mortality rates (2) 1958	U.S. mortality rates (2) 1966–1968	U.S. veteran cohort (1954–1962) (6)	ACS cohort (1960–1963) (5)
Male	13.3	22.8	12.7	13.4
Female	8.3	8.3	—	—

[a]Reproduced with permission from Ref(2)

Table 2. Lung cancer death rate by method of smoking and number of cigarettes smoked per day

	Death rate (per 100,000 standardized for age)[b]
Nonsmokers	10
Cigarette smokers	140
Number of cigarettes smoked per day	**Death rate**
1–14	78
15–24	127
25	251

[a]Reproduced with permission from Ref(7)
[b]Age-standardized age distribution of all British physicians.

Table 3. Lung cancer incidence rates in Utah and California Mormons (per 100,000) for males

Study	Years covered	Incidence ratio
Gardner and Lyon (8)	1966–1970	9.2[a]
Enstrom (2)	1967–1975	24.5[b]

[a]Age adjusted to total Mormon male population, ages 20 + only.
[b]Age adjusted to unknown standard.

Table 4. Age-adjusted lung cancer incidence rates in Utah (per 100,000) during 1967–1975 by religion for males[a]

Non-Mormon	Mormon	Active Mormon[b]
58.8	27.1	9.2[c]

[a]Reproduced with permission from Ref(8)
[b]Active = high priests and seventies group rate.
[c]Covers 1966-1970 only.

The higher estimates have all come uniformly from studies that have not ascertained directly the individuals' smoking status and likely are biased by the inclusion of ex-smokers in the nonsmoking population. This is likely true for the Enstrom data on Utah and California Mormons and for the two United States samples cited by Enstrom (2). Doll and Peto (7) have demonstrated a twofold increase in risk in ex-smokers which persists at least 15 years after cessation of cigarette smoking. This failure to eliminate ex-smokers in studies of nonsmokers has the effect of raising estimated nonsmoking lung cancer rates.

Unfortunately, estimates for the incidence of lung cancer in females are less frequent. Few studies have followed women in large enough numbers to provide estimates, and most that have have not chosen to publish their results in a form that permits the computation of rates (9). Estimates of the incidence of lung cancer in nonsmoking women, shown in Table 5, have usually been in the form of an SMR and vary from 14 to 37 (10). Enstrom (2) has estimated the mortality rate in women based on a United States national mortality sample; these data are contained in Table 1. They also are subject to the same bias in ascertainment of exposure mentioned above, although it is not known whether this bias has a sex-specific component. The rates for women reported by Enstrom are lower than those he has reported for men.

The question of whether the rate of lung cancer is rising in nonsmokers is important because it implies the possibility of the effect of other unrecognized carcinogens in the general environment acting independently of cigarettes. Enstrom (2) has presented data to support an increasing rate in nonsmokers. His argument has been challenged by Doll and Peto (3), and their data in Table 6 present time-trend data for lung cancer mortality in nonsmokers from the United States Veterans follow-up study. This analysis found no increase up to 15 years after entry into the study in men classified as nonsmokers at the outset of the study.

Enstrom's conclusions are based also on his finding of an increased mortality in Mormon men who were highly active, yet Gardner and Lyon (8), studying the same group of men living in Utah for the same time period, arrived at a much lower estimate of mortality, closer to that found in the United States Veterans study and the British Physicians study. The fact that different reference populations have been used by both investigators does not account for the differences.

Other factors that influence the incidence of lung cancer have come to the fore since the original hypotheses concerning its association with cigarettes and must

Table 5. Age and sex-adjusted lung cancer mortality ratios for white California Seventh-Day Adventists (1960–1970) and non-Seventh-Day Adventists (1960–1971) by sex and education[a]

	Male	Female
SDA vs non-SDA		
High school or less	0.19	0.37
Some college or more	0.14	0.14
Total		
SDA vs non-SDA	0.18	0.31
SDA vs United States whites (1960–1975)	0.17	0.34

[a]Reproduced with permission from Ref(10)

Table 6. Lack of apparent upward trend in cancer of the lung among male United States nonsmokers[a]

	Years since entry to study						
	1	2–4	5–7	8–10	11–13	14–16	All study years
Lung, observed	6.0	24.0	31.0	40.0	41.0	35.0	177.0
Lung, expected	6.5	23.6	30.9	39.2	43.9	33.0	177.0
Ratio: obs/exp	0.9	1.0	1.0	1.0	1.0	1.1	1.0

[a]Reproduced with permission from Ref(3)

also be considered. Virtually no study to date has adjusted its data for the following factors:

1. Occupational exposures that increase lung cancer risk independent of cigarette smoking
2. Passive smoking
3. Dietary factors, such as β-carotene, that may act to protect against lung cancer
4. Place of residence and the potential for exposure to other chemicals based on residence

Whereas all these factors are not of equal weight, they should be considered in any study of lung cancer in nonsmokers.

Occupation

Occupation has been the best studied factor and demonstrates the strongest association with lung cancer independent of cigarette smoking. Table 7 presents occupational data for two exposures that demonstrate an independent effect for an occupational exposure as a carcinogen. Asbestos exposure independent of cigarette smoking increases lung cancer risk in the asbestos workers by sevenfold (11). The addition of cigarette smoking has a multiplicative effect and increases risk 60 times over that of nonsmokers. The independent effect of asbestos on lung cancer mortality needs to be considered in estimating the incidence of lung cancer in nonsmokers.

Nonsmoking uranium miners demonstrate a 12-fold increase in lung cancer mortality compared to the nonexposed (13).

Workers exposed to bis-chloromethyl ethers who are also nonsmokers demonstrate a significant increase in lung cancer mortality that is actually greater than smokers, as shown in Table 8 (1). The reason for the protective effect of cigarette smoking in this industrial cohort is not clear, and the size of the relative risks must be viewed with caution because they are based on very small numbers, but it again demonstrates the need to consider occupation in estimating the true

Table 7. Other factors associated with lung cancer

	Asbestos exposure[a], rate ratios	
Smoking	**No**	**Yes**
No	1.0	7.1
Yes	10.9	61.4

		Uranium exposure[b] rate ratios		
Smoking	**No exposure**	**1**	**2**	**3**
Nonsmoker	1.0	1.8	7.6	12.3
20 per day	—	24.1	41.4	117.1

[a]Reproduced with permission from Ref(12)
[b]Reproduced with permission from Ref(13)

Table 8. Standardized mortality ratios (SMRs) for lung cancer among chemical workers with moderate to heavy cumulative exposure to chloromethyl ethers, 1963–1972, by cigarette smoking habit in 1963[a]

Cigarette smoking habit	Lung cancer: Observed number	Lung cancer: Expected number	SMR
Nonsmokers and ex-smokers	6	0.00222	2,703
Current	5	0.14090	35
<1 pack per day	4	0.08295	48
1 + packs per day	1	0.05795	17
Total	11	0.14312	77

[a]Reproduced with permission from Ref(1)

incidence of lung cancer mortality in nonsmokers. There are a number of occupational exposures (chromium, arsenic, coke oven exposure, etc) that increase a person's risk of lung cancer, but their effect independent of cigarette smoking has not been established.

Passive Smoking

Passive smoking is defined as inhaling cigarette smoke from another person, usually a spouse. Tables 9 and 10 present data on the occurrence of lung cancer in female spouses of men who are nonsmokers and smokers. The data come from Greece (14) and Japan (15). Both studies found at least a twofold increase in risk in lifelong, nonsmoking women married to smoking husbands compared to women married to nonsmoking men.

Garfinkel (16) did not confirm these findings in the United States; however, additional studies are required before we can conclude that passive smoking is not a risk factor for nonsmokers. Any study of lung cancer in nonsmokers should take this into account as a possible confounding factor.

Place of Residence

The question of the effect of urban–rural place of residence on risk of lung cancer is controversial. Table 11 presents data from Utah for Mormons and non-Mormons. For Mormons, no urban–rural gradient is noted, but for non-Mormon

Table 9. Passive smoking: relative risk of lung cancer among women by smoking habits of husbands in Greece[a]

Nonsmokers	Ex-smokers	Current smokers: 1–20	Current smokers: 21 +
1.0	1.8	2.4	3.4

[a]Reproduced with permission from Ref(14)

Table 10. Standardized mortality for lung cancer in women by age, occupation, and smoking habit of the husband (patient herself a nonsmoker)[a]

	Husband's smoking habit		
	Nonsmoker	Ex-smoker or 1–19 a day	≥20 a day
Husband's age 40–59			
Population of wives	14,020	30,676	20,584
Number of deaths from lung cancer	11	40	36
Occupation-standardized mortality per 100,000	5.64	9.34	13.14
Husband's age: ≥60 years			
Population of wives	7,875	13,508	4,877
Number of deaths from lung cancer	21	46	20
Occupation-standardized mortality per 100,000	15.79	24.44	29.60
Standardized risk ratio for all ages	1.00	1.61	2.08
Husband working in agriculture			
Population of wives	10,406	20,044	9,391
Number of deaths from lung cancer	17	52	24
Age-standardized mortality per 100,000	9.54	17.02	18.40
Husband working elsewhere			
Population of wives	11,489	24,140	16,070
Number of deaths from lung cancer	15	34	32
Age-standardized mortality per 100,000	9.13	10.46	17.78
Standardized risk ratio for all occupations	1.00	1.43	1.90

[a]Reproduced with permission from Ref(15)

Table 11. Age-adjusted incidence rates (per 100,000) 1967–1975 in Utah Mormons versus non-Mormons[a]

	Latter Day Saints		Non-Latter Day Saints	
Sex	Urban	Rural	Urban	Rural
Male	27.1	27.3	75.7	40.3
Female	4.8	4.4	11.2	9.4

[a]Reproduced with permission from Ref(17)

men a significant gradient exists (17, 18). Haenszel and Taeuber (19) noted a similar finding in their study, which raised the question between a synergistic effect of cigarette smoking and urban environment. It also brings up the question of passive smoking in both environments and the opportunity for synergistic effects between air pollution and cigarette exposure both directly and passively.

Dietary Factors

Recent studies (20–22) have indicated that foods rich in β-carotene may exert a protective effect on the incidence of lung cancer in cigarette smokers (see Table 12).

Table 12. Estimated vitamin A intake and risk of lung cancer[a]

	Relative risk by number of cigarettes smoked		
Level of vitamin A intake (1000 IU)	**<OR> 1 pack per day (176 patients, 600 controls)**	**>pack per day (98 patients, 122 controls)**	**Smoking adjusted (274 patients, 722 controls)**
<25	1.9	3.8	2.4
25–49	2.3	2.5	2.4
50–74	1.8	1.8	1.8
75–99	2.1	1.0	1.7
100–124	1.9	1.5	1.7
125–150	2.1	0.8	1.5
>150	1.0	1.0	1.0

[a]Reproduced with permission from Ref(22)

Additional unpublished data (Kolonel, presented to the National Cancer Institute, Surveillance, Epidemiology and End Results Meeting, Seattle, Washington, September 1983) also confirm this observation and raise the question of a dietary factor, previously unrecognized, that may exert at least a twofold protective effect on risk of lung cancer in smokers. The effect in nonsmokers has not been studied. Again, no investigator has attempted to adjust his estimates of lung cancer mortality for protective dietary factors. This should also be considered in studying the risk of lung cancer in both smokers and nonsmokers.

All of the above-mentioned factors demonstrate relative risks ranging from 1.5-to 12-fold independent of cigarette smoking, and all therefore could influence the incidence estimate of lung cancer in nonsmokers, although occupation is the strongest and best investigated. Relative risks estimated from epidemiologic studies that used comparison groups having a significant proportion of the comparison group exposed to any of these factors singularly or in combination would lead to substantial underestimates of the true risk.

Lung Cancer in Low-Incidence Populations

Table 13 presents data from Hawaii on lung cancer in women from three different ethnic groups (23). None of these data is adjusted for any of the additional factors mentioned. Yet the estimate of relative risk based on cigarette smoking varies from 1.8 to 10.5, and there appears to be little difference in the percentage smoking cigarettes. These data point out the need to establish more precisely a true, nonsmoking comparison group before embarking on the study of lung cancer and cigarette smoking and that lung cancer rates do vary substantially in different populations. Tables 3–5 also contain data on both the Latter-Day Saint (LDS) and Seventh-Day Adventist (SDA) populations (2, 8, 10), both of which experience substantially lower rates of lung cancer, and many other cancers, primarily related to less tobacco usage because of religious reasons.

Table 13. Age-adjusted lung cancer incidence rates, cigarette smoking experience, risk associated with cigarette smoking, and the population risk for lung cancer attributable to smoking for Japanese, Chinese, and Hawaiian women in Hawaii [a]

	Incidence rates (per 100,000)	Percentage ever smokers	Odds ratio	Population attributable risk (PAR) percent	Rate
Hawaiian	42	39	10.5	79	4
Japanese	12	20	4.9	44	2.4
Chinese	24	16	1.8	11	13.3

[a]Reproduced with permission from Ref(23)

Conclusions

Mortality rates as estimates of incidence rates of lung cancer vary by more than twofold and are difficult to assess because of differences in methods used to adjust for age and in the definition of a nonsmoker. The assumption that these rates have been increasing over time is not supported and is likely an artifact of failure to adjust for a number of other exposures that are carcinogenic to the respiratory mucosa of the lungs. The wide variation in relative risks for cigarette smoking is likely influenced by failure to adjust for these other factors in the nonsmoking comparison group used in the studies. Given the importance of some of these factors, particularly the passive smoking question, additional studies need to be mounted to determine the true incidence of lung cancer in nonsmokers.

References

1. Weiss W. The cigarette factor in lung cancer due to chloromethyl ethers. J Occu Med 1980;22:527-529.
2. Enstrom JE. Rising lung cancer mortality among non-smokers. JNCI 1979;62:755-60.
3. Doll R, Peto R. The causes of cancer. Oxford: Oxford University Press, 1981.
4. Enstrom JE, Godley FH. Cancer mortality among a representative sample of non-smokers in the United States during 1966-68. JNCI 1980;65:1175-83.
5. Hammond EC. Smoking in relation to the death rates of one million men and women. Natl Cancer Inst Monogr 1966;19:127-204.
6. Kahn HA: The Dorn study of smoking and mortality among U.S. veterans: Report on eight and one-half years of observation. Natl Cancer Inst Monogr 1966;19:1-126.
7. Doll R, Peto R. Mortality in relation to smoking: 20 years' observations on male British doctors. Br J Med 1976;2:1525-36.
8. Gardner JW, Lyon JL. Cancer in Utah Mormon men by lay priesthood level. Am J Epidemiol 1982;116:243-57.
9. Cederlöf R, Friberg L, Hrubec Z, Lorich U. The relationship of smoking and some social covariables to mortality and cancer morbidity. Stockholm Karolinska Institute, 1975.
10. Phillips RL, Garfinkel L, Kuzma JW, Beeson WL, Lotz T, Brin B. Mortality among California Seventh-Day Adventists for selected cancer sites. JNCI 1980;65:1097-1107.
11. Hammond EC, Selikoff IJ, Seidman H. Asbestos exposures, cigartette smoking and death rates. Ann NY Acad Sci 1979;274:473-90.
12. Frank AL. Public health significance of smoking-asbestos interactions. Ann NY Acad Sci 1979;274:791-4.
13. Archer VE, Gillam JD, Wagoner JK. Respiratory disease mortality among uranium miners. Ann NY Acad Sci 1976;271:280-93.

14. Trichopoulous D, Kalandidi A, Tzonou A. Incidence and distribution of lung cancer in Greece. In: Pontifex G, ed, Lung Cancer—etiology, epidemiology, prevention, early diagnosis, treatment. Amsterdam Excerpta Medica, 1982, 10–17.
15. Hirayama T: Non-smoking wives of heavy smokers have a higher risk of lung cancer: A study from Japan. Br J Med 1981;282:183–5.
16. Garfinkel L. Time trends in lung cancer mortality among nonsmokers and a note on passive smoking. JNCI 1981;66:1061–6.
17. Lyon JL, Gardner JW, West DW. Cancer incidence in Mormons and non-Mormons in Utah during 1967–75. JNCI 1980;65:1055–61.
18. Lyon JL, Gardner JW, West DW. Cancer in Utah: Risk by religion and place of residence. JNCI 1980;65:1063–71.
19. Haenszel W, Taeuber KE. Lung cancer mortality as related to residence and smoking histories. II. White females. JNCI 1964;32:803–38.
20. Graham S, Mettlin C. Fiber and other constituents of vegetables in cancer epidemiology. In: Newell GR, Ellison NE, eds, Nutrition and cancer: etiology and treatment. New York: Raven Press, 1981;189–215.
21. Hirayama T: Diet and cancer. Nutr Cancer 1979;1:67–81.
22. Mettlin C, Graham S, Swanson M. Vitamin A and lung cancer. JNCI 1979;62:1435–1438.
23. Hinds MW, Stemmerman GN, Yang HY, Kolonel LN, Lee J, Wigner E. Differences in lung cancer risk from smoking among Japanese, Chinese, and Hawaiian women in Hawaii. Int J Cancer 1981;27:297–302.

CHAPTER **11**

Ecogenetics of Lung Cancer: Genetic Susceptibility in the Etiology of Lung Cancer

JOHN J. MULVIHILL and ALLEN E. BALE

Clinical Epidemiology Branch, National Cancer Institute, Landow 5A21, Bethesda, Maryland 20205

ABSTRACT

The hope that the best known respiratory carcinogen, tobacco use, could be controlled has delayed the search for inborn determinants of lung cancer. Clues to significant host factors are seen for some cell types. Genetic differences may contribute to ethnic variations in rates, for example, of lung cancer in rural Louisiana, where inbreeding is increased, and of adenocarcinoma of the lung on Cantonese women in Hong Kong. Case–control studies revealed a 2.5-fold excess of lung cancer among relatives of patients with lung cancer compared to relatives of controls; the familial risk was more evident among nonsmokers than among smokers and was synergistic with the effect of smoking. Some published pedigrees suggest lung cancer is part of the Li-Fraumeni syndrome of familial soft-tissue sarcomas, breast cancer, and other neoplasms. Other pedigrees of lung cancer seem to be examples of ecogenetics: the interaction of environmental factors with susceptible hosts. Variations in carcinogen-metabolizing enzymes, such as aryl hydrocarbon hydroxylase, may alter lung cancer susceptibility in smokers. Finally, the finding of a chromosomal marker (3p-) in small-cell carcinoma of the lung gives reason to pursue the search for genetic variations in susceptibility to lung cancer.
Key Words: **Ecogenetics, lung cancer, susceptibility, Li-Fraumeni syndrome, AHH (aryl hydrocarbon hydroxylase), genetic markers, genotype, heredity, environment, immunodeficiency, demography, risk factors, chromosone, families, multiple primary neoplasms**

Introduction

Conventional approaches to understanding the etiology of lung cancer in human beings have focused effectively on environmental agents (1, 2). In particular, efforts to identify and control pulmonary carcinogens have been most successful with hazards of occupational inhalants, such as radioactive ores, mustard gas, asbestos, nickel, chromates, and arsenic (3, 4).

By contrast, the carcinogenic mechanisms of one of the most common human carcinogens, tobacco, are poorly characterized and poorly controlled through public education (5). The association between smoking and certain types of lung cancer is striking and beyond question (6). Most scientists agree smoking causes lung cancer, among other diseases; for them, remaining problems concern the origin and prevention of the smoking habit and, as an ironic but practical expedient, the development of less hazardous cigarettes or nicotine substitutes. A vocal minority doubts a causal relation between cigarette smoking and lung cancer and suggests that an inborn characteristic—a genotype—predestines an individual to cigarette smoking and independently to lung cancer. To understand this view, first advanced by the respected statistician-geneticist R.A. Fisher (7), one must appreciate the role of host factors in lung cancer and, in particular, the genetics of smoking behavior. Finally, genetic detection of oncogenes in human lung cancers (8) reinforces the notion that, regardless of the environmental determinants of lung tumors, genetic mechanisms, eg, mutant DNA, are likely a common mechanism in the genesis of clinical lung cancers and do provide knowledge of potential use in preventing or controlling lung cancer deaths.

The term "ecogenetics" may be applied to heritable variations in susceptibility to environmental agents (9). An appreciation of human ecogenetics avoids the deceptive dichotomy of considering environmental agents to the exclusion of genetic determinants in cancer etiology; otherwise, clues are lost to such questions as "Why do some heavy smokers not get lung cancer?" and "Why do women have a higher ratio of pulmonary adenocarcinoma to squamous cell carcinoma than men?" Exploration of ecogenetics may lead occupational health workers to identify susceptible individuals and may contribute further to knowledge of carcinogenesis. Pending advances in motivational research, identification of host factors that modify susceptibility to respiratory carcinogens seems worthwhile.

Demographic Variables

Standard epidemiologic data give few clues to host-related factors. Rapid changes in the incidence of lung cancer and its sex ratio are well explained by trends in tobacco use and not by large changes in mutation rates or gene pools (9); nonetheless, Belcher (10) suggested a genetic factor based on anomalies of sex ratios for lung cancer worldwide. The geographic distribution of lung cancer in the United States suggests variations from occupational exposures, except for a concentration in rural southern Louisiana, where inbreeding is conspicuous (11). Compared to whites, lung cancer in the United States is accelerating more rapidly in blacks, is higher in Americans of Chinese extraction, and is lower in Mexican-Americans and American Indians (9). Worldwide ethnic and geographic variations may arise from genetic and environmental factors, which sometimes can be distinguished by studying the cancer experience of migrants. For lung cancer, the observations are inconclusive: The migrant rates are either intermediate between the native rates in their former and new countries or, in the United States, appear to exceed both rates (12). As socioeconomic level rises, lung cancer death rates fall, an association not entirely explained by smoking habits (13).

Black Ohio residents with lung cancer had a twofold risk of being born in the South rather than in Ohio; this intracountry migrant effect suggested lung cancer determinants in early life, perhaps genetic or dietary (14). Ethnic comparisons in Texas showed that, compared with whites, rates were higher in Mexican-Americans over age 74 but much lower in those under 70 (15).

These studies were generally based on death certificates, which are numerous and available, but which often fail to specify cell type. Striking epidemiologic peculiarities are seen when cell types are distinguised. For example, Chinese women in Hong Kong have a peculiar predominance of adenocarcinoma of the lung, a relatively infrequent cell type elsewhere. In Singapore, the peculiar excess of adenocarcinoma of the lung in Cantonese females was associated not with smoking, but with low consumption of green vegetables and implicated susceptibility caused by relative deficiency of vitamin A (16).

Studies of twins have not shown a genetic factor because of inadequate numbers of cases, although one study of 10,945 twin pairs was large enough to demonstrate the influence of smoking on lung cancer (17).

Empiric Familial Risk

Where demography falls short, a more powerful tool, the case-control study, has shown significant familial influences that could be environmental, genetic, or both. In two separate studies, Tokuhata and Lilienfeld (18, 19) found 2.7 and 2.4 times more lung cancer among relatives of patients with lung cancer than among relatives of controls. The familial factor was more evident among nonsmokers than among smokers. Conversely, the effect of smoking was less evident among case relatives (who had the familial tendency already) than among control relatives. The familial and smoking effects were synergistic. In an uncontrolled study of 130 patients with lung cancer, 11% had two or more first-degree relatives with lung cancer (20).

Again, these data (18, 19) were not analyzed by histologic pattern, but lung cancer is a heterogeneous disease with a variety of cell types and suspected etiologies. As Anderson identified subgroups of women at very high risk of breast cancer (2), studies of specific pathologic types of lung cancer may reveal strong genetic factors that are undetectable when all cell types are combined.

Tokuhata (22) used his Baltimore study group to demonstrate that, irrespective of lung cancer, the smoking habit clearly ran in families. For both sexes, offspring were often smokers when both parents smoked, less so when only one smoked, and least when neither did. These empiric observations suggest a familial influence in determining smoking habits. The tendency may be inborn because three studies of twins, including one with twins separated since birth, showed a greater concordance for smoking among monozygous than dizygous twins (9).

Published Pedigrees

Six reported kindreds with carcinoma of the lung suggest an interaction between external agents and genetic susceptibility (9, 23–25). In most families the patients with lung cancer had been heavy smokers. In one the eldest brother worked in a copper smelter, the youngest affected brother had exposure to chromium fumes, and a sister had a second primary lung cancer. In the two National Cancer Institute families (24) an inborn determinant of risk was inferred from the coexistence of a birth defects syndrome in one family and the occurrence of two radiogenic cancers and one leukemia associated with chlorambucil use.

Lung cancer is occasionally seen as one of the diverse cell types in families. In one instance of the familial soft-tissue sarcoma–breast cancer syndrome of Li and Fraumeni [A in original report (26)], a man developed alveolar cell carcinoma of the lung, his daughter with Turner syndrome had anaplastic lung cancer, and a distant cousin had metachronous squamous cell carcinomas of the larynx and lung.

"Familial" does not mean "genetic", and lung cancer certainly may occur among relatives because of common environmental exposure to respiratory carcinogens. Pleural mesothelioma caused death in a 52-year-old daughter of a man with the same tumor type who had worked with asbestos for more than 13 years. The daughter's only exposure was secondary contact, as a child, to dust brought home in the father's clothing; more than 30 years passed before her malignancy appeared (27).

This instance of familial mesothelioma illustrates that long latent periods for a carcinogen may thwart efforts to distinguish genetic and environmental influences in familial cancer. However, it also shows the value of studying rare histologic types, where the origins often are clearer than in common cell types. For example, the report of a father and son with pulmonary histiocytosis reinforces evidence that histiocytoses of other organs may have a significant hereditary component (28). Host determinants may be seen most clearly in alveolar cell carcinoma and adenocarcinoma of the lung.

Reports of lung cancer and pleural mesothelioma in spouses and children of asbestos workers further emphasize the familial hazards of chemicals brought home on work clothes (29, 30). Peculiarities of alveolar cell carcinoma continued to appear, eg, a report of the tumor in identical twin brothers with similar ages of onset, histochemistry, and metastatic behavior (31).

Multiple Primary Neoplasms

An additional phenomenon useful in delineating etiologic factors is the occurrence of distinct, multiple primary malignancies in a patient. The families in the previous section and others (9) suggest that lung cancer may occur as a second primary neoplasm more often than expected by chance alone, although the frequency of pulmonary metastases makes proof of an independent primary tumor in the lung especially difficult. Among all patients with multiple primary neoplasms in the Connecticut Tumor Registry (32), the risk of developing lung cancer was significantly elevated in men with cancer of the lip, mouth, pharynx, and larynx, and in women with cervical cancer. The increased risk may be attributed to continued use of tobacco, which also may contribute to the risk following bladder cancer. (The converse strengthens this possibility: lung cancer patients have a significant risk for subsequent cancer of the mouth and upper respiratory tract.) Case reports suggest that environmental agents other than smoking may cause multiple primaries, eg, asbestos, and cancer therapy with radiation and drugs. Lung cancer was reported in association with antimetabolite therapy in a few patients with lymphoproliferative malignancies and psoriasis. This suggests that some multiple primary malignancies involving the lung may arise from impaired host immunity (9).

Immune Factors

In addition to the above observations, scattered evidence is converging that relates immune defects to the genesis of some lung tumors.

1. Immune evaluation of newly diagnosed lung cancer patients usually shows depressed cutaneous reactivity and T-cell counts, and normal B-cell levels (33–39), although there are series with normal responsivity to phytohemagglutinin (PHA) (37, 38, 40). Early studies failed to distinguish by cell type and clinical course, but recently severe immunodeficiency has been correlated with poor prognosis except in adenocarcinoma (37).
2. Uranium miners, known to be at high risk for lung tumors, had normal immunoglobulin levels at the time of employment; these levels fell after 1 year and remained low even 10 years later (41).
3. In one study, lung cancer has occurred in five renal transplant recipients on therapeutic immunosuppression, compared to 1.8 expected (42). Other studies of transplant recipients and patients with inborn immunodefiencies failed to show an excess of lung tumors (43, 44).
4. Certain disorders with diverse, poorly delineated immunologic abnormalities, such as dermatomyositis, sarcoidosis, and scleroderma, may be associated with lung cancer. A strong heritable tendency has been observed in each condition except dermatomyositis, which seems to be a paraneoplastic manifestation of lung cancer and not a disease predisposing to it (9). In 2544 patients with sarcoidosis seen in 10 years, nine lung tumors were observed compared to 2.8 expected (45). By 1980 over 44 patients with scleroderma (progressive systemic sclerosis) were reported with cancer of the lung, mostly alveolar cell carcinoma and adenocarcinomas (46). There is a striking positive correlation between alveolar cell carcinoma and the intensity of interstitial pulmonary fibrosis. The observed progression of fibrosing alveolitis to lung cancer in scleroderma is likely to be a common route by which various disorders predispose to cancer, especially alveolar cell carcinoma. This concept of pathogenesis, similar to that suggested for hepatocellular carcinoma after cirrhosis, unites under the rubric of

"scar carcinoma" such diverse pneumonic processes as pulmonary infarction, rheumatic mitral valve heart disease, and desquamative interstitial pneumonia. In these conditions, intermediary alveolar metaplasia and benign adenomatosis are frequent autopsy findings, and the tumors are thought to be multifocal in origin (9).

5. Early atypia is occasionally seen in lungs from individuals with nonpulmonary cancer treated with radiation or drugs, including methotrexate, cyclophosphamide, bleomycin, and busulfan. It would not be surprising, then, to see lung cancer, particularly alveolar cell carcinoma, as a late complication of cancer therapy (which, in general, suppresses immunity) (9, 47).

Chromosomal Abnormalities

A consistent deletion of the short arm of chromosome 3, [del 3p (14–23)], has been seen in karyotypes from fresh tumor specimens and tissue culture lines established from small-cell lung cancers (48).

No specific chromosome abnormalities have been seen in other cell types although lung tumor tissue tends to be hyperploid. Pleural effusions from lung cancers sometimes have cells with abnormal karyotypes that aid in diagnosing intrathoracic malignancy (49).

Patients with scleroderma have a second characteristic, besides immunologic defects that may contribute to their predisposition to cancer: excessive chromosomal breaks have been seen in their peripheral blood and bone marrow. Breaks were seen also when cells from normal controls were preincubated in sera from affected patients. One group related the abnormalities to cyclophosphamide therapy, but a larger controlled study of patients with progressive systemic sclerosis demonstrated aberrations that were not attributable to radiation or cytotoxic therapy (9).

Antecedent Familial Lung Disease (cf Ref 9)

Scleroderma may explain familial aggregations of lung tumors, such as the sisters reported by Petitjean et al (50); one of these had alveolar cell carcinoma. Another sibship of two brothers with alveolar cell carcinoma was probably explained by the concomitant familial diffuse interstitial pulmonary fibrosis (IPF), present also in a cousin without tumor (51). In a recent update of the family (52), alveolar cell carcinoma was seen in three of five family members with IPF; a sixth person had alveolar cell carcinoma without definite pulmonary fibrosis. An autosomal dominant form of congenital cystic disease of the lung (familial fibrocystic pulmonary dysplasia), indistinguishable from Hamman-Rich syndrome except by its chronicity and inheritance, was associated with lung cancer in two brothers and with sporadic lung tumors in members of other affected families.

Other autosomal dominant traits have IPF as an occasional feature and may in the future be associated with lung cancer. These syndromes include certain phakomatoses (neurofibromatosis, tuberous sclerosis, and von Hippel-Lindau disease), Marfan syndrome, and familial pulmonary alveolar microlithiasis.

The spectrum of the dominantly inherited multiple endocrine neoplasias (MEN) includes pulmonary neoplasms, such as bronchial carcinoid in MEN I and bronchial mucosal neuroma in MEN III (53). The existence of medullary carcinoma of the lung has been proposed as a counterpart of medullary thyroid carcinoma as seen in MEN II (54). Because oat cell carcinoma resembles carcinoid in morphology, histochemistry, and ability to produce ectopic hormones, it may prove to have neural crest origins and a considerable heritable component, as carcinoid does (55).

As for autosomal recessive traits, the occurrence of pulmonary liposarcoma in one of four sisters with congenital adrenal hyperplasia is probably a coincidence but may be iatrogenic, for hyperadrenocorticism can cause large mediastinal lipomas. Multiple leiomyomas, sometimes a recessive trait when it affects the skin, also can involve the lungs. A 52-year-old man was reported with Kartagener syndrome and bronchogenic carcinoma, again probably fortuitous despite the presence of immunodeficiency and pulmonary malformations that may predispose to lung cancer in other disorders (9).

Case reports suggest the association of peculiar lung tumors with congenital malformation of the lungs: undifferentiated carcinoma with ipsilateral hypoplasia of the pulmonary artery; rhabdomyosarcoma in congenital cystic adenomatoid malformation of the lung; and anaplastic carcinoma in a fibromyomatous hamartoma of the lung.

In one Swedish family, autosomal dominant inheritance of IPF and an abnormal hemoglobin (Malmö) was associated with anaplastic small-cell carcinoma. Although a subsequent American family with hemoglobin Malmö had no pulmonary disorder, in the Swedish family this hemoglobin can be considered a genetic marker for lung cancer.

Genetic Markers, Including Aryl Hydrocarbon Hydroxylase

A more controversial marker is the inducibility of aryl hydrocarbon hydroxylase (AHH). Aryl hydrocarbon hydroxylase is a multiple-component enzyme system that catalyzes endogenous and exogenous lipid-like molecules to more polar ones for better elimination. In experimental systems, it also converts polycyclic hydrocarbons, as found in cigarette smoke, to intermediate metabolities that are more potent mutagens and carcinogens than the parent molecules. Aryl hydrocarbon hydroxylase is found in human lungs (specifically alveolar macrophages), leukocytes, and most organs. In humans, cigarette smoking can induce sustained elevation of AHH. In mice, inducibility varies in many inbred strains—in some as an autosomal dominant, in others as a codominant trait (56).

Relating AHH to human lung cancer, Kellermann et al (57, 58) reported two simple but stunning observations 10 years ago. First, AHH inducibility in humans seemed to be controlled by a single locus with two alleles. Second, in a series of patients with lung cancer, 96% (compared to 55% in controls) had high or intermediate levels of inducibility; low levels were found in 4% of lung cancer patients but in 45% of controls.

Subsequently, twin studies suggested significant genetic determinants. Each study with findings of higher inducibility in lymphocytes of lung cancer patients, compared with controls, seemed balanced by negative reports. While difficulties with the lymphocyte assay were debated, others turned to assays of pulmonary alveolar macrophages or explants of bronchial mucosa (9).

Although improved studies continue to be done (59), it now seems the promise of the early findings has faded, with good reason:

1. Simple Mendelian inheritance was unlikely in humans because AHH is not one but several enzymes and because codominance occurs in inbred mice.
2. Evidence for one locus with two alleles came from a frequency distribution of inducibility that was said to have three modes, but the small number of cases made the interpretation tenuous.
3. The early Kellermann assay depended on lymphocytes stimulated by mitogens and might not have detected the metobolic activity of bronchial mucosa. T-cell function is depressed in many lung cancer patients who therefore would be unavailable for the Kellermann assay because their lymphocytes would not transform. The controls of Kellermann et al (58) were not matched for age, smoking habits, or degree of lymphocyte transformability (60). A more recent in vivo assay is even more cumbersome than the lymphocyte method (61). Future use of recombinant DNA technology to detect polymorphisms of the human AHH locus (or more appropriately the locus for cytochrome P_1-450) may provide a direct approach to resolving the conflicting evidence from functional bioassays (62).

Genetic deficiency of α_1-antitrypsin predisposes to emphysema of the panlobular type, and lung cancer may occur to excess in patients with emphysema but of the opposite variety, namely centrilobular. In any case, α_1-antitrypsin levels are increased in patients with lung cancer or abnormal sputum cytology. No unusual α_1-antitrypsin phenotypes were detected in 72 patients with lung cancer compared with 196 controls. Serum activity was doubled, consistent with the previous interpretation that genetic α_1-antitrypsin deficiency did not predispose to lung cancer as it did to emphysema. Lung cancer and chronic obstructive pulmonary disease may still have a common familial factor. First-degree relatives of patients with each disease have similarly impaired forced expiration, a pulmonary function test, compared with controls with nonpulmonary disease. In 12 "lung cancer families," a history of chronic obstructive pulmonary disease was found in more first- than second-degree relatives (9).

As for other genetic markers, blood group B has been associated with adenocarcinoma, and group O with undifferentiated cancer of the lung in males (63). In one study of the histocompatibility locus HLA and lung cancer (64), B44 was associated with a high risk of developing small-cell carcinoma, and other studies have shown increased survival with AW19 and B5, but not consistently (65,66).

Conclusions

In lung cancer, as in most human disease, pathologic heterogeneity signals important etiologic differences. In bronchogenic carcinoma, for example, cigarette smoking is the most important etiologic factor, and little evidence exists for inherited influences. On the other hand numerous peculiarities of alveolar cell carcinoma suggest familial factors: it is poorly related to smoking; is found in families with other tumors, acquired immune diseases, or heritable disorder of the lung (especially those associated with IPF and scleroderma); and occurs as an autosomal dominant trait in mice (67) and as a likely viral disease, called jaagsiekte, in sheep (68).

For even rarer cell types, genetic factors may emerge when sufficient cases are assembled. The syndromes of MEN include pulmonary neoplasms, such as bronchial mucosal neuroma in MEN III and bronchial carcinoid in MEN I (Wermer syndrome). Carcinoid alone can be an autosomal dominant trait and shares many histologic, histochemical, and endocrinologic features with oat cell carcinoma (9).

In the search for additional genetic factors, the area to examine may be the interaction of known environmental carcinogens with susceptible genotypes (69). This field may be termed ecogenetics, a word already used to apply to the long-term effects of the environment on the genome but that may tolerate a special use in medical genetics. By analogy to pharmacogenetics, the study of variations in the response to drugs, clinical ecogenetics could be the study of variations in the response to environmental agents in general. One challenge in ecogenetics in oncology may be the development of means for screening potential employees for abnormal genotypes that predispose them to neoplasia after occupational exposures that are harmless to normal genotypes.

References

1. Hueper WC. A quest into the environmental causes of cancer of the lung. Public Health Monogr 36, U.S. Public Health Service. Washington, DC.: U.S. Government Printing Office, 1956.
2. Fraumeni JF Jr. Respiratory carcinogenesis: an epidemiologic appraisal. JNCI 1975;55:1039–46.
3. U.S. Atomic Energy Commission. Inhalation carcinogenesis. In: Hanna MG Jr, Nettesheim P, Gilbert JR, eds, Proceedings of a Biology Division, Oak Ridge National Laboratory Conference. Oak Ridge, TN: U.S. Atomic Energy Commission, 1970.
4. Fraumeni JF Jr, Blot WJ. Lung and pleura. In: Schottenfeld D, Fraumeni JF Jr, eds, Cancer epidemiology and prevention. Philadelphia: W.B. Saunders, 1982:564–82.
5. Wynder EL, Hoffmann D. The tenth anniversary of the Surgeon General's report on smoking and health: have we made any progress? JNCI 1975;54:533–4.
6. Leading Article, Lung cancer and smoking: is there proof? Br Med J 1976;2:439–40.
7. Fisher RA. Dangers of cigarette-smoking. Br Med J 1957;2:297–8.
8. Pulciani S, Santos E, Lauver AV, Long LK, Aaronson SA, Barbacid M. Oncogenes in solid human tumors. Nature 1982;300:539–42.
9. Mulvihill JJ. Host factors in human lung tumors: an example of ecogenetics in oncology. Natl Cancer Inst Monogr 1979;52:115–21.
10. Belcher JR. Worldwide differences in the sex ratio of bronchial carcinoma. Br J Dis Chest 1971; 65:205–21.

11. Mason TJ, McKay FW, Hoover R, Blot WJ, Fraumeni JF Jr. Atlas of cancer mortality for U.S. counties: 1950–1969. U.S. Department of Health, Education and Welfare Publ (NIH) 75-780 Washington, DC: U.S. Government Printing Office, 1975.
12. Mancuso TE, Sterling TD. Lung cancer among black and white migrants in the U.S. J Natl Med Assoc 1975;67:106–11.
13. Brown SM, Selvin S, Winkelstein W Jr. The association of economic status with the occurrence of lung cancer. Cancer 1975;36:1903–11.
14. Mancuso TF. Lung cancer among black migrants. Interaction of host and occupational factors. JOM 1977;19:531–2.
15. Lee ES, Roberts RE, Labarth DR. Excess and deficit lung cancer mortality in three ethnic groups in Texas. Cancer 1976;38:2551–6.
16. MacLennan R, Da Costa J, Day NE, et al. Risk factors for lung cancer in Singapore Chinese, a population with high female incidence rates. Int J Cancer 1977;20:854–60.
17. Cederlof R, Floderus B, Friberg L. Cancer in MZ and DZ twins. Acta Genet Med Gemellol (Roma) 1970;19:69–74.
18. Tokuhata GK, Lilienfeld AM. Familial aggregation of lung cancer in humans. JNCI 1963;30:289–312.
19. Tokuhata GK, Lilienfeld AM. Familial aggregation of lung cancer among hospital patients. Public Health Rep 1963;78:277–83.
20. Guirgis HA, Lynch HT, Harris RE, et al. Familial aggregation of lung cancer and other pulmonary diseases (Abstract). Int Congress Series 397:77, Amsterdam, Excerpta Medica, 1976.
21. Anderson DE. Genetic study of breast cancer: identification of a high risk group. Cancer 1974;34:1090–7.
22. Tokuhata GK. Smoking habits in lung-cancer proband families and comparable control families. JNCI 1963;31:1153–71.
23. Jones FL Jr. Bronchogenic carcinoma in three siblings. Bull Geisinger Med Cent 1977;29:23–5.
24. Goffman TE, Hassinger DD, Mulvihill JJ. Familial respiratory tract cancer. JAMA 1982; 247:1020–3.
25. Ooi WI, Rothschild H, Chen VW, Bailey-Wilson JE, Corcoran KA, Elston RC. Familial risk and lung cancer. Clin Res 1981;29:862A.
26. Li FP, Fraumeni JF Jr. Soft-tissue sarcomas, breast cancer and other neoplasms: a familial syndrome? Ann Intern Med 1969;71:747–52.
27. Anderson HA, Lilis R, Daum SM, Fischbein AS, Selikoff IJ. Household-contact asbestos: neoplastic risk. Ann NY Acad Sci 1976;271:311–23.
28. Perry MC, Harrison EG Jr, Gilchrist GS. Familial erythrophagocytic lymphohistiocytosis. Report of two cases and clinicopathologic review. Cancer 1976;38:209–18.
29. Lillington GA, Jamplis RW, Differding JR. Conjugal malignant mesothelioma. N Engl J Med 1974;291:583–4.
30. Li FP, Lokich J, Lapey J, et al. Familial mesothelioma after intense asbestos exposure at home. JAMA 1978;240:467.
31. Joishy SK, Cooper RA, Rowley PT. Alveolar cell carcinoma in identical twins: similarity in time of onset, histochemistry, and site of metastasis. Ann Intern Med 1977;87:447–50.
32. Schoenberg BS. Multiple primary malignancies: the Connecticut experience, New York: Springer-Verlag, 1977.
33. Krusmann WF, Slanina J, Hennekeuser HH, Wahren C, Scholz R, Vorwerck H. Uber den Einfluss energiereicher Strahlen (60Co) auf PHA-Stimulierbarkeit und cytochemisches Verhalten von Lymphocyten bei Morbus Hodgkin und Bronchialcarcinom. Z Krebsforsch 1974;81:119–34.
34. Gross RL, Latty A, Williams EA, Newberne PM. Abnormal spontaneous rosette formation and rosette inhibition in lung carcinoma. N Engl J Med 1975;292:439–43.
35. Wanebo HJ, Rao B, Miyazawa N, et al. Immune reactivity in primary carcinoma of the lung and its relation to prognosis. J Thorac Cardiovasc Surg 1976;72:339–47.
36. Stefani S, Kerman R, Abbate J. Immune evaluation of lung cancer patients undergoing radiation therapy. Cancer 1976;37:2792–6.
37. Dellon AL, Potvin C, Chretien PB. Thymus-dependent lymphocyte levels in bronchogenic carcinoma: correlations with histology, clinical stage, and clinical course after surgical treatment. Cancer 1975;35:687–94.
38. Holmes EC, Golub SH. Immunologic defects in lung cancer patients. J Thorac Cardiovasc Surg 1976;71:161–8.

39. Olkowski ZL, McLaren JR, Mansour KA. Immunocompetence of patients with bronchogenic carcinoma. Ann Thorac Surg 1976;21:546-51.
40. Barnes EW, Farmer A, Penhale WJ, Irvine WJ, Roscoe P, Horne NW. Phytohemagglutinin-induced lymphocyte transformation in newly presenting patients with primary carcinoma of the lung. Cancer 1975;36:187-93.
41. Andrlikova J, Wagner V, Palek V. Investigation of immunoglobulin (IgG, IgA, IgM) levels in the blood serum of uranium miners after higher and lower exposure to ionizing radiation. Strahlentherapie 1975;149:212-8.
42. Hoover R. Effects of drugs—immunosuppression. In: Hiatt HH, Watson JD, Winsten JA, eds, Origins of human cancer: A. Incidence of cancer in humans. Cold Spring Harbor, NY: Cold Spring Harbor Laboratory, 1977:369-79.
43. Penn I. Depressed immunity and the development of cancer. Clin Exp Immunol 1981;46:459-74.
44. Kinlen LJ, Sheil AGR, Peto J, Doll R. Collaborative United Kingdom-Australasian study of cancer in patients treated with immunosuppresive drugs. Br Med J 1979;2:1461-6.
45. Brincker H, Wilbek E. The incidence of malignant tumours in patients with respiratory sarcoidosis. Br J Cancer 1974;29:247-51.
46. Talbott JH, Barrocas M. Carcinoma of the lung in progressive systemic sclerosis: a tabular review of the literature and a detailed report of the roentgenographic changes in two cases. Semin Arthritis Rheum 1980;9:191-217.
47. Harris CC. The carcinogenicity of anticancer drugs: a hazard in man. Cancer 1976;37:1014-23.
48. Whang-Peng J, Bunn PA Jr, Kao-Shan CS, et al. A nonrandom chromosomal abnormality, del 3p(14-23), in human small cell lung cancer (SCLC). Cancer Genet Cytogenet 1982;6:119-34.
49. Dewald G, Dines DE, Weiland LH, Gordon H. Usefulness of chromosome examination in the diagnosis of malignant pleural effusions. N Engl J Med 1976;295:1494-500.
50. Petitjean R, Burghard G, Stampfler G, Fievez M. Une nouvelle observation d'association sclerodermie et cancer alveolaire du poumon. J Fr Med Chir Thorac 1968;22:43-52.
51. Driessen APPM,Scherpenisse LA. Familiair voorkomende diffuse interstitiele longfibrose gecompliceerd door alveolaire-cellen carcinoom. Ned Tijdschr Geneeskd 1970;114:2041-5.
52. Beaumont F, Jansen HM, Elema JD, Ten Kate LP, Sluiter HJ. Simultaneous occurrence of pulmonary interstitial fibrosis and alveolar cell carcinoma in one family. Thorax 1981;36:252-8.
53. Schimke RN. Tumors of the neural crest system. In: Mulvihill JJ, Miller RW, Fraumeni JF Jr, eds, Genetics of human cancer. New York: Raven Press, 1977:179-97.
54. Gordon HW, Miller R Jr, Mittman C. Medullary carcinoma of the lung with amyloid stroma: a counterpart of medullary carcinoma of the thyroid. Hum Pathol 1973;4:431-6.
55. Smith LH. Oat cell carcinoma as a malignant apudoma. J Thorac Cardiovasc Surg 1975; 70:147-51.
56. Nebert DW, Atlas SA. Aryl hydrocarbon hydroxylase induction (Ah locus) as a possible genetic marker for cancer. In: Mulvihill JJ, Miller RW, Fraumeni JF Jr, eds, Genetics of human cancer. New York; Raven Press, 1977;301-18.
57. Kellermann GH, Luyten-Kellermann M, Shaw CR. Genetic variation of aryl hydrocarbon hydroxylase in human lymphocytes. Am J Hum Genet 1973;25:327-31.
58. Kellermann GH, Shaw CR, Luyten-Kellermann M. Aryl hydrocarbon hydroxylase inducibility and bronchogenic carcinoma. N Engl J Med 1973;289:934-7.
59. Kouri RE, McKinney CE, Slomiany DJ, et al. Positive correlation between high aryl hydrocarbon hydroxylases activity and primary lung cancer as analyzed in cryopreserved lymphocytes. Cancer Res 1982;42:5030-7.
60. Kellermann GH. Genetic control of carcinogen metabolism in man. In: Montesano R, Bartsch H, Tomatis L, eds, Screening tests in chemical carcinogenesis. Lyon: International Agency for Research on Cancer, 1976;297-317.
61. Harris CC, Autrup H, Haugen A, Lechner J. Studies of host factors in carcinogenesis using cultured human tissues and cells. In: Bartsch H, Armstrong B, eds, Host factors in human carcinogenesis. Lyon: International Agency for Reseach on Cancer, 1982:497-514.
62. Nebert DW. Pharmacogenetics and human cancer. In: Bartsch H, Armstrong B, eds, Host factors in human carcinogenesis. Lyon: International Agency for Research on Cancer, 1982:365-80.
63. Ashley DJB. Blood groups and lung cancer. J Med Genet 1969;6:183-6.
64. Markman M, Braine HG, Bias WB, Abeloff MD. Association between HLA Bw44 and small cell carcinoma of the lung. N Engl J Med 1982;307:1087.

65. Rogentine GN Jr, Dellon AL, Chretien PB. Prolonged disease-free survival in bronchogenic carcinoma associated with HLA-A19 and HLA-B5. Cancer 1977;39:2345–7.
66. Ford CHJ, Newman CE, MacKintosh P. HLA frequency and prognosis in lung cancer. Br J Cancer 1981;43:610–4.
67. Shimkin MB, Stoner GD. Lung tumors in mice. Adv Cancer Res 1975;21:1–58.
68. Perk K, Hod I. Sheep lung carcinoma: an endemic analogue of a sporadic human neoplasm. JNCI 1982;69:747–9.
69. Saccomanno G, Archer VE, Auerbach O, et al. Susceptibility and resistance to environmental carcinogens in the development of carcinoma of the lung. Hum Pathol 1973;4:487–95.

CHAPTER **12**

Trends in Histologic Types of Lung Cancer, SEER, 1973–1981

CONSTANCE PERCY, JOHN W. HORM, and
THOMAS E. GOFFMAN

National Cancer Institute, Landow 5B06, Bethesda,
Maryland 20205

ABSTRACT

Analysis of the National Cancer Institute's (NCI) Surveillance, Epidemiology and End Results (SEER) lung cancer data (1973–1981) by histologic type shows some interesting changes. The data were divided into the four major histologic groups of the World Health Organization's (WHO) classification scheme. The proportion of squamous cell carcinomas has remained about the same for both males and females. Adenocarcinomas are the predominant histologic type in women. In both males and females the proportion of all lung cancers that are adenocarcinoma has increased about 20% since 1973. This rapidly increasing number of adenocarcinomas in men and women has implications for lung cancer screening and treatment. Small (oat) cell carcinomas, the most lethal type, also have increased in frequency. Although large cell carcinomas were not coded separately before 1977, they represent about 8% of the lung cases. There has been a large decrease in carcinoma, NOS, from over 25% of the lung cases in 1973 to less than 10% in 1981. New treatment for small (oat) cell carcinoma requires that pathologists distinguish between small and large cell carcinomas.
Key Words: Lung cancer incidence, histology trends

Introduction

As discussed in a previous paper (1) the number of small (oat) cell carcinomas of the lung in women increased more than any other histologic type of lung cancer from the early 1950s to the 1970s. Recent data given in that paper were from the National Cancer Institute's (NCI) Surveillance, Epidemiology and End Results (SEER) program (2). Four years of data have been collected since that paper was presented. The purpose of this study is to examine trends of the principal histologic

Verlag Chemie International, Inc.
Lung Cancer: Causes and Prevention.

types of lung cancer for the 9 years 1973 through 1981. Histologic types of cancer in lung are more important than in many other sites because of the different etiologic, clinical, therapeutic, and prognostic features of each morphologic entity. New methods of treatment, especially for small (oat) cell carcinoma, by various combinations of chemotherapeutic agents (3) or of chemotherapy and radiation, have increased the survival of patients with small (oat) cell carcinoma, which has been the most lethal type of lung cancer (4). Because of such changes in therapy for specific cell types of lung cancer it is important that the pathologist be as specific as possible in making the histologic diagnosis.

Methods and Materials

The NCI SEER program was started in 1973 in seven geographic areas of the United States: San Francisco-Oakland, California, Standard Metropolitan Statistical Area (SMSA); Detroit, Michigan, SMSA; and five states: Hawaii, Connecticut, Iowa, New Mexico, and Utah. Although the SEER program has since expanded, the data for this study are only for original areas in order to have comparable data over time. These seven areas represent about 81% of the population of the present nine SEER registries, excluding Puerto Rico. This original group includes about 8% of the total United States white population. There was not a sufficient number of blacks in the original seven areas of the SEER program during these years to allow an assessment of trends in blacks. A future paper on histologic types in blacks covering all sites is in preparation.

All SEER cases are coded by the International Classification of Diseases for Oncology (ICD-O) (5), which embodies the World Health Organization's (WHO) International Histologic Classification of Tumours (6). The original lung classification published by Kreyberg et al (7) has been revised (8) and a comparison of the two is about to be published (9). The revised classification, which differs only slightly from the original, is reflected in the histologic groupings used in this study. Prior to 1977 when ICD-O was first published, the SEER program used the Manual of Tumor Nomenclature and Coding (MOTNAC) (10) for coding the site and histologic type of all cancers. MOTNAC did not have a separate code number for "large cell carcinoma"; therefore, separate data for large cell carcinoma are not available before 1977.

Because this is a study involving histologic types, only microscopically proved cases have been used. Overall in the SEER program 92% of the cases are microscopically confirmed; for lung this figure is slightly lower—87%. In addition, cases diagnosed only at autopsy or by death certificate only were excluded from this analysis. In the early years of the SEER program only 85% of the lung cancers were histologically proved, by 1981, 91% had microscopic proof.

These trends represent changes in the percentage that the number of each histologic type represents of the total number of lung cancers and are not rates of histologic types.

Results

For the 9 years of this study 54,165 microscopically proved lung cancers were reported to the SEER program, 72% were males and 28% females. However, with the rising incidence of female lung cancer, this male–female ratio is decreasing. In 1981 68% of the lung cases were males and 32% were females. Although each final pathologic diagnosis is coded exactly and is available, we have grouped the data according to the four most frequent histologic types of the WHO classification plus carcinomas, not otherwise specified (NOS), and all "other specific types." These four principal categories account for nearly 85% of the cases.

Table 1 and Figure 1 present the data for white males. The relative frequency of squamous cell carcinoma, the predominant histologic type in males, has not changed over this 9-year period and represents about 36% of all lung cancers. The proportion of the total that are small (oat) cell carcinoma has been increasing slightly, from about 13% in the early SEER years to 17% during the last few years. The percentage of adenocarcinoma has increased from 20% in 1973 to 24.6% in 1981, an increase of about 3% per year. The adenocarcinoma group includes bronchiolo-alveolar carcinoma (17%), mucinous or mucin-producing carcinoma (10%), papillary adenocarcinoma (3%), and acinar adenocarcinoma (2%), as well as adenocarcinoma, NOS (68%). As explained earlier separate data on large cell carcinoma were not available until the inception of ICD-O in 1977. In the 5 years from 1977 to 1981 there has been a slight increase in the proportion of large cell carcinoma from 7 to 9% of all lung cancers in males. The largest decrease has been in the category carcinoma, NOS which includes such nonspecific terms as bronchogenic carcinoma, undifferentiated or anaplastic carcinoma, as well as carcinoma, NOS. In order to have comparable figures for carcinoma, NOS from 1973 to 1981, large cell carcinoma was combined in this study with carcinoma, NOS. This group represented over a quarter of the cases in the years 1973, 1974, and 1975. In 1981 this unspecified group was 18%. However, 9% are large cell carcinoma and 9% are carcinoma, NOS. Therefore, there was about a 33% decrease since 1973 in the proportion of carcinoma, NOS including large cell carcinoma. The percentage of other specific histologic types remained at about 2% of the total throughout the years, and the ill-defined group of malignant neoplasms around 1% for nearly all years.

Table 2 and Figure 2 show the histologic distribution for female lung cancers. Again squamous cell carcinoma remains at a fairly constant percentage—about 20–22%. However, it is not the predominant type in females as it is in males. Adenocarcinomas are the most frequent histologic type in females and their proportion of the total has been increasing at about 1.5% annually. Included in this group are bronchiolo-alveolar adenocarcinomas, papillary adenocarcinoma, and mucinous adenocarcinoma, which are all proportionately higher in females. Small (oat cell) carcinoma is also increasing in frequency in females and represents a slightly greater proportion in females than in males. Large cell carcinomas represent about 8% of the total cases, as they do in males. Again the carcinoma, NOS group has shown a large decrease from 26% in 1973 to 17% in 1981. As in males for 1981, half of this figure is large cell carcinoma (8%) and 8.9% are carcinoma, NOS. The differences in the distribution of histologic types for each sex can be seen easily in Figure 3.

Table 1. Percentage distribution of lung cancers[a] from the SEER areas[b], 1973–1981, white males

	Year of diagnosis								
Histology	**1973**	**1974**	**1975**	**1976**	**1977**	**1978**	**1979**	**1980**	**1981**[c]
No. of cases	3736	3871	4046	4155	4336	4511	4601	4787	4742
Squamous cell carcinoma	36.6	37.9	37.7	36.9	37.6	37.8	36.7	35.9	36.2
Small cell carcinoma	13.2	13.8	14.4	14.2	15.8	16.2	16.3	17.2	17.4
Adenocarcinoma	19.9	20.8	19.2	22.2	21.7	23.2	23.5	23.9	24.6
Large cell[d] carcinoma	—	—	—	—	6.8	7.5	8.5	9.4	9.0
Carcinoma, NOS	27.4[d]	24.1[d]	25.5[d]	23.7[d]	14.7	12.4	12.1	10.0	9.0
Neoplasm, NOS	1.1	1.1	1.1	1.0	1.1	0.9	0.8	1.5	1.6
Other specific histologies	1.4	2.0	1.6	1.6	2.0	1.7	1.8	1.7	2.0

[a] Microscopically confirmed cases only.
[b] Seven original SEER areas.
[c] Preliminary data.
[d] Large cell carcinoma was coded with carcinoma, NOS until the inception of ICD-O in 1977.

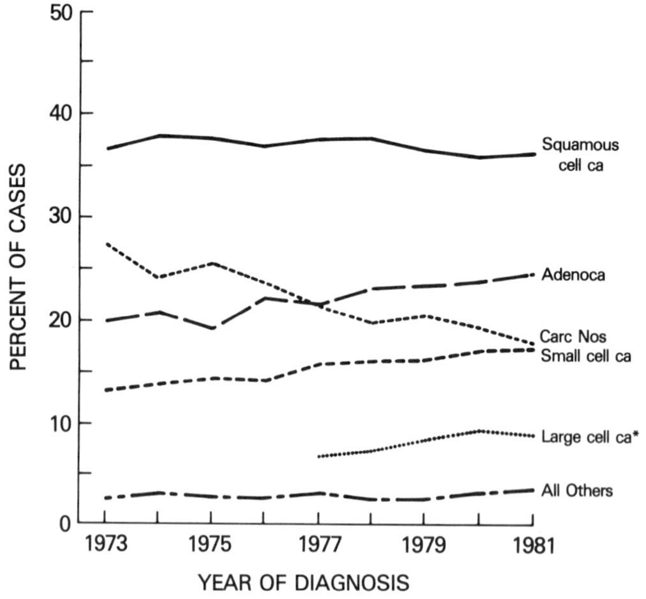

Figure 1. Trends in lung cancer histology, white males, 1973-1981*, Large cell carcinoma is also included with carcinoma, NOS.

Table 2. Percentage distribution of lung cancers[a] from the SEER areas[b], 1973-1981, white females

	Year of diagnosis								
Histology	**1973**	**1974**	**1975**	**1976**	**1977**	**1978**	**1979**	**1980**	**1981[c]**
No. of cases	1163	1298	1479	1551	1696	1878	2038	2046	2231
Squamous cell carcinoma	22.3	22.1	19.8	19.8	20.6	20.8	21.6	20.3	21.5
Small cell carcinoma	16.7	16.4	18.2	16.3	17.1	18.7	18.6	18.3	20.6
Adenocarcinoma	29.4	32.3	34.5	37.4	36.6	35.0	33.4	36.6	34.8
Large cell[d] carcinoma	—	—	—	—	6.9	8.8	9.1	9.4	8.2
Carcinoma, NOS	25.8[d]	24.6[d]	21.9[d]	22.1[d]	14.3	12.5	12.7	11.2	8.9
Neoplasm, NOS	1.2	0.8	1.1	0.9	1.0	0.8	1.2	1.5	2.7
Other specific histologies	4.2	3.5	4.1	3.2	3.2	3.0	3.1	2.4	3.0

[a] Microscopically confirmed cases only.
[b] Seven original SEER areas.
[c] Preliminary data.
[d] Large cell carcinoma was coded with carcinoma, NOS until the inception of ICD-O in 1977.

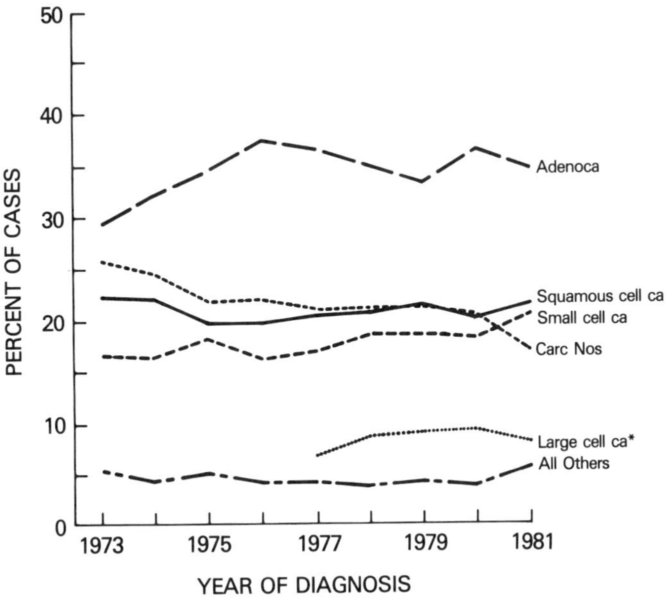

Figure 2. Trends in lung cancer histology, white females, 1973-1981.*, Large cell carcinoma is also included with carcinoma, NOS.

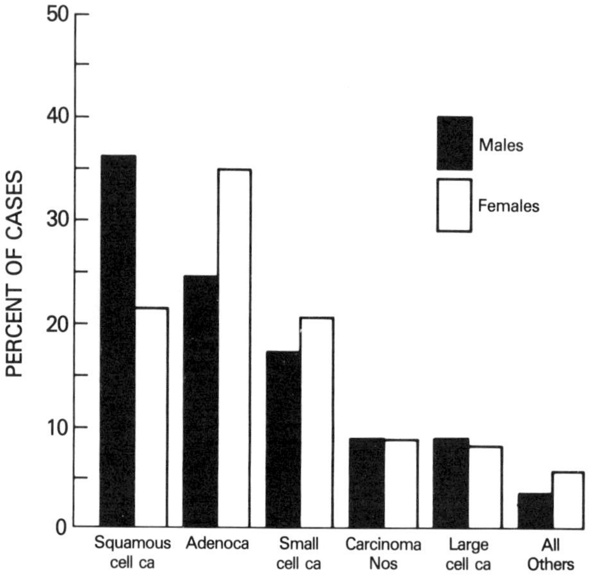

Figure 3. Distribution of SEER lung cancer cases by histology, whites, 1981.

The bottom lines of each table show percentages for other specific histologic types. Although these are a very minor percentage of the total, it is interesting to note that the proportion of female lung cancers classified as other specific histologies is nearly twice that of the males. An examination of the content of this group shows this principally results from malignant carcinoids, which have a greater relative frequency in women than in men.

Although New Orleans is no longer part of the SEER program the distribution of histologic types for the years they participated, 1974–1977, are very similar to those for the rest of the SEER program for both sexes for the corresponding years.

Discussion

Prior to the 1970s small cell carcinoma was a rapidly fatal disease. Considerable progress was made in the early 1970s in the treatment of small cell carcinoma by various combinations of chemotherapeutic agents with or without radiation or other types of treatment. Because the selection of therapy has become more specifically related to the histologic type of lung cancer, some of the observed changes in the relative frequencies of morphologic types can be attributed to the clinician requesting the pathologist to be as specific as possible, ie, to distinguish between small and large cell carcinoma. With a large group of unspecified carcinomas, determining trends for specific histologic types is difficult. The carcinoma, NOS group in the SEER program has decreased significantly over the 9-year period of this study and by 1981 was down to 9% in both men and women as is shown in Figures 1-3. The decrease in unspecified bronchogenic carcinoma, NOS has been noted in individual hospitals before (11), and certainly the SEER data show that a similar trend is also found throughout the country. The average annual percentage increase in the proportion of small (oat) cell carcinoma of the lung in men has been over 3% between 1973 and 1981; women over 2%. A similar increase, but not quite as large, was observed for adenocarcinoma, 3% in males and 1.5% in females. Because squamous and large cell carcinoma are staying fairly constant, it is assumed that those cases formerly diagnosed as carcinoma, NOS are now more specifically diagnosed as small (oat) cell carcinoma or adenocarcinoma.

It should be kept in mind that all changes presented are in terms of percentage of total. The trends in lung cancer, in general, have been increasing, as noted by Dr. Devesa in Chapter 3 of this volume. Analysis is now being completed to assess trends in incidence rates for specific lung cancer cell types.

References

1. Berg JW, Percy C, Horm, J. Recent changes in the pattern of occurrence of oat cell carcinoma of the lung. In: Magnus, K, ed, Trends in cancer incidence. Washington, DC: Hemisphere Publishing, 1982:215-21.
2. Young JL Jr, Percy CL, Asire AJ, eds. Surveillance, Epidemiology, and End Results: incidence and mortality data, 1973-1977. NIH Publ 81-2330, National Cancer Institute Monograph 57, 1981.
3. Greco FA, Einhorn LH, Richardson RL, Oldham RK. Small cell lung cancer: progress and perspectives. Semin Oncol 1978;5:323-35.
4. Weiss RB, Minna JD, Glatstein E, Martini N, Ihde DC, Muggia FM. Treatment of small cell undifferentiated carcinoma of the lung: update of recent results. Cancer Treat Rep 1980;64:539-48.
5. World Health Organization. International classification of diseases for oncology 1976. Geneva: WHO, 1976.
6. World Health Organization. International histological classification of tumours, Nos. 1-25. Geneva: WHO, 1967-1981.
7. Kreyberg L, Leibow AA, Uehlinger EA. Histological typing of lung tumours. International histological classification of tumours, No. 1. Geneva: WHO, 1967.
8. World Health Organization. Histological typing of lung tumours. International histological classification of tumours, No. 1, 2nd ed. Geneva: WHO, 1981.
9. Percy C, Sobin L. Surveillance, Epidemiology and End Results' lung cancer data applied to the World Health Organization's classification of lung tumors. JNCI 1983;70:4.
10. Percy CL, Berg JW, Thomas LB, eds. Manual of tumor nomenclature and coding, 1968 ed. American Cancer Soceity, 1968.
11. Vincent RG, Pickren JW, Lane, WW, et al. The changing histopathology of lung cancer: a review of 1682 cases. Cancer 1977;39:1647-55.

CHAPTER **13**

Screening for Lung Cancer: The Mayo Lung Project

ROBERT S. FONTANA and WILLIAM F. TAYLOR

Department of Medicine, Mayo Medical School, Rochester, Minnesota 55905
Department of Biostatistics, Mayo Medical School, Rochester, Minnesota 55905

ABSTRACT

Screening for lung cancer by chest roentgenography and sputum cytology testing could best be managed in a clinical setting. Cytology testing alone detects fewer than 20% of lung cancers, but sputum-detected cancers have an excellent prognosis. Chest roentgenography may be a more effective detector of early-stage lung cancers than published reports have suggested.

The resectability of lung cancers detected by the Mayo Lung Project (MLP) screening program has been twice that observed in clinical practice at the Mayo Clinic. The proportion of resectable (postsurgical AJC stage 1 or 2) lung cancers detected by the screening program has been more than twice that encountered in clinical practice.

The 5-year lung cancer survival in the MLP screened group has been 40%, compared to 15% in the control group. Although there is no significant difference now in lung cancer mortality rates between the two groups, further observation and evaluation are indicated.
Key Words: **Cancer, lung cancer, screening, sputum, cytology, chest, x-ray**

In 1970 there were 68,000 cases of lung cancer in the United States and 62,000 deaths from the disease. Lung cancer was the leading cancer killer among men, and among women it was exceeded only by breast cancer and colorectal cancer (1).

The great majority of lung cancers in this country could be ascribed to cigarette smoking. Lung cancer was rare among nonsmokers. Therefore, it was largely preventable. Antismoking programs were achieving some success, although not as much as had been hoped (1).

Lung Cancer: Causes and Prevention.

Lung cancer was uncommon among male smokers under 45 years old, but the incidence increased rapidly with age. The "high-risk" group for developing lung cancer consisted primarily of middle-aged and older men who had been chronic, heavy smokers of cigarettes.

Surgical resection was considered the treatment of choice. Other measures were thought to be of little value. Chemotherapy for lung cancer was still in its infancy in 1970.

Lung cancer remains an insidious and frustrating condition. Its early symptoms are nonspecific and simulate chronic bronchial irritation induced by smoking. By the time specific symptoms, such as chest pain, develop the disease is usually advanced and incurable. "Curative" surgical resection has been possible in fewer than 25% of all cases, and the overall 5-year survival rate is 10% or fewer (1–3).

Lung cancer is not one disease but several, each with its own histopathology, clinical manifestations, treatment, and prognosis (4). However about 90% of all lung cancers can be classified pathologically into one of four different cell types, collectively designated "bronchogenic carcinoma" (5). These are squamous (epidermoid) carcinoma, adenocarcinoma, large-cell undifferentiated carcinoma, and small-cell undifferentiated carcinoma. In 1970 at Mayo the squamous type accounted for 40–50% of all bronchogenic carcinomas and each of the other three cell types accounted for 15–20%.

About 60% of squamous cell carcinomas are located centrally, that is, in the hilar regions of the lungs. The remainder are peripheral and exhibit a tendency to cavitate. Of the four major cell types, squamous cancer responds best to surgical treatment and has the best prognosis (2, 6).

Adenocarcinomas and large-cell carcinomas have similar clinical characteristics. Both tend to arise in the peripheral portions of the lungs. Their prognosis is less favorable than the prognosis for squamous cancer (2, 6).

Most small-cell cancers arise in the hilar regions. Only 20% are peripheral. This cell type has a dismal prognosis because of its propensity to disseminate early and widely. Surgical resection alone is rarely helpful. Radiation therapy can provide only palliation. Recently, clinical trials have demonstrated that survival with small-cell cancer can be improved by chemotherapy, but survival time is dreadfully brief (2, 6).

In 1970 it was recognized that if lung cancer could be detected while still apparently localized within the lung it might be resected and that among such cases the 5-year survival following resection approximated 30% (7). It remained to be determined whether mortality rates from lung cancer were actually lower among patients whose tumors were "localized," but detection of lung cancer at a time when it was asymptomatic and apparently localized and resectable was generally viewed as advantageous.

Then as now there were only two tests capable of detecting asymptomatic, "localized," potentially curable lung cancer. These were the chest roentgenogram and the sputum cytology test (8). There was evidence that the two tests tended to complement one another, the chest roentgenogram being better for detecting peripheral tumors and the cytology test better for hilar tumors, especially squamous cell cancers (8). There were anecdotal series of cases that seemed to demonstrate the ability of both tests to detect relatively small, apparently localized lung cancers that were successfully resected, as judged by 5-year survival rates (8–10).

Yet attempts to apply these tests as periodic screening procedures for early detection of lung cancer had not been successful. In 1970 it was widely held that annual chest roentgenography was of no value in detecting curable lung cancer. Results of several uncontrolled evaluations of screening for lung cancer by semiannual photofluorograms were regarded as equivocal at best (11–13).

Only one screening program utilizing both chest roentgenography and sputum cytology testing had been published prior to 1970, and its results were discouraging (14). Moreover, it was difficult to localize roentgenographically unapparent, cytologically detected lung cancers. As noted, these cancers are usually squamous cancers arising in the centrally located bronchi, especially the upper lobe bronchi. Fortunately, the flexible bronchofiberscope, developed in Japan by Ikeda, was introduced into the United States in 1969 (15). This instrument greatly extended the endoscopic field of vision, particularly in the upper lobe areas, thus enabling localization and sampling of small, roentgenographically "occult" bronchial tumors.

In 1970 a preliminary study was conducted at Mayo to evaluate routine cytologic testing of sputum in high-risk patients. Three-day "pooled" collections of sputum were obtained from 58 Mayo Clinic outpatients who were over 45 years old, had negative chest x-ray films, and smoked at least one package of cigarettes daily. Three of these men were found to have cancer cells in the sputum. Two of the three had localized squamous cell cancers that were subsequently resected. The third had a small-cell cancer (L.B. Woolner, unpublished observations, 1970).

Mayo is a clinical center where more than one-quarter million patients are examined each year. Many of these patients come for general medical examinations and are concerned about cancer. Many are cigarette smokers and ask to be checked for lung cancer. In May of 1970, in response to these requests, Mayo's Division of Thoracic Diseases formally recommended that "any man aged 45 years or more who smokes one package of cigarettes or more each day should have a sputum cytology examination as well as a chest x-ray at least once a year" (16). This was and is an empiric recommendation unsupported by statistical proof. However, it was made with the knowledge that the chest x-ray film and the sputum cytology examination were the only tests proved capable of detecting asymptomatic, potentially curable lung cancer. It was also made after results of the preliminary study of sputum cytology testing were known.

At this same time, we became interested in evaluating, under controlled conditions, both chest roentgenography and sputum cytology as screening procedures for early detection of lung cancer. Based upon available data, we were not satisfied that either the 3-day "pooled" sputum cytology examination or the full-size (36 × 43 cm) chest roentgenogram had been adequately tested. Accordingly, a proposal was submitted to the National Cancer Institute (NCI) for a long-term study of screening for early-stage lung cancer using these modalities. The study, designated the Mayo Lung Project (MLP), was funded in 1971 (17).

Similar, but not identical, lung cancer screening programs were sponsored by NCI at the Johns Hopkins Medical Institutions and at the Memorial Sloan-Kettering Cancer Center. Data from all three centers, collectively described as the NCI Cooperative Early Lung Cancer Group, have been monitored at the University of Cincinnati (18).

The goal of the MLP has been to determine whether chest roentgenography and sputum cytology testing, offered every 4 months for 6 years to a group of high-risk Mayo Clinic outpatients undergoing general medical examinations can appreciably reduce the lung cancer death rate in this group compared with a control group not offered regular testing (17).

This report considers the features of an ideal cancer screening program (see Table 1) and comments on how these apply to the MLP. The report also examines certain aspects of the MLP as observed on July 1, 1982, relating them to what was known in 1970.

Feature 1: The Cancer of Concern Should Be Common and Serious

This feature was true for lung cancer in 1970. In 1983 there are predicted to be 135,000 new cases of lung cancer in the United States and 117,000 lung cancer deaths (19). These are double the figures for 1970. Lung cancer now accounts for 25% of all cancer deaths and 5% of total deaths. Deaths from lung cancer approximate those from all accidents, and accidents are the fourth leading cause of death in this country (behind heart disease, cancer, and stroke). Of the more than $27 billion recently estimated as the annual cost of smoking-related illnesses in the United States lung cancer accounted for more than 4 billion (20). Feature 1 was quite certain in 1970, and it is even more so today.

Feature 2: The Cancer Should Have a Prolonged Detectable Preclinical Phase

It is presumed that early (presymptomatic) detection of cancer enables earlier application of treatment and that the earlier treatment is applied, the more likely it is to be effective. In 1970 this was assumed for lung cancer, but the evidence was flimsy (21). It still is. Direct evaluation would have required an unethical experiment in which a random half of patients with early cancers would have received prompt treatment, whereas the remainder would have had treatment delayed.

As with all cancers, there are three phases in the evolution of lung cancer. These are: (a) asymptomatic and undetectable, (b) asymptomatic and detectable (by chest

Table 1. Features of an ideal cancer screening program

1. The cancer of concern should be common and serious.
2. The cancer should have a prolonged detectable preclinical phase.
3. Any new screening program should be applied easily and must be evaluated.
4. The cancer should be concentrated within a high-risk group.
5. Screening must be acceptable and reliable.
6. During their evaluation, screening procedures should not be available to the control group.
7. It should be possible to rapidly localize and treat suspected cancers.
8. Screening should detect significantly more cancers, especially early-stage cancers, than would have been observed if screening had not been undertaken.
9. There should be tangible benefits for those who are screened.
10. The cost-benefit ratio of the screening program should be favorable.

roentgenography and sputum cytology), and (c) symptomatic (that is, clinically evident). By definition, there is no way of accurately measuring the asymptomatic, undetectable phase. It may last several years, considering the usual long interval between the onset of cigarette smoking and the development of overt lung cancer. The asymptomatic detectable phase varies considerably among the four major cell types of lung cancer, being shortest (weeks to months) for most small-cell cancers and longest (years) for most roentgenographically occult squamous cancers and some peripheral, roentgenographically visible adenocarcinomas (9, 11).

Feature 3: Any New Screening Program Should Be Applied Easily and Must Be Evaluated

Careful evaluation is essential. Otherwise we may simply perpetuate erroneous concepts. Lacking direct experimental evaluation of early treatment of cancer, the next best thing is a randomized clinical trial of screening for early cancer, utilizing controls, with death as the endpoint. Those persons identified by screening tend to receive earlier treatment than do unscreened controls; hence an evaluation of screening is an evaluation of early treatment. A randomized clinical trial of screening as a test of early treatment has numerous drawbacks. Notwithstanding, it constitutes the best experiment available for evaluating the effectiveness of early treatment (22). Without concomitant controls it would be impossible to determine whether earlier detection of cancer (and earlier treatment) truly prolonged life or simply identified cancer at an earlier date without affecting total lifespan. In the MLP the need for controls was a paramount consideration.

The MLP used Mayo Clinic outpatients as study and control subjects. There were several reasons for this, including their availability and willingness to cooperate (17). The most important reason for choosing to use Mayo patients was our firm belief that any program aimed at early detection of lung cancer could best be implemented through existing health facilities and primary physicians. In this way patients with proved lung cancer would have their treatment expedited and patients with equivocal test results could be evaluated with a minimum of delays and worries.

Feature 4: The Cancer Should Be Concentrated within a High-Risk Group

For lung cancer, smoking habits, age, and sex constitute an excellent "pre-screen," because middle-aged and older men who are heavy smokers have a much higher incidence of lung cancer than any other available population. Other risk factors are acknowledged, including heredity and environmental and occupational exposures, but these are minor compared to the hazard of cigarette smoking (23).

The design of the MLP is as follows: 10,933 Mayo outpatients who were men over 45 years old without known lung cancer and who were smokers of at least one package of cigarettes daily received 36 × 43 cm chest roentgenograms and 3-day "pooled" sputum cytology tests. If either test proved positive for lung cancer on this initial screening the patient became a "prevalence" case. There were 91 such cases, a prevalence rate of 8.3 per thousand offered the screening. The rate increased rapidly with age, from 1.1 per thousand among men 45–49 years old to 17.1 per thousand among those 65 and older. (These prevalence cases are not considered further in this presentation, which concerns itself primarily with "incidence" cases, detected after initial screenings that were regarded as satisfactory and negative.)

There were 9211 men who completed the initial screen with results that were reported as satisfactory and negative and who met certain other criteria for continued screening (life expectancy at least 5 years, mentally competent, pulmonary resection—at least lobectomy—possible). These men were subsequently studied in two randomized groups.

The screened group of 4618 patients was asked, and reminded, to have chest roentgenograms and 3-day "pooled" sputum cytology tests at 4-monthly intervals for a period of 6 years. Intensive efforts were made to secure compliance. After the 6 years of screening, contact with each patient in the group was made yearly by letter.

The control group of 4953 patients received only the standard 1970 Mayo recommendation concerning yearly chest x-ray films and sputum tests. No reminders about tests were sent, but contact was maintained by annual followup letter.

Feature 5: Screening Must Be Acceptable and Reliable

Each patient in the 4-monthly screened group was considered with respect to the length of time he had been participating in the MLP. A determination was then made of the number of chest roentgenograms and sputum tests he should have completed during this time. The number of expected completed tests was then compared with the actual number completed. During the first year of the MLP 85% of tests expected were completed, but by the fifth year the figure had dropped to 75%. It subsequently leveled off between 70 and 75%. The response of the controls to the annual followup letter was a constant 98% (22). Although these findings compare quite favorably with the compliance observed in other screening programs, noncompliance diluted the difference between the screened and the control groups.

It was of interest that in the MLP the death rates from lung cancer and from all other causes were much higher among the noncompliant than among the compliant patients. This phenomenon also has been observed in other cancer screening programs (24, 25).

Mention has been made of the fact that the chest x-ray film and the sputum cytology test complement each other in detecting asymptomatic lung cancer. Sufficiently advanced, roentgenographically visible lung cancers of any of the four major cell types may be associated with the presence in the sputum of cancer cells of that same type. Roentgenographically occult lung cancers, on the other hand, almost invariably are squamous cancers originating in the subsegmental or larger central bronchi (15).

Both tests are painless and safe. The radiation exposure secondary to a well-collimated 36 × 43 cm chest x-ray examination obtained at 140 kV is insignificant (18). Both tests are relatively inexpensive when compared to the cost of a 4-months' supply of cigarettes. Both tests are simple to perform, but the interpretations can be difficult. Control of quality is essential. Dual readings of chest films enhance accuracy (26).

Sensitivity and specificity, the traditional measures of the effectiveness of screening procedures, are difficult to measure in the MLP. The chest roentgenogram is a very versatile test, accounting for approximately half of all radiologic procedures. It is considerably more sensitive for lung cancer than is sputum cytology, but cytology is highly specific for squamous cancer. Combined, the two tests have a reasonable positive predictive value for lung cancer in the high-risk group (W.F. Taylor, unpublished observations, 1983).

Feature 6: During Their Evaluation, Screening Procedures Should not Be Available to the Control Group

This has become a source of particular concern to the MLP. The value of any cancer screening test can be more easily determined if, during the period of assessment, that test is not available to control subjects through other sources, such as private physicians. During the controlled study of mammography as a screening device for breast cancer, this procedure was not widely utilized in clinical practice (25). Even now there is little sputum cytology testing of asymptomatic patients with negative chest x-ray films. However, nearly 100 million chest x-ray examinations are performed in the United States each year, and middle-aged and older men who have been heavy smokers undoubtedly receive more than their share (27). Such men are candidates not only for lung cancer, but also for a variety of other common conditions for which chest roentgenography is indicated, including coronary artery disease, hypertension, obstructive pulmonary disease, and respiratory infections (27).

We have estimated that at least 50% of MLP control patients receive chest roentgenograms each year. About one-third of all lung cancers in the control group have been detected in the asymptomatic phase by "accidental" chest films. "Contamination" of this sort further reduces the contrast between the controls and the screened group.

Feature 7: It Should be Possible to Rapidly Localize and Treat Suspected Cancers

Vital to any lung cancer screening program is the presence of easily accessible, highly qualified medical facilities where patients with suspected cancer can receive prompt diagnostic workups, appropriate treatment, and adequate followup. It is for this reason that we endorse the concept of early detection of lung cancer within the framework of the general medical examination, with referral as indicated. This allows maximal utilization of existing medical resources and insures continuity of care.

In the MLP the control cases of lung cancer tended to be more advanced when detected and consequently were treated faster than the cancers in the screened group. About half of the control cancers were treated within 2 weeks of detection and 90% within 1 month. Among the cancers in the screened group, half were treated within 1 month and 90% within 3 months (22). The time from detection of the tumor to its localization and treatment was particularly long for those cases in the screened group that were roentgenographically occult. Recently, hematoporphyrin derivative, a photoactive compound that concentrates within cancer cells and acts as an endobronchial tumor marker, has greatly expedited localization of these occult cancers (28).

Feature 8: Screening Should Detect Significantly More Cancers, Especially Early-Stage Cancers, Than Would Have Been Observed If Screening Had not Been Undertaken

An effective cancer screening program should detect early-stage, asymptomatic, curable cancers which, without screening, would in time become advanced, symptomatic, and incurable.

A successful randomized clinical trial of cancer screening would proceed as follows: (a) During the screening period the number of cancers in the screened group would become progressively larger than the number in the control group. The excess number in the screened group would be composed primarily of early-stage cancers detected by the screen. (b) During the postscreening period the numbers of cancers in the two groups eventually would equalize, mainly because of the appearance of larger numbers of advanced, symptomatic cancers in the control group. (c) Ultimately, there would be significantly more cancer deaths in the control group than in the screened group. However, at any time during the course of the trial, data would be more current and complete for the screened group than for the controls, because the screened group would be under closer surveillance.

The MLP randomized clinical trial of screening for early lung cancer has now been in progress for more than a decade. Disregarding lead time bias, it is evident that data concerning the patients in the 4-monthly screened group, who have become conditioned to notify us of any change in status, are considerably more current than are data on the controls, with whom contact is made only once a year. To compensate for this difference we have "backdated" by a year all information relating to MLP "incidence" lung cancers (those detected among the 9211 randomized patients whose initial, or "prevalence," screens were considered negative). Thus incidence data reported July 1, 1982, refer only to cancers discovered prior to July 1, 1981, but include all information about these cancers known to us on July 1, 1982.

From the beginning of the MLP the incidence cases of lung cancer in the 4-monthly screened group have outnumbered the cases in the control group. On July 1, 1982, when MLP statistics were backdated to July 1, 1981, 145 incidence cases had been documented in the 4-monthly screened group, a rate of 4.8 per thousand man-years of surveillance. In the control group there were 124 cases, or 4.1 per thousand man-years.

Unfortunately, 32 (22%) of the cancers in the 4-monthly group and 33 (27%) of the cancers in the control group were of the small-cell type, which has an extremely poor prognosis that is not helped by screening. Only 50 (35%) of the 4-monthly cancers and 40 (32%) of the control cancers were of the more favorable squamous type. This distribution is quite different and much less encouraging than that anticipated in 1970.

In the 4-monthly group 80 (55%) of the 145 cancers were detected by the screening tests. There were 58 cancers detected by roentgenography alone, 16 by cytology alone, and 6 by both modalities, confirming that the two screening tests do complement each other in the detection of asymptomatic lung cancer. Of the remaining 65 cancers in the 4-monthly group, approximately one-third were detected between screening ("interval" cases), one-third occurred in men who were noncompliant with screening ("dropouts"), and one-third in men who had completed their 6 years of screening.

Almost 90% of the incidence cancers that were detected cytologically were resected (all cytologically detected cancers were squamous). Of greater significance, perhaps, was the observation that two-thirds of the 85 cancers in the 4-monthly group who were detected roentgenographically, either by screening films or "accidentally" (by nonstudy films), were resectable.

Nearly one-third of the control cancers were detected by "accidental" chest films, and three-fourths of these were resectable. This "contamination" of the control group does not appear to be the result of deliberate "self-screening" by control patients, as may be suspected in this highly motivated population. Instead, there is evidence that control patients tend to receive chest films because of other circumstances, including noncancerous illnesses that tend to occur with increasing frequency as these smokers grow older (17).

There were 44 cancers in the 4-monthly group and 86 in the control group that were discovered after patients developed symptoms of lung cancer. Only 11% of these cancers were resectable. Symptomatic lung cancer is almost always fatal.

The overall resectability of the 4-monthly incidence cancers was 52%. The resectability of the control cancers was 31%. In clinical practice at Mayo, lung cancer resectability is between 25 and 30% or about half the resectability observed among the 4-monthly incidence cancers (29).

Considering deaths from lung cancer only, the 5-year survival of the cytologically detected cases was more than 80%, and the 5-year survival of the roentgenographically detected cases, almost 50%. The survival of the symptomatic cases at 4 years was about 5%. As a group, the asymptomatic patients whose cancers were detected by one of the testing procedures did well, whereas the symptomatic patients did very poorly. This observation applies not just to the MLP. but to all lung cancers observed at Mayo (29) (J.H. Pemberton, D.M. Nagorney, J.C. Gilmore, W.F. Taylor, P.E. Bernatz, unpublished observations, 1982).

In the 4-monthly group nearly half the cancers were localized and resectable, that is, they were classified as postsurgical stage 1 or 2 according to the staging system of the American Joint Committee for Cancer Staging and End-Results Reporting (AJC) (6). Only one-fourth of the cancers in the control group were postsurgical stage 1 or 2. In contemporary Mayo experience less than 20% of all lung cancers have been so classified (29).

The 5-year survival rate (lung cancer deaths only) of patients in the 4-monthly group who had postsurgical AJC stage 1 or 2 cancers was approximately 70% (it was somewhat lower in the control group, possibly because of less detailed surgical staging in this group). The 5-year survival of patients with stage 3 or unresected cancers in both groups was less than 10%. Staging (especially postsurgical–pathologic staging) seems to be a fairly accurate procedure for estimating survival.

Yet it will be recalled that in a successful cancer screening program one should find not only more early-stage cancers in the screened group but also, eventually, more advanced cancers in the control group. On July 1, 1982 (backdated to July 1, 1981) there were 78 cases of AJC stage 3 (and unresectable) cancers in the 4-monthly screened group and 92 in the control group.

The failure to observe a substantial difference in the advanced and unresectable cancers in the two groups has been a disappointment. There are still 21 fewer cancers in the control group, and some of these ultimately should surface as advanced and unresectable, but time may be running out. It would appear that there may be two populations of lung cancers in the MLP, a larger one for which screening (or treatment) is of little value and a smaller one for which screening and treatment may be helpful. This concept has been advanced by others (30). Regardless of that, the proportion of MLP incidence cases surviving lung cancer at 5 years was 40% in the 4-monthly group and 15% in the control group. These results might have been predicted from the distribution of the various AJC stages of the cancers in the two groups.

Feature 9: There Should Be Tangible Benefits for Those Who Are Screened

The benefits of screening for lung cancer would be a reduction in morbidity or mortality from the disease. In this presentation only mortality is considered.

According to MLP data available on July 1, 1982 (backdated to July 1, 1981) both the 4-monthly screened group and the control group had been under observation for approximately 30,000 man-years. The death rate (per thousand man-years) from all causes was 23 in the 4-monthly group and 22.5 in the control group. The death rate from lung cancer was 2.6 in the 4-monthly group and 2.7 among the controls. These differences are insignificant.

When considered from the standpoint of duration of participation in the MLP, the yearly lung cancer death rates in the two groups were almost identical during each of the first 6 years. In the seventh and eighth years of the study, the lung cancer death rates in the control group were somewhat higher. Further observation should resolve this issue.

Feature 10: The Cost–Benefit Ratio of the Screening Program Should Be Favorable

Screening must not only reduce lung cancer morbidity or mortality, but also it must do so at an acceptable cost. At present this aspect of screening for lung cancer is irrelevant to the MLP, because the screening program itself has not yet been shown to be beneficial. However, if it finally proves to be effective, then we believe that it can be made cost effective by implementing it in a clinical setting.

Discussion

It has been stated that randomized clinical trials are time consuming, tedious, expensive, and often outdated by the time they are completed and reported. Nevertheless, if they are well conceived and conducted, they provide reliable information (not always the desired information, but reliable). Moreover, if the data are meticulously collected and collated, the truth will out.

The MLP is entering its followup period, and in many respects its most active phase. As it does, the truth is beginning to unfold and the data are becoming understandable. This applies particularly to the persistent failure to demonstrate a significant difference in lung cancer mortality between the 4-monthly screened group and the control group. An appreciable difference may yet develop, for there is still a discrepancy between the total number of lung cancer cases in the two groups. Furthermore, the predicted sequence of events in the MLP screening has proceeded at a much slower pace than was anticipated at the outset.

However, it must also be acknowledged that there have been other factors, not all foreseen, that have exerted a negative influence upon the study. There have been frustrations associated with the 25% noncompliance of the 4-monthly group with the screening program, the "contamination" of the control group, the higher than expected incidence of small-cell cancer, and the lower than assumed incidence of squamous cancer. There have been uncertainties surrounding the "information lag" in ascertaining the status of the control group. There have been worries over the effect of competing death risks, especially heart disease, on an aging smoking population. There have been reservations about the precision of the AJC cancer staging system and the degree of effectiveness of treatment, including surgical resection. There have been concerns regarding the occurrence of multiple primary cancers and the possibility that some cancers, notably roentgenographically occult cancers, do not behave in a very malignant fashion.

Fortunately, because the MLP has been conducted conscientiously, the relative importance of most of these factors ultimately will be determined. At present, the following observations seem pertinent.

1. Screening for lung cancer by chest roentgenography and sputum cytology testing has been conducted unobtrusively and effectively in a clinical setting.
2. Screening by these modalities has been accepted by Mayo Clinic patients.
3. Sputum cytology testing detects fewer cancers than had been expected (less than 20%), but sputum detected cancers tend to have an excellent prognosis.
4. Chest roentgenography may be a more effective detector of early-stage lung cancer than published reports have suggested.
5. The resectability of cancers detected by the MLP screening program has been twice that observed in clinical practice at Mayo.
6. The proportion of postsurgical AJC stage 1 or 2 cancers in the MLP 4-monthly screened group has been more than twice that encountered in clinical practice.
7. The 5-year lung cancer survival in the 4-monthly screened group has been 40%, compared to 15% in the control group.
8. While as yet there is no significant difference in lung cancer mortality between the MLP 4-monthly screened group and the control group, further observation seems indicated.

Now is obviously not the time to recommend large-scale radiologic or cytologic programs of screening for lung cancer. Because these programs usually are initiated by those who conduct the screening, they should benefit the screened by reducing lung cancer morbidity or mortality. It has not yet been demonstrated that screening can do this.

Neither does it seem appropriate now to withhold the only two tests proved capable of detecting asymptomatic lung cancer from patients who request general medical examinations, particularly patients in the high-risk category. To do so should require clear-cut evidence of lack of benefit, and this has not been demonstrated, either.

It seems reasonable now to allow application of the two tests to rest in the hands of the individual physician caring for the individual patient. The physician may obtain the tests during the examination of a high-risk patient if he or she believes they are indicated and the patient agrees. Advantages and disadvantages of testing should be discussed with the patient, as should all aspects of the medical examination. At the same time, any patient still smoking cigarettes should be informed of the risks of continuing and strongly advised to quit. Assistance in quitting also should be offered.

Acknowledgments

Work reported here was supported by Research Contract CN-53886 from the National Institutes of Health.

References

1. American Cancer Society. 1970 Cancer Facts and Figures. New York, ACS, 1969.
2. Fontana, RS. A national correspondence course on lung cancer and asbestos-related pulmonary disease. Chicago: American College of Chest Physicians, 1981.
3. Vincent RG, Takita H, Lane WW, Gutierrez AC, Pickren JW. Surgical therapy of lung cancer. J Thorac Cardiovasc Surg 1976;71:581–91.
4. Sobin LH. The WHO histological classification of lung tumors: rev ed. In: Wilkinson PM, ed, Advances in medical oncology, research and education, vol. II. Oxford: Pergamon Press, 1979:5–8.
5. Clagett OT, Allen TH, Payne WS, Woolner LB. The surgical treatment of pulmonary neoplasms: a 10-year experience. J Thorac Cardiovasc Surg 1964;48:391–400.
6. American Joint Committee for Cancer Staging and End-Results Reporting. Staging of lung cancer 1979. Chicago, 1979.
7. National Cancer Institute. Cancer patient survival report No. 5. Publ 77–992. U.S. Department of Health, Education and Welfare, Besthesda, Md: NCI, 1976
8. Davies DF. A review of detection methods for the early diagnosis of lung cancer. J Chronic Dis 1966;19:819–45.
9. Woolner LB, David E, Fontana RS, Andersen HA, Bernatz PE. In situ and early invasive bronchogenic carcinoma: report of 28 cases with postoperative survival data. J Thorac Cardiovasc Surg 1970;60:275–90.
10. Jackman RJ, Good CA, Clagett OT, Woolner LB. Survival rates in peripheral bronchogenic carcinomas up to four centimeters in diameter presenting as solitary pulmonary nodules. J Thorac Cardiovasc Surg 1969;57:1–8.
11. Weiss W, Boucot KR, Seidman H. The Philadelphia Pulmonary Neoplasm Research Project. Clin Chest Med 1982;3:243–56.
12. Brett GZ: Earlier diagnosis and survival in lung cancer. Br Med J 1969;4:260–2.
13. Nash FA, Morgan JM, Tomkins JG. South London lung cancer study. Br Med J 1968;2:715–21.
14. Lilienfeld A, Archer PG, Burnett CH, et al. An evaluation of radiologic and cytologic screening for the early detection of lung cancer: a cooperative pilot study of the American Cancer Society and the Veterans Administration. Cancer Res 1966;26:2083–121.
15. Fontana RS. Editorial. The needle in the haystack. Mayo Clin Proc 1978;53:616–7.
16. Mayo Staff Newsletter, May 22, 1970;7:1.
17. Fontana RS, Sanderson DR, Woolner LB, et al. The Mayo Lung Project for early detection and localization of bronchogenic carcinoma: a status report. Chest 1975;67:511–22.

18. National Cancer Institute. Manual of procedures, National Cancer Institute Cooperative Early Lung Cancer Group, 2nd ed, rev. NIH Publ 79-1972. Bethesda, Md: National Institutes of Health, 1972.
19. American Cancer Society 1983 Cancer Facts and Figures. New York: ACS, 1982.
20. Luce RB, Schweitzer SO. Editorial. Smoking and alcohol abuse: a comparison of their economic consequences. N Engl J Med 1978;298:569-71.
21. Ball WC Jr. Editorial. The effect of surgical treatment on the natural history of lung cancer. Am Rev Respir Dis 1983;127:1.
22. Taylor WF, Fontana RS, Uhlenhopp MA, Davis CS. Some results of screening for early lung cancer. Cancer 1981;47:1114-20.
23. Doll R, Peto R. The causes of cancer: quantitative estimates of avoidable risks of cancer in the United States today. JNCI 1981;66:1191-308.
24. Boucot KR, Seidman H, Weiss W. The Philadelphia Pulmonary Neoplasm Research Project: the risk of lung cancer in relation to symptoms and roentgenographic abnormalities. Environ Res 1977;13:451-69.
25. Fink R, Shapiro S, Lewison J. The reluctant participant in a breast cancer screening program. Public Health Rep 1968;6:479-90.
26. Yerushalmy J. The statistical assessment of the variability in observer perception and description of roentgenographic pulmonary shadows. Radiol Clin North Am 1969;7:381-92.
27. Population exposure to x-rays, U.S. 1970. Washington DC: U.S. Department of Health, Education and Welfare. Public Health Service, Food and Drug Administration, 1970.
28. Cortese DA, Kinsey JH, Woolner LB, Sanderson DR, Fontana RS. Hematoporphyrin derivative in the detection and localization of radiographically occult lung cancer. Am Rev Respir Dis 1982;126:1087-8.
29. Williams DE, Pairolero PC, Davis CS, et al. Survival of patients surgically treated for stage I lung cancer. J Thorac Cardiovasc Surg 1981;82:70-6.
30. Rossing TH, Rossing RG. Survival in lung cancer: an analysis of the effects of age, sex, resectability and histopathologic type. Am Rev Respir Dis 1982;126:771-7.

CHAPTER **14**

Lung Cancer in Japan: Effects of Nutrition and Passive Smoking

TAKESHI HIRAYAMA

Epidemiology Division, National Cancer Center, Research Institute, Tsukiji 5-chome, Chuo-ku, Tokyo 104, Japan

ABSTRACT

Lung cancer is on a sharp increase in both men and women in Japan. Nonsmoking wives with smoking husbands were found to carry an elevated risk of lung cancer and ischemic heart disease by a large-scale cohort study, 1966-1981, for 265,118 adults in 29 Health Center Districts in Japan, the risk steadily going up with the increase in number of cigarettes smoked by the husband. In major cancers other than lung, no such risk elevation was observed. A nonsmoking husband with a smoking wife also showed an elevated risk of lung cancer. The risk-reducing effect of daily intake of green–yellow vegetables on lung cancer was observed for passive smoking just as for active smoking. Those women eating green–yellow vegetables daily showed a significantly lower risk of lung cancer from the passive influence of their husbands' smoking. Such risk reduction was not observed for ischemic heart disease. The observed results suggest that the influence of husband's smoking on nonsmoking wives in raising the risk of lung cancer is as a cancer promoter rather than a cancer initiator. This promoter hypothesis may explain why such continuous but low-dose exposure of passive smoking, which starts after adult age is reached, significantly elevates lung cancer risk in nonsmoking wives.

Key Words: **Japan, cohort study, passive smoking, lung cancer, ischemic heart disease, green–yellow vegetables, β-carotene, promoter, promoter–inhibitor**

Lung Cancer: Causes and Prevention.

Introduction

The mortality from lung cancer has been increasing rapidly in Japan (Figure 1). The number of deaths among males was 520 in 1947 and 17,555 in 1982, the corresponding number for females was 248 and 6661.

There exists little sign of a slowing down of the rate of increase, and the number of deaths from lung cancer are expected to exceed the number of deaths from stomach cancer in the near future. In parallel to this trend the number of cigarettes sold in Japan also has been on a sharp rise (Figure 1). The random sample survey conducted by the Tobacco Monopoly Corporation in 1982 revealed that currently 70.1% of adult males and 15.4% of adult females smoke in Japan.

The purpose of this chapter is to study the causative factors of lung cancer in Japan with special reference to the effect of passive smoking relative to the effect of active smoking. The possible influence of nutrition, β-carotene-rich green–yellow vegetables in particular, on the risk enhancing effect of active and passive smoking also is studied.

Methods

The materials of our ongoing large-scale cohort study for 265,118 adults aged 40 years and above in Japan were analyzed in detail to discover factors altering the

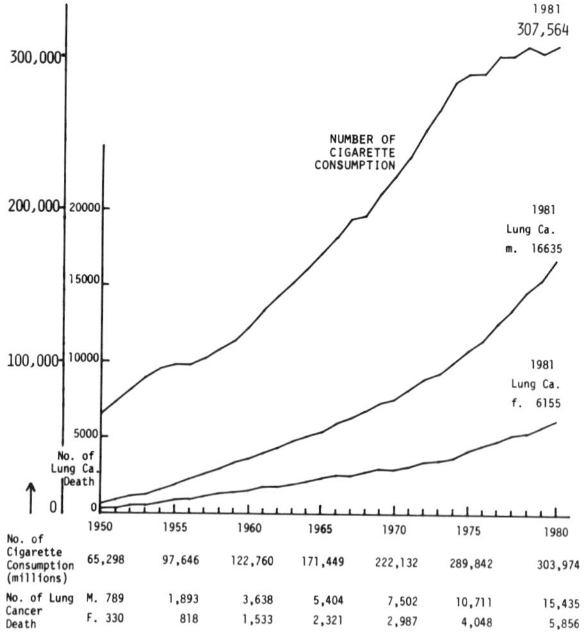

Figure 1. Trends in cigarette consumption and lung cancer deaths in Japan (1950–1981).

risk of lung cancer in both men and women. For statistical analysis, programs included in the book *Epidemiologic Analysis with a Programmable Calculator* (U.S. Department of Health, Education and Welfare, 1979) mainly were used.

Results

Active Smoking and Lung Cancer Risk

Cigarette smoking was identified by far the most important cause of lung cancer in Japan, both by case-control studies conducted by the author and other researchers and by a large-scale cohort study (1-6) being conducted by the author for 265,118 adults (122,261 men and 142,857 women) aged 40 and above (95% of census population) in 29 Health Center Districts in Japan. These subjects were surveyed in October-December 1965 and followed up from January 1966 until December 1981. A clear-cut dose-response relationship was observed between the number of cigarettes ever smoked and the age-standardized mortality rate of lung cancer. The mortality rate of lung cancer also was found to be higher the earlier smoking was begun when age and total number of cigarettes ever smoked were standardized (Figure 2). The lung cancer-standardized mortality rate was observed

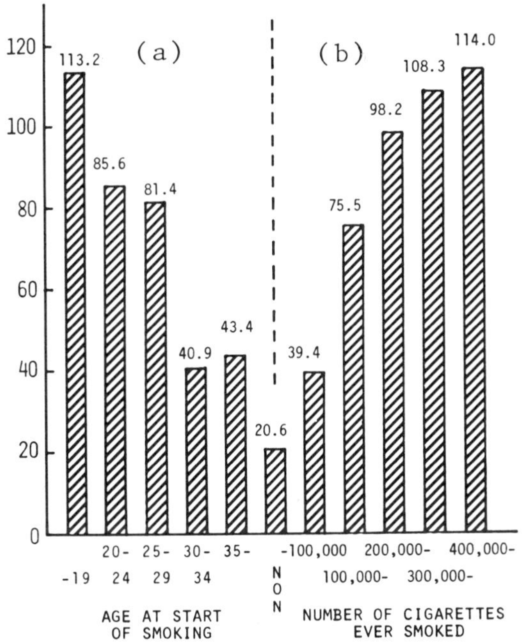

Figure 2. Lung Cancer. (a) Attained age- and amount of smoking-standardized mortality rate by age at start of smoking. (b) Attained age- and age at start of smoking-standardized mortality rate by total amount of cigarettes ever smoked. (Prospective study, 1966–1978 Japan.)

to be 18.3% lower in smokers who do not inhale compared to regular deep inhalers, and 48.9% lower in smokers of filtertip cigarettes compared to smokers of nonfiltertip cigarettes, according to our cohort study. The risk of lung cancer in daily smokers also was noted to approach gradually that of nonsmokers with the lapse of years after smoking cessation, risk difference diminishing by 41.6% in 5 years after stopping the habit. This strongly suggests the major part of the influence of smoking during adulthood is the promoter action of substances included in mainstream smoke.

Effect of Nutrition on Active Smokers

Daily intake of green-yellow vegetables, rich in β-carotene, was found significantly to lower the risk of lung cancer (7, 8), particularly when the total amount of cigarettes ever smoked was less than 300,000 (6) (Figure 3). No other dietary habit showed such risk reduction. Risk reduction after smoking cessation appeared to be more pronounced in case of daily consumers of green-yellow vegetables. Taking similar evidence in laboratory studies into consideration, a promoter-inhibitor interaction model was conceptualized.

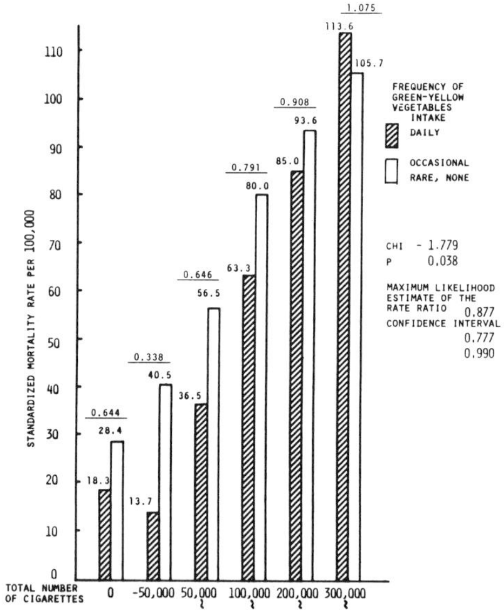

				0	-50,000	50,000	100,000	200,000	300,000
OBSERVED PERSON-YEARS				185433	16123	69253	276835	217364	148883
				61380	4965	25946	107886	87944	68999
LUNG CANCER DEATHS	GREEN-YELLOW VEGETABLES INTAKE	DAILY	OBS.	34	3	25	175	185	169
			EXP.	39.2	3.0	28.0	174.5	190.2	155.1
		OTHERS	OBS.	17	2	15	86	82	73
			EXP.	14.8	1.0	12.0	77.5	87.8	81.9

THE HETEROGENECITY CHI-SQUARE 5.925 N = 5
TWO-SIDED P = 0.314

Figure 3. Standardized mortality rate for lung cancer by total number of cigarettes ever smoked and by frequency of green-yellow vegetable intake; males. (Prospective study, 1966–1978.)

Passive Smoking and Lung Cancer

In the present cohort study (1966–1981), 427 deaths from lung cancer in women were recorded during 16 years of followup (1966–1981). Of these women, 269 were married, and 200 of these also were nonsmokers. These cases occurred among 91,540 nonsmoking married women whose husbands' smoking habits were studied. The risk of lung cancer was carefully measured, taking into consideration possible confounding variables. There was a statistically significant increased risk in relation to the extent of the husband's smoking (Figure 4), which confirmed the validity of previous reports (9, 10). The association was significant when observed by age of husbands (Table 1, Figures 1 and 5) and also by age of wives (Table 2). The further detailed analysis on materials cross-tabulated by age and occupation of the husband also confirmed the association (Table 3). The husband's drinking habits were noted to have no effect in raising the risk of lung cancer in nonsmoking wives (Table 4).

Similar significant risk elevation of lung cancer with the increase in the extent of husband's smoking also was observed with ischemic heart disease when observed by husband's age and occupation (Tables 5 and 6). The significant risk elevation of cancer of the nasal sinus also was observed in nonsmoking wives with husband's smoking. The risk elevation of emphysema and chronic bronchitis with spouse's smoking also was noted with borderline significance. However there was no tendency of risk elevation at all in major cancers other than lung (total of cancers of stomach, cervix, and breast), the standardized mortality rate in nonsmoking wives being almost exactly the same regardless of the husband's smoking habit (Table 7, Figure 6).

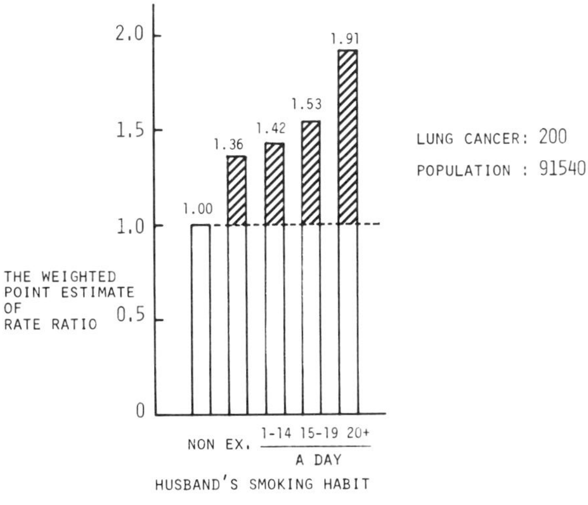

Figure 4. Age-standardized mortality rate ratio for lung cancer in nonsmoking wives by smoking habits of their husbands. (Prospective study, 1966–1981, Japan.)

Table 1. Mortality rate for lung cancer in women by age group and by smoking habit of husband (patient herself a nonsmoker): prospective study, 1966–1981, Japan[a]

Husband's age group	Husband's smoking habit: Nonsmoker		Ex-smoker		Number of cigarettes a day: 1-14/d		15-19/d		20+/d		Total	
	No.	Pop.	No.	Pop.	No.	Pop.	No.	Pop.	No.	Pop.	No.	Pop.
40–49	4	6,229	1	1,255	8	8,621	6	5,158	16	10,764	35	32,027
50–59	10	7,791	3	1,922	20	9,668	8	4,052	24	9,820	65	33,253
60–69	18	7,120	11	2,687	28	7,243	9	2,513	23	4,651	89	24,214
70–79	5	755	2	348	2	612	1	105	1	226	11	2,046
Total	37	21,895	17	6,212	58	26,144	24	11,828	64	25,461	200	91,540

	Nonsmoker	Ex-smoker	1-14/d	15-19/d	20+/d	
[a]The weighted point estimate of rate ratio and test-based 90% confidence limits		2.18	2.01	2.38	2.71	
	1.00	1.36	1.42	1.58	1.91	
		0.85	1.01	0.98	1.34	
(1-19/d)				2.02		Mantel extension χ^2 2.915
			1.45			one-tail
				1.04		p value 0.00178
Mantel-Haenszel χ^2	—	1.0855	1.8290		3.0295	
one-tail p value		0.1389	0.0337		0.0012	

Table 2. Mortality rate for lung cancer in nonsmoking wives by smoking habit of husbands and by age group of wife: prospective study; 1966-1981, Japan[a]

Wife's age group	Husband's smoking habit: Nonsmoker		Ex-smoker / Number of cigarettes a day: 1-19/d		20+/d		Total	
	No.	Pop.	No.	Pop.	No.	Pop.	No.	Pop.
40–49	4	7.918	21	17,492	21	12,615	46	38,025
50–59	14	7,635	46	15,640	31	8,814	91	32,089
60–69	16	6,170	31	10,381	10	3,793	57	20,344
70–79	3	172	1	671	2	239	6	1,082
Total	37	21,895	99	44,184	64	25,461	200	91,540

	Nonsmoker	Ex-smoker 1-19/d	20+/d	
[a]The weighted point estimate of rate ratio and test-based 90% confidence limits		2.01	2.55	
	1.00	1.43	1.74	
		0.99	1.19	Mantel extension χ^2 2.424
Mantel-Haenszel χ^2	—	1.6042	2.3731	one-tail
one-tail p value		0.0543	0.0088	p value 0.00768

Table 3. Mortality rate for lung cancer in women by age, occupation, and smoking habit of husbands (patient herself a nonsmoker)[a]

Husbands age (year)	Occupation[b]	Nonsmoker		Ex-smoker or 1–19/day		≥ 20/day	
		No.	Pop.	No.	Pop.	No.	Pop.
40–49	Total	4	6,229	15	15,034	16	10,764
	1		324		653	1	566
	2		90		231		293
	3	1	908	2	2,247	3	1,867
	4	1	476	1	993		1,044
	5	1	2,502	6	5,941	9	3,636
	6		46		165		108
	7		177	1	486	1	426
	8		1,112	3	3,431	2	2,241
	9		162	1	345		243
	10	1	432	1	542		340
50–59	Total	10	7,791	31	15,642	24	9,820
	1	1	345		593	2	446
	2		175		253	1	319
	3	1	817	5	1,764	1	1,324
	4	1	653	2	1,133	5	1,092
	5	4	3,497	16	6,812	9	3,514
	6		35		89		50
	7		120		273	1	234
	8	3	1,375	6	3,478	2	2,155
	9		164		378	1	251
	10		610	2	869	2	435
60–69	Total	18	7,120	48	12,443	23	4,651
	1		227	1	327	1	179
	2	1	91		143		124
	3		305	2	594	2	327
	4	2	508	5	822	1	500
	5	13	4,084	33	6,845	10	2,152
	6		9		31		14
	7		45		82		55
	8	1	805	5	1,784	4	736
	9		121	1	208		92
	10	1	925	1	1,607	5	472
70 +	Total	5	755	5	1,065	1	226
	1		32		30		5
	2		21		14		4
	3		18	1	36		8
	4		48		73		20
	5	3	323	1	446		89
	6		1		1		0
	7		1		5		1
	8		87	2	119	1	36
	9		11		19		2
	10	2	213	1	322		61
[a] Standardized Risk Ratios		1.000		1.436		1.872	

Mantel extension χ^2: 3.124; one-tail p value: 0.00089.

[b] Occupation: 1, Professional and technical workers; 2, managers and officials; 3, clerical and related workers; 4, sales workers; 5, farmers, lumbermen, and fishermen; 6, workers in mining and quarrying occupations; 7, workers in transport and communication occupations; 8, craftsmen, production process workers, and laborers; 9, service workers; 10, not classifiable and not reported.

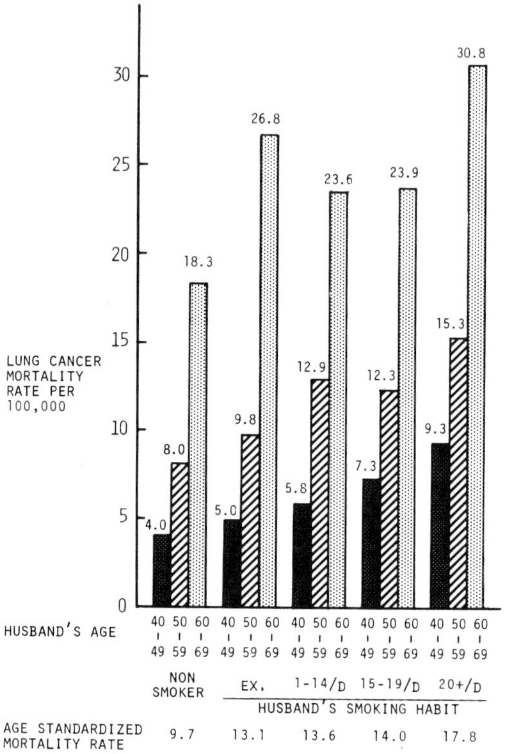

Figure 5. Age-specific mortality rate for lung cancer per 100,000 in nonsmoking wives by smoking habits of their husbands. (Prospective study, 1966–1981, Japan.)

Table 4. Mortality rate for lung cancer in women by age group and by alcohol drinking habits of husband: (patient herself a nonsmoker): prospective study, 1966–1981, Japan

Husband's age group	Husband's drinking habits								Total	
	Nondrinker		Occas. Rare		Daily		Obscure			
	No.	Pop.	No.	Pop.	No.	Pop.	No.	Pop.	No.	Pop.
40–49	12	6,141	10	15,877	13	9,935	0	74	35	32,027
50–59	12	7,437	29	14,666	24	10,786	0	364	65	33,253
60–69	23	6,741	35	9,234	27	7,606	4	633	89	24,214
70–79	1	686	5	666	4	589	1	105	11	2,046
Total	48	21,005	79	40,443	68	28,916	5	1,176	200	91,540
The weighted point estimate of rate ratio and test-based 90% confidence limits	1.00		1.03	1.61 0.66	1.11	1.59 0.77				
Mantel-Haenszel χ^2 one-tail p value	—			−0.1019 0.4594		0.4564 0.3240			Mantel extension χ^2 0.626 one-tail p value 0.26566	

Table 5. Mortality rate for ischemic heart diseases in women by age group and by smoking habits of husband: prospective study, 1966–1981, Japan

Husband's age group	Husband's smoking habit							
	Nonsmoker		Number of cigarettes a day: Ex-smoker 1-19/d		20+/d		Total	
	No.	Pop.	No.	Pop.	No.	Pop.	No.	Pop.
40–49	13	6,229	40	15,034	33	10,764	86	32,027
50–59	26	7,791	56	15,642	49	9,820	131	33,253
60–69	65	7,120	125	12,443.	47	4,651	237	24,214
70–79	14	755	19	1,065	7	226	40	2,046
Total	118	21,895	240	44,184	136	25,461	494	91,540
The weighted point estimate of rate ratio and test-based 90% confidence limits	1.00		1.10 (1.33, 0.91)		1.31 (1.63, 1.06)		Mantel extension χ^2 2.073	
Mantel-Haenszel χ^2 one-tail p value	—		0.8504 0.1976		2.0723 0.0191		one-tail p value 0.01909	

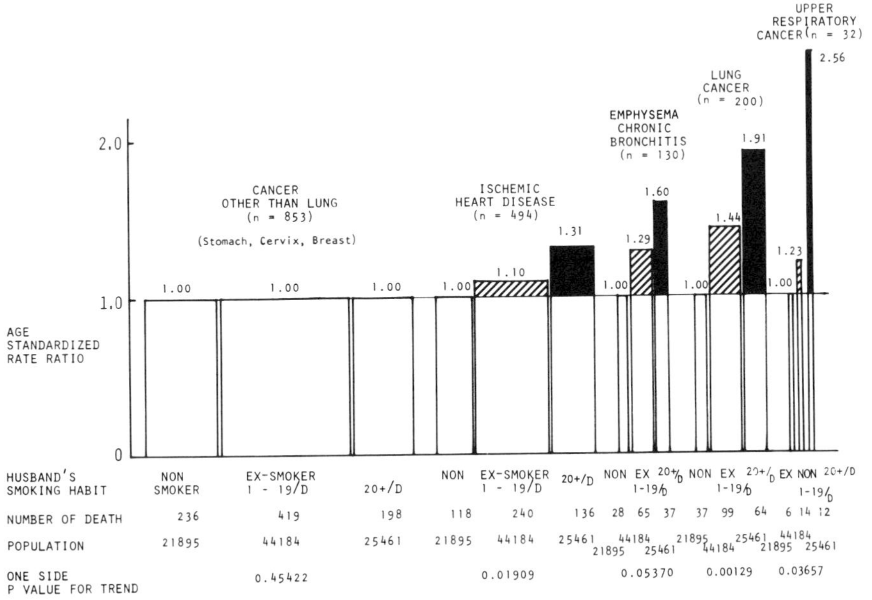

Figure 6. Standardized mortality rate ratio for selected causes of death in 91,540 nonsmoking women by smoking habits of their husbands. (Prospective study, 1966–1981, Japan.)

Table 6. Mortality rate for ischemic heart disease in women by age, occupation, and smoking habit of husbands (patient herself a nonsmoker)[a]

Husbands age (years)	Occupation[b]	Nonsmoker		Ex-smoker or 1-19/day		≥ 20/day	
		No.	Pop.	No.	Pop.	No.	Pop.
40-49	Total	13	6,229	40	15,034	33	10,764
	1	1	324		653	1	566
	2		90	1	231		293
	3		908	4	2,247	1	1,867
	4		476	1	993	5	1,044
	5	8	2,502	25	5,941	18	3,636
	6		46		165		108
	7	1	177	2	486		426
	8		1,112	7	3,431	6	2,241
	9		162		345	1	243
	10	3	432		542	1	340
50-59	Total	26	7,791	56	15,642	49	9,820
	1	1	345	3	593		446
	2	2	175		253		319
	3	2	817	5	1,764	6	1,324
	4		653	6	1,133	4	1,092
	5	15	3,497	27	6,812	26	3,514
	6		35	1	89		50
	7		120	1	273	2	234
	8	5	1,375	8	3,478	11	2,155
	9		164	1	378		251
	10	1	610	4	869		435
60-69	Total	65	7,120	125	12,443	47	4,651
	1	2	277	2	327	1	179
	2	1	91	2	143	1	124
	3	2	305	5	594	1	327
	4	10	508	8	822	5	500
	5	36	4,084	79	6,845	27	2,152
	6		9	1	31		14
	7	1	45	1	82	1	55
	8	7	805	13	1,784	6	736
	9	1	121	2	208		92
	10	5	925	12	1,607	5	472
70+	Total	14	755	19	1,065	7	226
	1	2	32	1	30		5
	2	2	21		14	1	4
	3		18	1	36		8
	4	1	48	1	73		20
	5	5	323	11	446	2	89
	6		1		1		0
	7		1		5		1
	8		87	1	119	3	36
	9		11	2	19		2
	10	4	213	2	322	1	61
[a] Standardized Risk Ratios		1.000		1.103		1.359	

Mantel extension χ^2: 2.351; one-tail p value: 0.00936.

[b] Occupation: 1, Professional and technical workers; 2, managers and officials; 3, clerical and related workers; 4, sales workers; 5, farmers, lumbermen, and fishermen; 6, workers in mining and quarrying occupations; 7, workers in transport and communication occupations; 8, craftsmen, production process workers, and laborers; 9, service workers; 10, not classifiable and not reported.

Table 7a. Mortality rates for major cancers other than lung in women by age group and by smoking habit of husband (patient herself a nonsmoker): prospective study, 1966–1981, Japan[a]

Husband's age group	Husband's smoking habit (cigarettes a day)							
	Nonsmoker		Ex-smoker 1–19		20+		Total	
	No.	Pop.	No.	Pop.	No.	Pop.	No.	Pop.
40–49	44	6.229	117	15,034	71	10,764	232	32,027
50–59	97	7,791	191	15,642	119	9,820	407	33,253
60–69	160	7,120	274	12,443	106	4,651	540	24,214
70–79	14	755	20	1,065	8	226	42	2,046
Total	315	21,895	602	44,184	304	25,461	1,221	91,540

	Nonsmoker	Ex-smoker 1–19	20+	Total
[a]The weighted point estimate of rate ratio and test-based 90% confidence limits	1.00	1.00 (1.11; 0.90)	1.00 (1.05; 0.95)	Mantel extension χ^2 0.115
Mantel-Haenszel χ^2 one-tail p value	—	−0.0015 0.4994	0.0449 0.4821	one-tail p value 0.4542

Table 7 b. Mortality rates for major cancers other than lung in women by age, occupation, and smoking habit of the husband (patient herself a nonsmoker)[a]

Husbands age (years)	Occupation[b]	Nonsmoker No.	Nonsmoker Pop.	Ex-smoker or 1–19/day No.	Ex-smoker or 1–19/day Pop.	≥20/day No.	≥20/day Pop.
40–49	Total	45	6,229	120	15,034	74	10,764
	1	2	324	1	653	3	566
	2		90	1	231	2	293
	3	9	908	17	2,247	12	1,867
	4	3	476	8	993	8	1,044
	5	17	2,502	59	5,941	35	3,636
	6		46		165		108
	7	1	177	6	486		426
	8	10	1,112	21	3,431	13	2,241
	9	1	162	4	345	1	243
	10	2	432	3	542		340
50–59	Total	98	7,791	195	15,642	122	9,820
	1	13	345	2	593	3	446
	2	2	175	1	253	1	319
	3	14	817	16	1,764	10	1,324
	4	1	653	18	1,133	9	1,092
	5	49	3,497	81	6,812	56	3,514
	6		35		89		50
	7	2	120	4	273	2	234
	8	12	1,375	49	3,478	31	2,155
	9		164	7	378	4	251
	10	5	610	17	869	6	435
60–69	Total	161	7,120	227	12,443	106	4,651
	1	5	227	5	327	2	179
	2	5	91	3	143	3	124
	3	7	305	11	594	5	327
	4	5	508	28	822	12	500
	5	102	4,084	158	6,845	58	2,152

Table 7 b. (cont.)

Husbands age (years)	Occupation[b]	Nonsmoker No.	Nonsmoker Pop.	Ex-smoker or 1–19/day No.	Ex-smoker or 1–19/day Pop.	≥ 20/day No.	≥ 20/day Pop.
	6		9	1	31		14
	7	1	45	3	82	2	55
	8	10	805	40	1,784	17	736
	9	2	121	3	208		92
	10	24	925	25	1,607	7	472
70 +	Total	14	755	21	1,065	8	226
	1		32		30		5
	2	1	21		14		4
	3	1	18		36		8
	4		48	1	73	2	20
	5	7	323	15	446	4	89
	6		1		1		0
	7		1		5		1
	8	1	87	2	119	1	36
	9		11		19		2
	10		4	213	3	322	1	61
[a] Standardized Risk Ratios		1.000		0.969		1.034	

Mantel extension χ^2: -0.129; one-tail p value: 0.44868.

[b] Occupation: 1, Professional and technical workers; 2, managers and officials; 3, clerical and related workers; 4, sales workers; 5, farmers, lumbermen, and fishermen; 6, workers in mining and quarrying occupations; 7, workers in transport and communication occupations; 8, craftsmen, production process workers, and laborers; 9, service workers; 10, not classifiable and not reported.

Comparison of the Effects of Active Smoking and Passive Smoking

When the risk of lung cancer in nonsmokers with nonsmoking spouses was taken as a unit, a definite dose–response relationship was observed, the highest risk being in heavy active smokers, followed by mild active smokers, then heavy passive smokers, and then mild passive smokers (Figure 7). The risk gradient was similar both in men and in women (Figure 8). A significantly elevated risk of lung cancer also was noted for nonsmoking husbands with smoking wives.

Because the size of population exposed to passive smoking is quite large in the case of women, the effect of passive smoking because of the husband's smoking was estimated as 65% of that of active smoking. Our recent survey showed that 47.5% and 32.6% of Japanese adult women were being exposed to passive smoking at home and at the workplace, respectively (Figure 9). Therefore it must be a sound estimate that the total effect of passive smoking is approximately equivalent to that of active smoking in women. However, as a majority of adult men are still smokers, the total effect of passive smoking relative to active smoking must be on

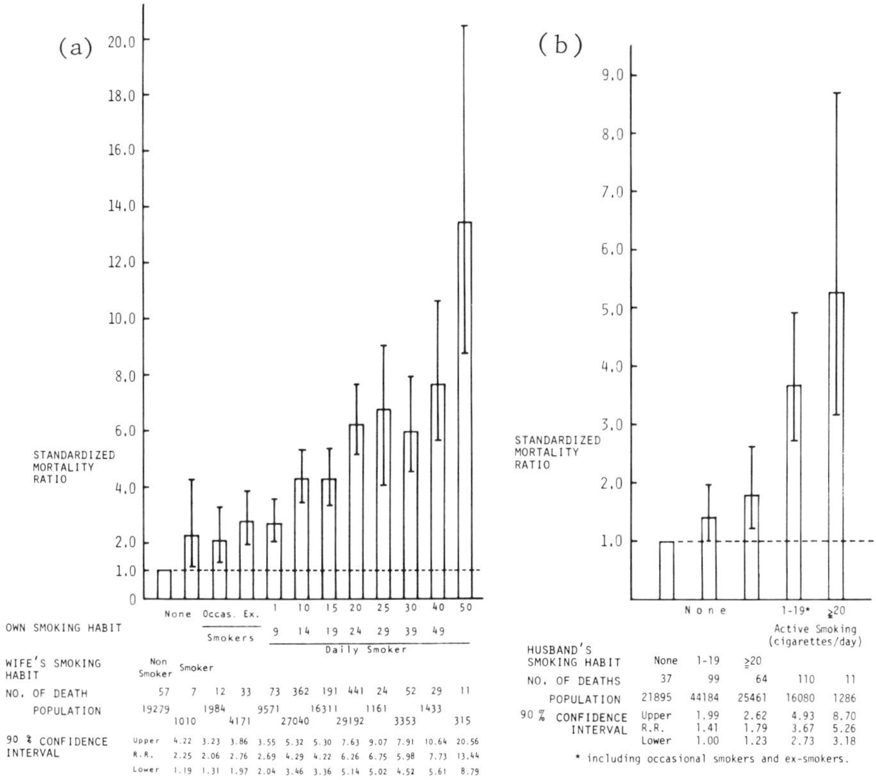

Figure 7. (a) Active and passive smoking and lung cancer mortality: relative risks (RR) with 90% confidence intervals; males.(Prospective study, 1966–1981, Japan.) (b) Active and passive smoking and lung cancer mortality: relative risks (RR) with 90% confidence intervals; females. (Prospective study, 1966–1981, Japan.)

the order of a few percent. The effect on lung cancer risk of passive smoking at home in relation to active smoking for men was calculated as 0.4% in our series.

Effect of Nutrition on Passive Smokers

A significantly lower risk of lung cancer was observed when nonsmoking wives with smoking husbands consumed green-yellow vegetables daily (Tables 8 and 9, Figures 10 and 11) suggesting that the promoter-inhibitor interaction model also applied to passive smoking just as in active smoking (Figure 9). Such risk reduction caused by daily intake of green-yellow vegetables was not observed for ischemic heart disease (Table 10, Figure 12).

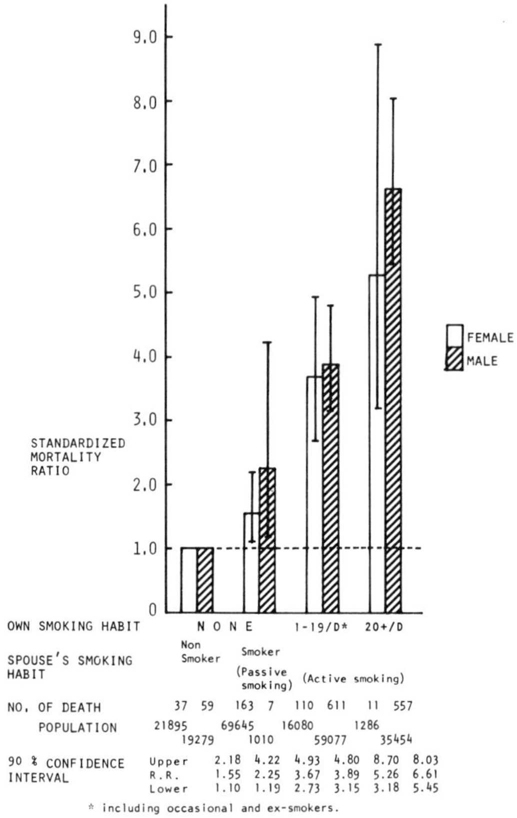

Figure 8. Active and passive smoking and lung cancer mortality: relative risks (RR) with 90% confidence intervals. (Prospective study, 1966–1981, Japan.)

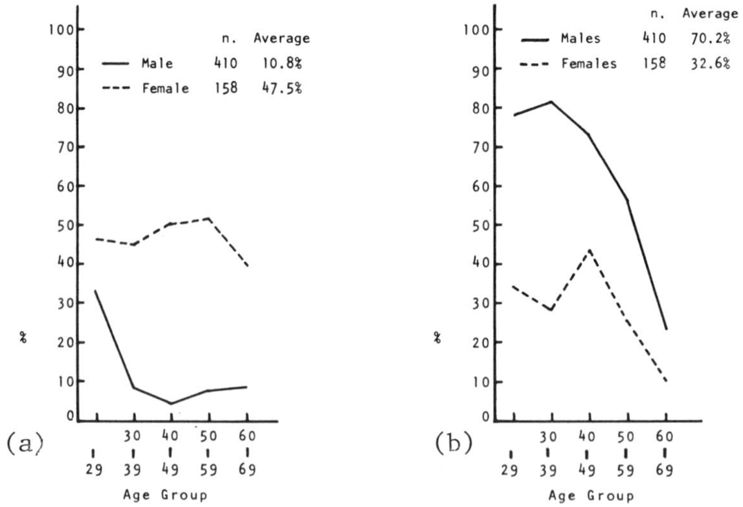

Figure 9. (a) Percentage of nonsmokers exposed to sidestream smoke at home, Japan, 1983. (b) Percentage of nonsmokers exposed to sidestream smoke at the workplace, Japan, 1983.

Table 8. Lung cancer mortality rate in nonsmoking wives by smoking habit of the husband: comparison between daily and non daily intake of green-yellow vegetables

Husband's smoking habits		Nonsmoker				Ex-smoker on 1-19 day				≥ 20/day			
Wife's eating habits		Green-yellow vegetables											
		Daily		Nondaily		Daily		Nondaily		Daily		Nondaily	
Husband's		Pop.	Lung Ca.	Pop.	Lung Ca.	Pop.	Lung Ca.	Pop.	Lung Ca.	Pop.	Lung Ca.	Pop.	Lung Ca.
Occupation	**Age**												
Agriculture	40–49	1,958	1	544	0	5,050	5	891	1	3,037	7	599	2
	50–59	2,805	4	692	0	5,196	11	1,616	5	2,588	9	926	0
	60–69	3,359	7	725	6	5,106	22	1,739	11	1,588	6	564	4
	70–79	258	3	65	0	287	1	159	0	45	0	44	0
Others	40–49	2,422	3	1,305	0	7,288	8	1,805	1	5,377	5	1,751	2
	50–59	3,181	5	1,113	1	6,732	12	2,098	3	4,633	5	1,673	10
	60–69	2,266	4	770	1	4,088	9	1,510	6	1,906	10	593	3
	70–79	216	2	216	0	371	1	248	3	81	1	56	0
Total		16,465	29	5,430	8	34,118	69	10,066	30	19,255	43	6,206	21

Grand total	**Population: 91540**	**Lung cancer: 200**
Green-yellow vegetables	Mantel-extension χ^2	P-value (two tailed)
Daily	2.072	0.03827
Nondaily	2.487	0.01288
Total	3.090	0.00200

Table 9. Effect of daily intake of green–yellow vegetables on lung cancer mortality in nonsmoking wives with smoking husbands[a]

Husband's smoking habit		Ex-smoker or 1–19/day				≥ 20/day			
Wife's eating habit		Green-yellow vegetables							
		Daily		Nondaily		Daily		Nondaily	
Husband's		Pop.	Lung Ca.	Pop.	Lung Ca.	Pop.	Lung Ca.	Pop.	Lung Ca.
Occupation	Age								
Agriculture	40–49	5,050	5	891	1	3,037	7	559	2
	50–59	5,196	11	1,616	5	2,588	9	926	0
	60–69	5,106	22	1,739	11	1,588	6	564	4
	70–79	287	1	159	0	45	0	44	0
Others	40–49	7,288	8	1,805	1	5,377	5	1,751	2
	50–59	6,732	12	2,098	3	4,633	5	1,673	10
	60–69	4,088	9	1,510	6	1,906	10	593	3
	70–79	371	1	248	3	81	1	56	0
Total		34,118	69	10,066	30	19,255	43	6,206	21

[a]Mantel-Haenszel χ^2: −1,986; p (two-tailed 0.047). Odds ratio: Nondaily green–yellow vegetable intaker, 1,000; daily green–yellow vegetables intake, 0.707 (standardized rate ratio); 90% confidence limits, 0.538–0.943.

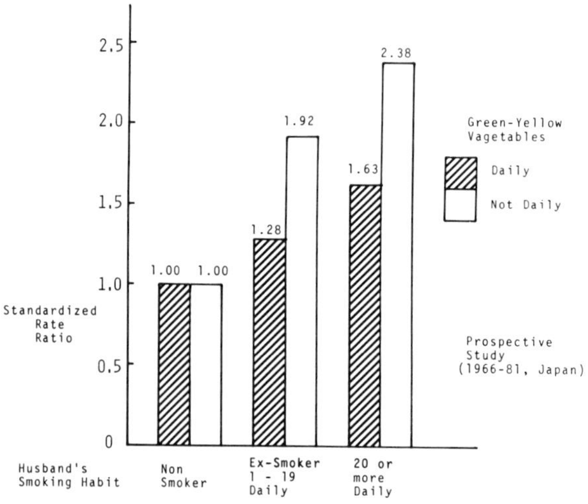

Green-Yellow Vegetables	Mantel-Extension Chi	p value (two-tailed)
Daily	2.072	0.03827
Others	2.487	0.01288

Figure 10. Lung cancer mortality ratio in nonsmoking wives by smoking habits of their husbands. Comparison between daily and nondaily intake of green–yellow vegetables.

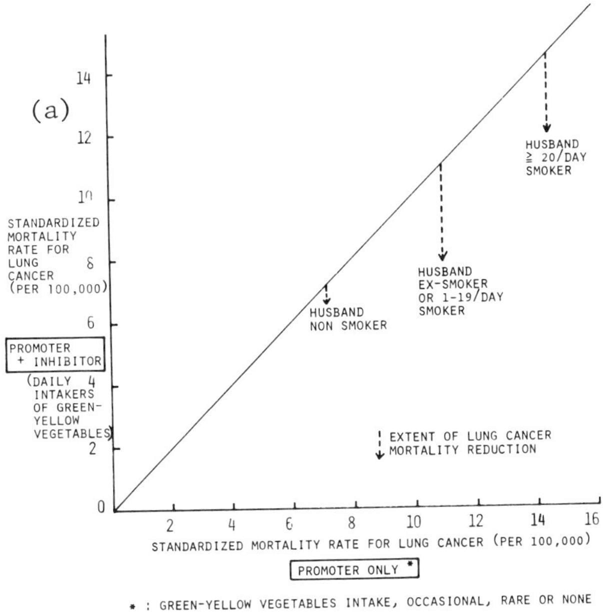

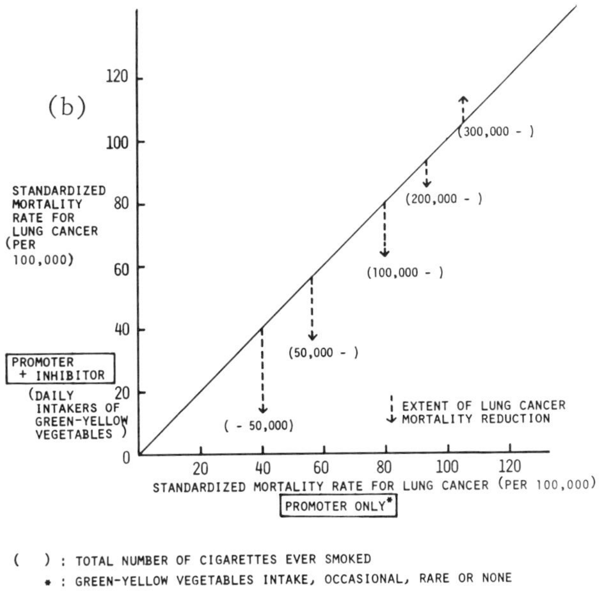

Figure 11. (a) Standardized mortality rate for lung cancer in nonsmoking wives by smoking habit of the husband. Comparison between daily and nondaily intake of green-yellow vegetables. (Prospective study, 1966–1981, Japan.) (b) Standardized mortality rate for lung cancer according to total number of cigarettes smoked and frequency of consumption of green-yellow vegetables; males. (Prospective study, 1966–1978, Japan.)

Table 10. Ischemic heart disease mortality rate in nonsmoking wives by smoking habit of the husband: comparison between green–yellow vegetables intake daily and nondaily

Husband's smoking habit		Nonsmoker				Ex-smoker or 1–19/day				≥ 20/day			
Wife's eating habit		Green–yellow vegetables											
		Daily		Nondaily		Daily		Nondaily		Daily		Nondaily	
Husband's		Pop.	Ischemic Heart D.	Pop.	Ischemic Heart D.	Pop.	Ischemic Heart D.	Pop.	Ischemic Heart D.	Pop.	Ischemic Heart D.	Pop.	Ischemic Heart D.
Occupation	Age												
Agriculture	40–49	1,958	6	544	2	5,050	18	891	7	3,037	14	599	4
	50–59	2,805	11	692	4	5,196	25	1,616	2	2,588	21	926	5
	60–69	3,359	30	725	6	5,106	55	1,739	24	1,588	21	564	6
	70–79	258	2	65	3	287	10	159	1	45	2	44	0
Others	40–49	2,422	3	1,305	2	7,288	10	1,805	5	5,377	12	1,751	3
	50–59	3,181	8	1,113	3	6,732	18	2,098	11	4,633	17	1,673	6
	60–69	2,266	21	770	8	4,088	33	1,510	13	1,906	11	593	9
	70–79	216	7	216	2	371	6	248	2	81	3	56	2
Total		16,465	88	5,430	30	34,118	175	10,066	65	19,255	101	6,206	35
Grand total		**Population: 91540**						**Ischemic heart disease: 494**					

Green-yellow vegetables	Mantel-extension χ^2	P value (two tailed)
Daily	2.307	0.02105
Nondaily	0.820	0.41222
Total	2.406	0.01613

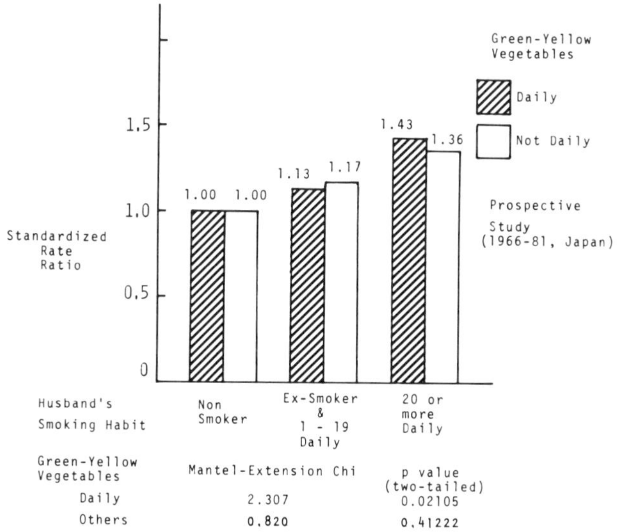

Figure 12. Ischemic heart disease mortality ratio in nonsmoking wives by smoking habits of their husbands. Comparison between daily and nondaily intake of green–yellow vegetables .

Discussion

The age-adjusted mortality rates for lung cancer have been sharply increasing both for men and for women in Japan. As only a fraction of Japanese women with lung cancer smoke cigarettes, the reasons for the trend of their mortality from lung cancer have been unclear. The present study appears to explain at least a part of this long-standing riddle.

This observation also questions the validity of the conventional method of assessing the relative risk of developing lung cancer in smokers by comparing them with nonsmokers. This study shows that nonsmokers are not a homogeneous group and should be subdivided according to the extent of previous exposure to indirect or passive smoking. Although the relative risk of indirect smoking was smaller than that of direct smoking, the absolute excess deaths from lung cancer resulting from passive smoking must be important because of the large size of the exposed group. Therefore, these results of our current study must be of public health importance, strengthening already existing evidence for a health hazard from passive smoking (11–13) (Table 11).

As shown in Figure 9, 47.5% and 32.6% of 158 nonsmoking adult women surveyed recently are noted to be exposed to sidestream smoke at home and at the workplace, respectively. One survey conducted in Aichi prefecture in Japan showed that nonsmoking wives are exposed to their husband's smoking 6.7 times a day on the average.

Because sidestream smoke contains varieties of cancer promoters at higher concentration than does mainstream smoke, it must be reasonable to consider the

Table 11. Passive smoking is harzardous to health

1. Existence of toxic substances (including carcinogens) in sidestream smoke mostly at higher concentration than in mainstream smoke.
2. Existence of a large number of nonsmokers who have to inhale sidestream smoke frequently and intensively for long years at home and/or at the workplace.
3. Existence of sidestream smoke component in blood and urine of nonsmokers exposed to passive smoking, (eg, nicotine, CO-Hb in blood and Mutagens in urine.).
4. Existence of functional abnormalities in nonsmokers exposed heavily to passive smoking (eg, respiratory or circulatory function).
5. Lung tissue damage and destruction in chronic passive smokers as shown by elevated hydroxyproline excretion in urine.
6. Higher incidence of selected diseases in nonsmokers exposed heavily to passive smoking (eg, pneumonia, bronchitis, asthma, ischemic heart disease, lung and nasal sinus cancer).
7. Experimental evidence.

main effect of passive smoking on lung cancer risk results from the prolonged exposure to such promoters in sidestream smoke. The risk-inhibitory effect of a daily intake of green–yellow vegetables that are rich in β-carotene must be considered as an additional evidence for such a promoter action hypothesis of passive smoking. The hypothesis also explains why exposure to passive smoking that starts after reaching adult age can significantly influence the risk of lung cancer.

The histology of 21 cases of lung cancer in nonsmoking wives of smoking husbands was not essentially different from that in smoking women (adenocarcinoma 57.1%, squamous cell carcinoma 19.0%, and small-cell carcinoma 4.8%). A case–control study conducted within our cohort study revealed a significant dose–response relationship between adenocarcinoma of the lung and the number of cigarettes smoked daily, relative risk being 1.39 and 5.75 for smokers of 1–14 and 15 or more cigarettes daily, the chi square for the trend being 6.848 with a one-tail p value of 0.004. Therefore the predominance of adenocarcinoma of the lung in nonsmoking women with smoking husbands should not be considered unfavorable evidence for promoter action hypothesis of passive smoking. In passive smoking, sidestream smoke usually is inhaled through the nose, whereas in active smoking mainstream smoke always is inhaled through the mouth. This difference could be a reason for the elevated risk of nasal sinus cancer in passive smokers. The mechanism of the action of passive smoking on the risk of ischemic heart disease, however, must be explained in different ways (eg, a combined action of carbon monoxide and nicotine).

In summary, to reduce the effect of active and passive smoking and to encourage the effect of nutrition, in particular β-carotene intake, would be the most productive course for lung cancer prevention. For selected persons exposed to other known carcinogens, eg, those related to occupation or radiation, such environmental exposure also must be minimized in addition to the preventive measures focused on lifestyle variables given above.

References

1. Hirayama T. Prospective studies on cancer epidemiology based on census population in Japan. In: Bucalossi P, Veronesi U and Cascinelli N, eds, Proceedings of the XIth international cancer

congress. Cancer Epidemiology, Environmental Factors, Vol. 3. Amsterdam: Excerpta Medica, 1975:26–35.
2. Hirayama T. Epidemiology of lung cancer based on population studies. In: Finkel A J and Duel W C, eds, Clinical implications of air pollution research. Chicago: The American Medical Association, 1976:69–78.
3. Hirayama T. Smoking and cancer. A prospective study on cancer epidemiology based on census population in Japan. In: Steinfeld J, Griffiths W, Ball K, and Taylor RM, eds, Proceedings of the 3rd world conference on smoking and health 1975. U.S. Department of Health, Education and Welfare Publ (NIH)77-1413 Washington, DC: 1977:65 – 72.
4. Hirayama T. Prospective studies on cancer epidemiology based on census population in Japan. In: Nieburgs HE, ed, Third international symposium on detection and prevention of cancer, Pt 1, Vol 1. New York: Marcel Dekker, 1977:1139–48.
5. Hirayama T. Smoking and cancer in Japan. A prospective study on cancer epidemiology based on census population in Japan. Results of 13 years follow up. In: Tominaga S, Aoki K, eds, The UICC Smoking Control Workshop, 1981. Nagoya: University of Nagoya Press, 1982:2–8.
6. Hirayama T. Epidemiological aspects of lung cancer in the Orient. In: Ishikawa S, Hayata Y, Suemasu K, eds, Lung cancer 1982. Amsterdam: Excerpta Medica, 1982:1–13.
7. Hirayama T. Diet and cancer. Nutr Cancer 1979;1(3):67–81.
8. Hirayama T. Does daily intake of green-yellow vegetables reduce the risk of cancer in man? An example of the application of epidemilogical methods to the identification of individuals at low risk. In: Bartsch H, Armstrong B, Davis W, eds, Proceeding of symposium on host factors in human carcinogenesis. International Agency for Research on Cancer Scientific Publ 39. Lyons: World Health Organization, 1982:531–40.
9. Hirayama T. Non-smoking wives of heavy smokers have a higher risk of lung cancer: a study from Japan. Br Med J 1981;282:183–5.
10. Trichopoulos D, Kalandidi A, Sparros L, MacMahon B. Lung cancer and passive smoking. Int J Cancer 1981;27(1):1-4.
11. Brunnemann KD, Adams JD, Ho DPS, et al. The influence of tobacco smoke on indoor atmospheres. II. Volatile and tobacco specific nitrosamines in main- and sidestream smoke and their contribution to indoor pollution. In: Proceedings of the 4th joint conference on the sensing of environmental pollutants. New Orleans, 1977. Washington, DC: American Chemical Society, 1978:876–80.
12. Brunnemann KD, Hoffmann D. Chemical studies on tobacco smoke LIX. Analysis of volatile nitrosamines in tobacco smoke and polluted indoor environments. In: Walter EA, Griciute L, Gastegnaro M, eds, Environmental aspects of N-nitroso compounds. International Agency for Research on Cancer Scientific Publ 19. Lyons: World Health Organization, 1978:343–56.
13. White RJ, Froeb FH. Small-airways dysfunction in nonsmokers chronically exposed to tobacco smoke. N Engl J Med 1980;302:720–3.

CHAPTER **15**

Nutritional Status and Chemoprevention in Relation to Lung Cancer

PETER GREENWALD and WILLIAM D. DeWYS

Division of Cancer Prevention and Control,
National Cancer Institute, National Institutes of Health,
Bethesda, Maryland 20205

ABSTRACT

Chemoprevention is a new area of research emphasis at the National Cancer Institute. Chemoprevention is the introduction of selected micronutrients, synthetic analogs, or other substances for the purposes of reducing cancer incidence. The rationale is based on a convergence of laboratory evidence of carcinogenesis inhibition together with epidemiologic data suggesting an inverse correlation between measures of vitamin A and other micronutrients and the incidence of lung and other cancers. Several human intervention trials have begun that aim to test the hypothesis that these agents can lower cancer incidence, and further trials are planned.
Key Words: **Diet, chemoprevention, cancer prevention, lung cancer**

The National Cancer Institute (NCI) is sponsoring preventive research in nutrition relevant to lung cancer through two related programs. One is a new program, the Chemoprevention Program; the other, the Diet and Nutrition Program, has been at NCI since 1975 and is now receiving increased emphasis. Both programs are the administrative responsibility of the recently reorganized Division of Cancer Prevention and Control (DCPC) and both programs are being implemented under the same basic planning model. In this chapter we (a) define the goals and areas of both programs, (b) explain the program model, and (c) summarize research studies pertinent to lung cancer. Understanding the model and where current and proposed research fits into the model is important to NCI for planning purposes and to the research community for initiation of future studies.

This discussion of chemoprevention and nutritional status in relation to lung cancer in no way should detract from the overwhelming importance of cigarette smoking as the main cause of preventable cancer deaths in the United States. As noted in the latest U.S. Surgeon General's report, there is no single, more effective action an individual can take to reduce the risk of cancer than to avoid smoking, particularly cigarettes.

Program Descriptions

Chemoprevention is based on the idea, from a public health point of view, that it is easier to add than to subtract; that is, it may be easier to add some constituent to the diet for preventive purposes than to modify dietary aspects of lifestyle in a major way. Chemoprevention is the introduction of selected micronutrients, synthetic analogs, or other substances for the purpose of reducing cancer incidence.

The Chemoprevention Program has as its rationale the mounting and converging laboratory and epidemiologic data that indicate that various agents can halt or reverse cancer progression in animals and reduce cancer risk in humans. An extensive body of research on carcinogenesis inhibition shows that selected compounds have a consistent inhibitory effect in many model systems and in different species. The consistency in different animal models in different species and dose–response gradients and other features of these carcinogenesis inhibition studies provide convincing evidence that it is likely that human benefit may be derived from this laboratory research.

The Program specifically deals with natural and synthetic agents that are chemically defined and can be administered in precise, specified dosages. Potential agents to be tested include vitamin A and its precursor β-carotene, ascorbic acid (vitamin C), α-tocopherol (vitamin E), the trace metal selenium, synthetic retinoids, phenolic inhibitors, protease inhibitors, and prostaglandin synthesis inhibitors.

The goals of the NCI Chemoprevention Program are to develop agents that are nontoxic at acceptable levels and that show significant inhibitory effects against one or more types of human neoplasia and/or related disorders in clinical trials. The three major objectives are:

1. To determine, in epidemiologic studies, the consumption and usage of micronutrients and chemopreventive agents and, in laboratory research, to identify and test the efficacy of potential new agents
2. To determine the effectiveness of selected agents in at-risk populations
3. To examine the safety and toxicity of various substances and their application both prior to initiating human intervention studies and during their course

Whereas the basic approach of chemoprevention is to add substances to the diet, the approach of the Diet and Nutrition Program is to add or subtract dietary substances. Instead of focusing on defined agents in precise dosages, the Nutrition Program chiefly emphasizes classes of foods described in rough percentages. The goal of the program is to develop dietary interventions effective in reducing cancer incidence. The objectives are:

1. To identify food constituents and dietary patterns
2. To determine which constituents are helpful and which are harmful
3. To determine which dietary modifications can reduce cancer incidence
4. To determine bioavailability
5. To identify metabolic and other host factors
6. To elucidate environmental interactions

The Basic Program Model

Although the program model applies to both the Chemoprevention and the Nutrition Programs, for convenience we describe and illustrate it here only in terms of the Chemoprevention Program. To apply the model to the Nutrition Program, simply replace the concept of a chemical agent with the concept of diet prescription (addition or omission to the diet).

Components and Process

The model, shown in Figure 1, is actually an outline of a process with four interrelated components of activity: research, methods development, operations, and

NCI Chemoprevention Program		
Research	Laboratory Human Intervention Studies Epidemiology	Description of research judged necessary to achieve program objective(s) sequentially ordered, by stages, with decision points controlling movement from stage to stage
Methods Development	Laboratory Human Intervention Studies Epidemiology	Identification of the methods required to conduct the research described in each of the stages for laboratory, human intervention, and epidemiological studies
Operations	Description of the managerial, administrative and informational requirements judged necessary for the efficient and effective operation of the program	
Resources	Personnel Facilities Materials Funds	Identification of resource requirements for each stage of each flow in terms of the four resource categories

Figure 1. Basic program model.

resources. As a process it involves dynamic interaction among its components, and ongoing evolution prompted by input from scientific advances and the scientific community. The process involves formulating program goals. For chemoprevention the goal includes identifying leads from laboratory research and from epidemiologic research and then bringing these leads through an orderly progression of research logic to clinical application. The process also involves defining program boundaries. For example, the program does not include studies of basic mechanisms relative to carcinogenesis, but picks up leads that are relative to chemoprevention. Finally, the process involves developing and implementing each of four components. The first of these components relates to organizing the research logic within the broad scientific area; the second, to assessing the methods available, required, and in need of development; the third, to putting into place the necessary managerial, administrative, and informational supports; and the fourth, to provide for the personnel, facilities, materials, and funds required to implement the program plan. The model was developed using the planning methods developed by Louis Carrese and his colleagues of the National Cancer Institute (1).

Flow of Research Logic

All four components, including operations and resources, are organized around three research categories: laboratory research, epidemiologic research, and human intervention studies. The flow of this research logic is shown in Figure 2. We envision a sequence of stages in laboratory research, a sequence of stages in epidemiologic research, and leads from either of these to be brought into human intervention studies that may lead to broad prevention application.

The sequence of stages in laboratory research is illustrated in Figure 3. The first stage is a review process in which we look at available information and research currently in progress throughout the world for the purpose of selecting potential inhibitors for further evaluation. The "DP" in the figure stands for "decision point." A decision point is established at the end of each stage and requires establishing criteria for evaluating the leads at that stage.

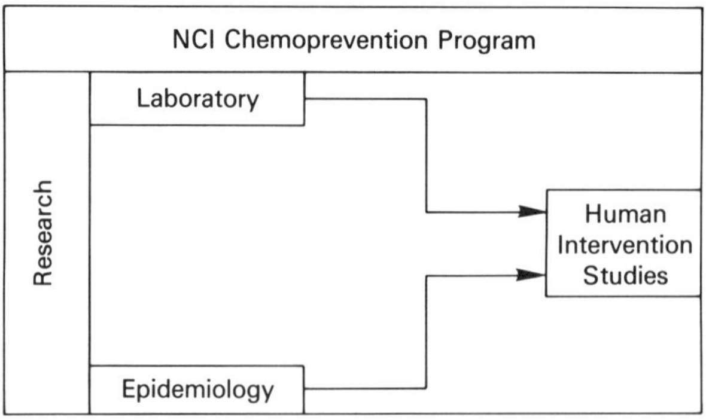

Figure 2. Research flow design.

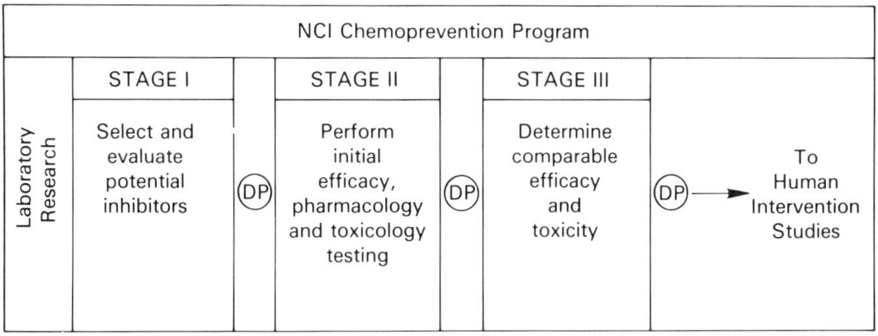

Figure 3. Laboratory research stages.

If the lead meets the criteria for transition from stage I, it is carried into stage II, in which initial studies are aimed at expanding the information about the efficacy of the inhibitor. Pharmacology studies in animal models and animal toxicology testing are implemented in that stage. When transition from stage II criteria are met, stage III animal studies are done, which include (1) comparison with other agents and evaluation of the new agent in combination with other agents, and (2) additional toxicity studies, particularly long-term toxicity studies, which are prerequisites to human intervention studies. At the third decision point, these results are evaluated in preparation for advancing to human intervention studies.

Parallel to this laboratory sequence is a sequence of epidemiologic studies (Figure 4). Again the sequence begins with a review of available literature and current research. However, in addition to identifying potential agents for further study, the objective is to identify populations for epidemiologic studies and for

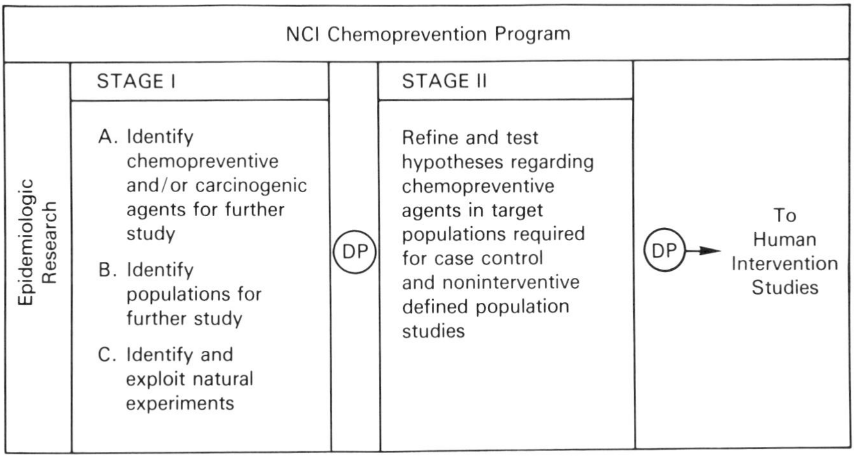

Figure 4. Epidemiologic research stages.

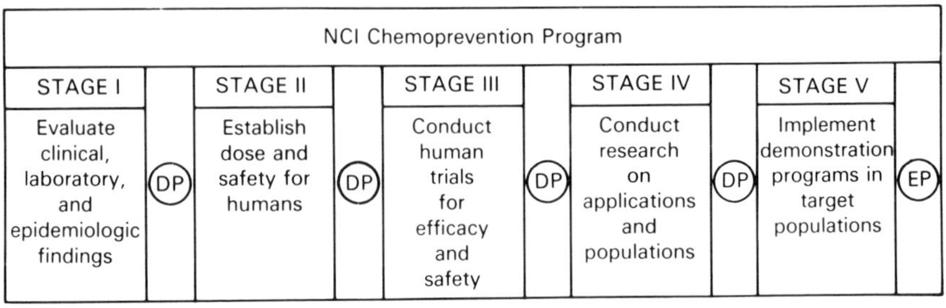

Figure 5. Human intervention studies stages.

clinical intervention studies. The third activity in this initial stage is a monitoring function, of identifying and evaluating natural experiments. For example, populations may change their lifestyles unexpectedly, particularly with respect to diet or environmental aspects, and we must be prepared to monitor those experiments. At the stage I decision point, there are two possible directions. One possibility is to bring the lead forward by additional epidemiologic studies that are more focused than the initial leads. The second possibility is that the lead so strongly fulfills the decision criteria that it may be reviewed against the next set of decision criteria without additional studies. The lead, then, could move to human intervention studies.

The human intervention sequence involves five stages (Figure 5). In the initial stage, combined information from laboratory and epidemiologic sequences is evaluated. A lead may enter clinical studies if it is very strong in terms of laboratory data or epidemiologic data, or moderately strong in both. The objective in stage II is to establish the dose and safety levels for humans. In stage III the agent enters human trials aimed at evaluating efficacy, expanding the data base in terms of safety, and evaluating risk–benefit issues in the eventual outcome of the trial. If the trial is positive and meets the DP criteria, cancer control applications (stage IV) undergo trials. Applications may require that additional research questions be answered; for example, how can an agent tested in capsule form be added in some way to the food supply? Or which populations would most benefit from the agent? After all criteria are met, the final stage is a demonstration program in larger target populations, followed by an evaluation point, which requires ongoing monitoring of the population to document the anticipated effect of the intervention.

Planning Dimensions of Operations and Resources

In addition to planning for the actual research flow, the program model incorporates other planning dimensions. An important dimension in operations is the assignment of responsibilities and focus among branches of the Division so that efforts can be concentrated in specific areas. A second dimension is calendar time because some of the concepts we propose take considerable time from proposal to actual initiation; typically, we are working on concepts that are relevant to several fiscal years. Research now in progress either is investigator-initiated or stems from a series of workshops held by a subcommittee of our NCI Board of Scientific

Counselors. We currently are planning for activities that we anticipate implementing over the next several years.

During the past year and a half, DCPC has been focusing strongly on the strategy and planning of various aspects of the Division's programs. Developing the basic program model has been a major activity. Implementing the model poses a double challenge to planning for operations and resources. The process model we have described above can be applied systematically in the present and future to all new research projects; we have the advantage in that aspect of the challenge. The second aspect is to fit into our planning those research projects that have a history; in other words, the Division has inherited many studies that may or may not adapt comfortably to the process of the research flow. If a project in a later stage of the model has not been judged rigorously by the decision point criteria, how are we to assess its value to the program?

For these planning activities we have used extensively our Board of Scientific Counselors, the National Cancer Advisory Board, and various task forces. We now have separate task forces for chemoprevention; diet, nutrition, and cancer; detection and diagnosis; smoking; and national cancer control objectives. The planning effort has been extensive, rigorous, and time consuming. For example, we spent 24 full or part days developing and critiquing the logic of the Chemoprevention Program alone.

The purpose of planning for program operations and resources is to identify the types and amounts of research and services that must be provided in order to achieve the goals and objectives of the program. This is an organizational initiative that seeks input from advising experts and attempts to remain flexible and able to adapt to new findings. As the program priorities become clear, we must plan for adequate funding and other resources to pursue the priorities.

An example from our Chemoprevention Program may be instructive. In chemoprevention, we surveyed ongoing research to identify current research in the scientific community regardless of the institution, mechanism, or source of funding. Our analysis led to the formulation and announcement of a request for application, entitled "The Role of Natural Inhibitors in the Prevention of Cancer," which invites investigator-initiated research proposals for observational studies and human intervention trials.

We currently are involved in developing our plan for the Diet, Nutrition and Cancer Program and hope to present it to the full Board of Scientific Counselors this year.

Summary of Research Studies Pertinent to the Prevention of Lung Cancer

During the past decade, major strides have been made in our knowledge about how diet can affect cancer risk. Several plausible hypotheses derive from a convergence of evidence from various fields and epidemiologic studies of human populations, complemented by parallel mechanistic studies with animals and other laboratory research. In this section, we highlight several historically important studies and present an extensive table of other relevant research categorized by study type.

Carcinogenesis Inhibition Studies in Animals

A historically important study in chemoprevention was done by Lasnitzki (2). She developed a method for growing mouse prostate cells on a watch glass containing a clot of mixed plasmas and chick embryo extract. Addition of the carcinogen, 20-methylcholanthrene, transformed these cells to hyperplasia or squamous metaplasia. Adding vitamin A inhibited the transformation. She also studied promotion by culturing the cells with the carcinogen and 9 days later adding vitamin A; inhibition still could be demonstrated.

Harris et al (3) observed that vitamin A deficiency caused squamous metaplasia in the tracheal epithelium of hamsters. That metaplasia is morphologically similar to that caused by the administration of carcinogens.

Boutwell and his colleagues (4) developed a two-stage model of mouse skin carcinogenesis. They shaved the skin on the mouse and induced papillomas through the use of an initiator followed by a promoter. Boutwell then demonstrated that administration of retinoic acid would inhibit cancer promotion and result in fewer papillomas per mouse or fewer mice with papillomas.

Dr. Sporn's group at NCI uses a model for mouse bladder tumors that induces tumors in about 40% of mice by the administration of butylhydroxybutyl nitrosamine via gastric intubation. In one study (5) 13-*cis*-retinoic acid was shown to reduce the bladder tumor incidence from 38% in the control group (given the carcinogen alone) to 5% in the study group (which also received 13-*cis*-retinoic acid). In another study from Sporn's group (6) mammary tumors were induced in almost 100% of the rats by administering the carcinogen methylnitrosourea. Subsequently, the most potent synthetic retinoid reduced the tumor incidence from 100% to 20%. Present efforts are aimed at developing retinoids with less toxicity than naturally occurring vitamin A and with a structure that helps the retinoids to reach those body tissues where most tumors arise.

Human Studies Related to Diet and Nutrition, Chemoprevention, and Lung Cancer

Research that bears upon the potential relationship of diet and chemoprevention to lung cancer is summarized in Table 1. Peto et al (7) have reviewed the hypothesis of an inverse relationship between β-carotene ingestion and its related retinoids. Migrants to cities in the United States from farms or foreign countries had a somewhat higher risk for lung cancer (8), an observation that might be explained in part by different dietary intakes. Several case–control epidemiologic studies (see Table 1) were consistent in showing lower vegetable consumption or lower estimates of vitamin A intake among patients than among controls. This relationship is supported by three cohort studies that observed a negative association between lung cancer and an index of vitamin A, the first by Bjelke (9). Hirayama (10) made a similar observation in Japan (see Chapter 14), and suggested that ex-smokers might particularly benefit from daily vegetable consumption. Shekelle et al (11) found the benefit to be limited to carotene. Three studies of serum or plasma vitamin A in lung cancer patients as compared to controls (Table 1) showed mixed results, but two prospective studies were very consistent in demonstrating an inverse relationship between retinol in stored sera and subsequent occurrence of lung cancer. The number of lung cancer patients in these latter two studies was small: 14 and 12.

Table 1. Selected human studies related to diet and nutrition, chemoprevention, and lung cancer

Investigator, year, title	Study design	Results
Descriptive epidemiologic studies		
Haenszel et al, 1962. Lung-cancer mortality as related to residence and smoking histories. I. White males. JNCI April 1962;28:947-1001.	10% sample of 1958 United States lung cancer deaths compared to census sample. Residence and smoking history from family informants. Analysis included residence history, controlled for smoking history.	Nonsmokers showed almost no differences in death rates by residence. United States farm-born and foreign migrants to cities had high lung cancer risks.
Case/control epidemiological studies		
MacLennan et al, 1977. Risk factors for lung cancer in Singapore Chinese. A population with high female incidence rates. Int J Cancer 1977; 20:854-860.	147 male and 86 female lung cancer patients and matched hospital controls were interviewed.	Persons with a low consumption of green vegetables were at higher risk for lung cancer. Adenocarcinoma in Cantonese women was unrelated to smoking.
Smith and Jick, 1978. Cancers among users of preparations containing vitamin A—A case-control investigation. Cancer 1978; 42:808-811.	800 cancer patients and 3,433 hospitalized control patients were interviewed about regular vitamin A use. The case group included 93 male and 17 female bronchus cancer patients.	8 of 93 (9%) of the male patients regularly used vitamin A as compared to 11% of the total male control group. 2 of 17 (12%) of the female patients used vitamin A versus 14% of controls. Overall results were not statistically significant, but among men a negative association was suggested.
Mettlin et al, 1979. Vitamin A and lung cancer. JNCI June 1979;62:1435-1438.	292 male lung cancer patients and 801 hospital controls were interviewed about diet and other epidemiologic factors. A vitamin A index was derived from vegetable and milk intake.	Lung cancer patients had a lower index of vitamin A than did controls. A dose-response gradient was found, with a relative risk of 2.4 for the lowest index values.

Table 1. (cont.)

Investigator, year, title	Study design	Results
Gregor et al, 1980. Comparison of dietary histories in lung cancer cases and controls with special reference to vitamin A. Nutr. Cancer 1980;2:93–97.	78 male and 22 female lung cancer patients and 110 rheumatology and medical outpatient controls were questioned about dietary sources of vitamin A and vitamin A pill use. Vitamin A intake was estimated in μg retinol equivalents per week.	Men ingested significantly less vitamin A than did controls, mainly because of lower liver and vitamin pill consumption. Women showed no significant difference, although liver consumption was somewhat higher among the patients.
Hinds et al, 1983. Dietary cholesterol and lung cancer risk among men in Hawaii. Am J Clin Nutr February 1983;37:192–193.	188 male lung cancer patients and 294 matched controls were questioned about diet. Eggs, dairy products, and organ meats were chief contributors to cholesterol intake.	Lung cancer patients had significantly higher cholesterol intake, with dose-response gradient. All five ethnic groups studied showed the increase.
Cohort epidemiologic studies		
Bjelke, 1975. Dietary vitamin A and human lung cancer. Int J Cancer 1975; 15:561–565.	Postal questionnaires on smoking and diet were sent to a general population sample of Norwegian men, and to siblings living in Norway of migrants to the United States. Five-year followup results for 8278 men for whom sufficient data were available are reported. Subsequent cancer was ascertained by record linkage with the cancer registry of Norway.	36 bronchus or lung cancers were found in followup of the study groups. An index of vitamin A was associated negatively with lung cancer incidence, with stratification by smoking habit. The association was greater with adenocarcinomas excluded.
Hirayama, 1979. Diet and cancer. Nutr. Cancer 1979;1:67–81.	Prospective study of 265,118 Japanese adults interviewed about diet and smoking at time of 1965 census. Ten-year followup through record linkage.	611 men and 196 women died with lung cancer. Consumers of green-yellow vegetables showed lower risk of lung cancer in each smoking status stratification. Among ex-smokers lung cancer reduction was greatest in daily vegetable consumers.
Shekelle et al, 1981. Dietary vitamin A and risk of lung cancer in the Western Electric study. Lancet November 28, 1981; 1185–1190.	2107 male employees were examined and received detailed dietary interviews. Intake of 26 separate foods or food groups was used to estimate retinol and carotene. Followup included annual reexamination through the ninth year and later mailed questionnaires and death certificate searches. 19 years of followup reported.	33 men developed lung cancer. A dose-response gradient was seen with the highest lung cancer rate in lowest quartile of carotene intake, independent of smoking. Retinol intake was not related to lung cancer rates.

Table 1. (cont.)

Investigator, year, title	Study design	Results
Serum/plasma vitamin A in lung cancer patients and controls		
Basu et al, 1976. Plasma vitamin A in patients with broncial carcinoma. Br J Cancer 1976; 33:119-121.	28 lung cancer patients were compared to 10 healthy persons and 9 non-cancer lung disease patients. Plasma vitamin A was determined by the antimony trichloride method.	Lung cancer patients had mean plasma vitamin A of 45.6 μg per 100 ml $\pm$ 5.8 standard error. Other patients were 64.3 $\pm$ 4.6 and healthy persons 68.4 $\pm$ 5.0
Cohen et al. 1977. Vitamin A serum levels and dietary vitamin A intake in lung cancer patients. Cancer Lett 1977;4:51-54.	64 male and 3 female patients in Veterans Administration Hospital had serum vitamin A measured by modified method of Sobel and Snow. Source of controls not stated.	Serum vitamin A level did not correlate with histologic subtype and was similar to "control population."
Atukorala et al, 1979. Vitamin A, zinc, and lung cancer. Br J Cancer 1979; 40:927-931.	22 male and 4 female lung cancer patients were compared to 7 male and 3 female noncancer lung disease patients and 8 male and 3 female other patients. Vitamin A was measured by a modification of the fluorometric method of Hansen and Warwick. Serum, β-carotene, retinol-binding protein, copper, and zinc also were measured.	Lung cancer patients had significantly lower serum vitamin A than either control group. Vitamin A in the cases correlated with retinol-binding protein and zinc.
Prospective Studies of Cancer and Retinol in Stored Blood		
Wald et al, 1980. Low serum-vitamin A and subsequent risk of lung cancer; preliminary results of a prospective study. Lancet Oct 1980; 18,813-815.	Serum of about 16,000 men receiving a health screening exam was stored at $-40°C$. After 1-4 years followup, sera of 86 men who developed cancer (14 lung cancers) were compared to 172 sera from controls. Retinol was measured by high pressure liquid chromatography similar to the method of De Ruyter and De Leenheer.	Low retinol levels were associated with an increased risk of cancer, independent of age, smoking habits, or serum cholesterol. The risk in the lowest quintile was 2.2. times higher than that in the highest quintile.
Kark et al, 1981. Serum vitamin A (retinol) and cancer incidence in Evans County, Georgia. JNCI 1981;66:7-16.	Serum from a community sample of 3102 people was stored at $-18°C$ and the population followed for 12-14 years. During followup, 85 persons developed cancer (12 lung	Low retinol levels were associated with an increased risk of cancer, after controlling for age, smoking, and other variables. The risk in the lowest quintile was 5.3 times higher than that in

Table 1. (cont.)

Investigator, year, title	Study design	Results
	cancers). Sera from these persons were compared to those of 174 matched controls, using a fluorometric method after alumina column separation similar to the method described by Futterman et. al.	the highest quintile. Retinol appeared quite stable to light, thawing, and refreezing.
Intervention trial		
Gouveia et al, 1982. Degree of bronchial metaplasia in heavy smokers and its regression after treatment with a retinoid. Lancet March 27, 1982; 710–712.	70 heavy smokers had bronchoscopy and bronchial biopsy and were classified according to a histopathologic index of metaplasia. The 34 with the most severe metaplasia were given a 6-month course of the retinoid, Etretrinate, at a dose of 25 mg/day.	Index of metaplasia scores dropped significantly in the 12 subjects who completed 6 months of treatment. 11 of the 12 had not modified their smoking habits.

In the only intervention trial reported to date, Gouveia et al (12) examined the effect of the synthetic retinoid Etretinate on 34 heavy smokers with bronchial metaplasia. The index of metaplasia scores dropped significantly in the 12 study subjects who completed 6 months of treatment. This preliminary study needs confirmation because the number of cases is small and the precision of the metaplasia score is uncertain.

Observations about the relationship of dietary cholesterol and lung cancer differ from those about serum cholesterol and colon cancer. Hinds et al (13) at the University of Hawaii Cancer Center observed an increased risk of lung cancer associated with high dietary cholesterol for all five major ethnic groups in Hawaii. In contrast, the Framingham Heart Disease Study (14) does not appear to show any particular relationship between low serum cholesterol and lung cancer. However, a somewhat inconsistent, weak relationship has been reported between very low serum cholesterol levels and cancer of the colon (14).

Chemoprevention and diet, nutrition, and cancer research are promising areas that shall receive increased research emphasis. In conclusion, we wish to emphasize again that, although it is hoped the chemoprevention area will be useful against many types of cancer, including lung cancer, the best we can all do about lung cancer is to encourage people not to smoke.

References

1. Carrese LM, Baker CG. The Convergence Technique: a method for the planning and programming of research efforts. Manag Sci 1967;13:B420–38.

2. Lasnitzki I. The influence of a hypervitaminosis on the effect of 20-methylcholanthrene on mouse prostate glands grown in vitro. Br J Cancer 1955;9:438–9.
3. Harris CC, Sporn MB, Kaufman DG, Smith JM, Jackson FE, Saffiotti U. Histogenesis of squamous metaplasia in the hamster tracheal epithelium caused by vitamin A deficiency or Benzo[*a*]pyrene-ferric oxide. JNCI 1972;48:743–61.
4. Verma AK, Shapas BG, Rice HM, Boutwell RK. Correlation of the inhibition by retinoids of tumor promoter-induced mouse epidermal ornithine decarboxylase activity and of skin tumor promotion. Cancer Res 1979;39:422.
5. Becci PJ. Inhibitory effect of 13-*cis*-retinoic acid on urinary bladder carcinogenesis induced in C57BL/6 mice by *N*-Butyl-*N*-(4-hydroxybutyl) nitrosamine. Cancer Res 1978;38(12):4464.
6. Thompson HJ, Becci PJ, Moon RC, et al. Inhibition of 1-methyl-1-nitrosourea-induced mammary carcinogenesis in the rat by the retinoid axerophthene. Arzneimittelforsch/Drug Res 1980;30-2(7):1128.
7. Peto R, Doll R, Buckley JD, Sporn MB. Can dietary beta-carotene materially reduce human cancer rates? Nature 1981;290:201–8.
8. Haenszel W, Loveland DB, Sirken MG. Lung-cancer mortality as related to residence and smoking histories. I. White males. JNCI 1962;28:947–1001.
9. Bjelke E. Dietary vitamin A and human lung cancer. Int J Cancer 1975;15:561–5.
10. Hirayama T. Diet and Cancer. Nutr Cancer 1979;1:67–81.
11. Shekelle RB, Lepper M, Liu S, Maliza C, Raynor WJ, Rossof AH. Dietary vitamin A and risk of cancer in the Western Electric study. Lancet 1981;November 28.1185–90.
12. Gouveia J, Mathe G, Hercend T, Gros F, Lemaigre G, Santelli G. Degree of bronchial metaplasia in heavy smokers and its regression after treatment with a retinoid. Lancet 1982.March 27.710–2.
13. Hinds MW, Kolonel LN, Lee J, Hankin JH. Dietary cholesterol and lung cancer risk among men in Hawaii. Am J Clin Nutr 1983;37:192–3.
14. Feinleib M: Summary: workshop on cholesterol and non-cardiovascular disease mortality, May 11–12, 1981. Bethesda, MD: National Heart, Blood and Lung Institute, National Institutes of Health.

CHAPTER 16

Vitamin A and Lung Cancer in Louisiana

BARBARA Y. LEGARDEUR, ALFREDO LOPEZ-S, and WILLIAM D. JOHNSON

Departments of Medicine and Biometry, Louisiana State University Medical Center, New Orleans, Louisiana 70112

ABSTRACT

To study the association of vitamin A and β-carotene with lung cancer incidence in Louisiana, we used two different approaches. In the first, we compared vitamin A nutritional status with age-adjusted mortality rates for respiratory system cancers in 19 Louisiana parishes. A case–control study of patients with lung cancer in a large metropolitan area was begun in which serum levels and dietary intake of retinol and β-carotene were determined along with other nutritional, environmental, and occupational factors. The correlation coefficients, calculated for the comparison of vitamin A nutritional status, showed a negative association between dietary vitamin A and mortality rates in white men. Although a trend toward a negative association between serum β-carotene and mortality was noted, the association was not statistically significant. In the case–control study, preliminary analysis showed that serum values of β-carotene, serum retinol, and retinol-binding protein were significantly lower for lung cancer patients than for persons in either of the two control groups. The findings of this report suggest that nutritional differences may be one of the contributory factors for the differences in mortality rates for lung cancer in certain geographic areas of Louisiana.
Key Words: **Vitamin A, β-carotene, lung cancer**

Introduction

The number of deaths attributed to lung cancer each year in Louisiana is relatively higher than in other areas of the United States. During 1950-1969, Louisiana had the highest rates in the country for white men, and 10 of Louisiana's 64 parishes ranked in the top 18 counties nationally for deaths from lung cancer (1). Furthermore, when shown on a map, the highest mortalities are concentrated in the south-southeastern portion of the state (2). The distribution of lung cancer in Louisiana and the diverse cultural and ethnic differences of the state suggest environmental factors may contribute to this high incidence of lung cancer (see

Lung Cancer: Causes and Prevention.

Chapter 6). Local studies have suggested that the industries of shipbuilding, fishing (3), and sugarcane farming (4) may increase lung cancer risk, whereas national correlation studies have implicated exposure in the shipbuilding, chemical, petroleum, and paper manufacturing industries (5, 6). However, according to a survey of employment in industry, as indicated on death certificates, no one industry was found to account for the excess mortality in southern Louisiana (3).

Nutritional factors have been postulated to contribute to lung cancer development, as reported in both epidemiologic (7, 8) and experimental studies (9, 10). In particular, a deficiency of vitamin A has been associated with lung cancer incidence. Recent reports (11, 12) show that persons consuming fruits and vegetables rich in β-carotene, a precursor of vitamin A, have a lower risk for lung cancer even after adjustment is made for cigarette smoking. For this reason, we thought that information on the nutritional status of a large sample of the Louisiana population, obtained during the Ten-State National Nutrition Survey (13), might provide clues as to the role of nutrition in the development of lung cancer in Louisiana. The results of that survey show that Louisiana has a large percentage of households in general, and of older persons in particular, consuming less than 50% of the recommended dietary intake of vitamin A. The survey also shows that Louisiana, when compared with other states, had an above average percentage of persons with unacceptable levels of serum retinol (preformed vitamin A) (13).

Here we report our findings on the correlation between vitamin A nutritional status and lung cancer incidence in Louisiana, by using the results of the Ten-State Nutrition Survey in comparison with Mason and McKay's reported mortalities for cancer (1). In addition, we present preliminary data from a case-control study of persons with lung cancer in the largest metropolitan area in the southern part of Louisiana (New Orleans).

Methods

Dietary intakes and biochemical indices of nutritional status in a sample of Louisiana residents were obtained during the Ten-State Nutrition Survey (13). That survey was done under the auspices of the U.S. Department of Health, Education and Welfare (DHEW) with the aim of estimating the prevalence, magnitude, and distribution of malnutrition in this country. Louisiana was one of the ten states surveyed. Nineteen representative parishes (counties) of Louisiana, involving a total of 1161 families and 5033 persons, participated in the study. Extensive information on nutrient intake and blood levels was obtained. However, for this study we focused our attention only on the intake and blood levels of retinol (preformed vitamin A) and β-carotene of those persons 18 years or older at the time of the survey. The mean intake and serum levels of retinol and β-carotene for black and white men were calculated for each of the 19 parishes. The mean nutrient levels for each sex-race group in the parish were then compared with the lung cancer mortality data for that parish. We used the average annual age-adjusted death rates of respiratory system cancers per 100,000 population for the period 1950–1969 as reported by Mason and McKay (1). Pearson's product-moment correlation coefficients were calculated for nutrient means versus the age-adjusted mortality.

In addition, we have begun a case-control study of patients with lung cancer in two New Orleans hospitals. Participants are persons newly diagnosed as having lung cancer and other hospitalized persons without cancer matched by race, sex, age, and parish of residency. Criteria for the control group included the exclusion of diseases that might affect vitamin A nutritional status. A second noninstitutionalized free-living control group of normal persons is also being compared. We are evaluating serum levels and dietary intakes of retinol, β-carotene, and related nutritional factors along with other environmental factors. Blood specimens are drawn after primary lung cancer has been confirmed by a histologic report and before treatment is begun. Blood samples also are obtained at the time of the interview from the hospital and free-living control groups. Retinol and β-carotene levels were determined spectrophotometrically by the trifluoroacetic acid method of Neeld and Pearson (14). Retinol-binding protein levels are determined by the radial immunodiffusion method of Mancini et al (15).

Using a 28-day dietary history, we ascertained the frequency of consumption, serving size, and method of preparation for an extensive list of foods that was then reduced to 80 different nutrients and related factors by a computerized method availble in our laboratory (16, 17). Finally, information on environmental exposures and smoking habits was obtained by trained interviewers, and pertinent information was taken from the patient's chart. Body mass index (18) was calculated from the patient's weight and height, obtained at the time of interview. The study followed the ethical standards of the Institutional Review Board of Louisiana State University Medical Center.

Results

Figure 1 shows a crude estimate of the average vitamin A intake for men in the northern and southern parishes of Louisiana who participated in the Ten-State Nutrition Survey. The approximate intake in the north was 5886 IU of vitamin A activity, whereas the approximate intake in the south was 2526 IU for vitamin A activity.

The correlation coefficients for average nutrient levels in each parish as compared with the death rates from respiratory system cancers in that parish are shown in Table 1. For both white and black men, a negative association between serum β-carotene and mortality was noted, whereas a positive association was seen for serum vitamin A levels and mortality. Because vitamin A levels have been suggested to increase with age (19), our analysis was repeated using age-adjusted serum vitamin A levels. In black men no change was seen; however, for white men the direction of the association changed from a positive to a negative correlation. The correlation coefficients were not statistically significant. A statistically significant association between dietary intake of vitamin A and mortality was observed for white men.

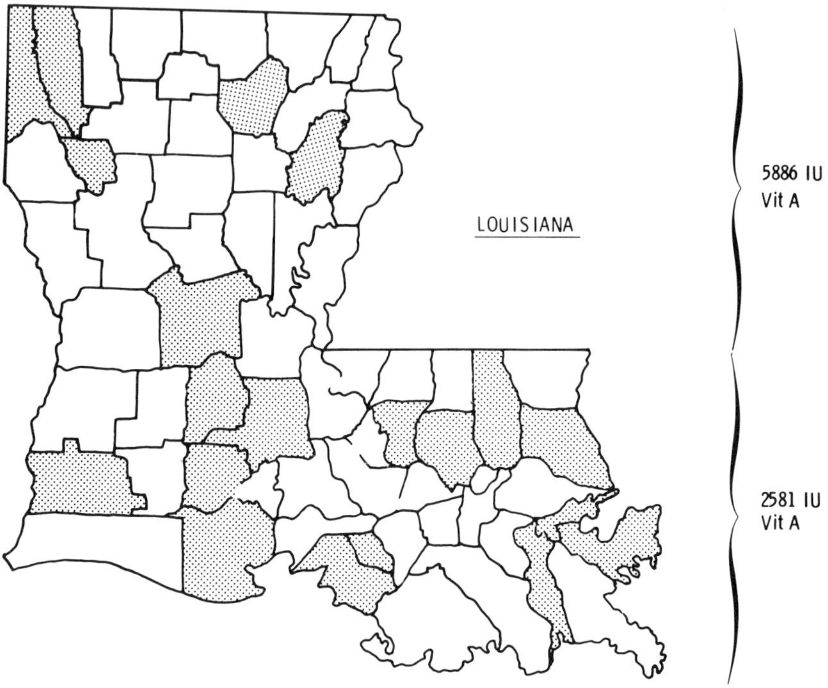

Figure 1. Vitamin A intake in Louisiana parishes participating in Ten-State Nutrition Survey (13).

Table 1. Pearson's correlation coefficients between vitamin A and β-carotene levels and mortality rates for respiratory system cancers in Louisiana

Groups	Mortality rates correlated with: Serum vitamin A	Age-adjusted vitamin A	Serum β-carotene	Dietary vitamin A
White males	0.37	−0.26	−0.23	−0.63[a]
Black males	0.20	0.17	−0.22	−0.21

[a]P < 0.05.

Table 2. Mean and standard deviation for serum vitamin A, β-carotene, retinol-binding protein, and body mass index in lung cancer cases and matched controls

Subjects	Serum levels (n = 31): Retinol (μg/dl)	β-carotene (μg/dl)	RBP[a] (μg/dl)	Body mass index (n = 19)
Lung cancer cases	48 + 18[b]	63 + 33[b]	4.5 + 1.8[b]	24.2 + 4.2
Hospital controls	58 + 20	92 + 61	5.3 + 1.8	25.2 + 4.9
Free-living controls	63 + 17	112 + 52	6.1 + 1.6	24.8 + 3.2

[a]RBP = retinol-binding protein.
[b]P < 0.05.

Table 2 shows the serum levels of β-carotene, retinol, and retinol-binding protein and the body mass index for lung cancer patients and matched controls. The difference in serum levels between the persons with lung cancer and both the hospitalized patients and the free-living controls was statistically significant. No difference for body mass index was found in a random selection of the lung cancer patients and the two control groups.

Discussion

The results of the investigation of vitamin A status in the northern and southern parishes of Louisiana suggest that nutritional factors may contribute to the excess mortality of lung cancer in south Louisiana. Recognizing that the data derive from two independent sources having different and unrelated purposes, a trend is still apparent. The more consistent association of mortality with serum β-carotene rather than serum retinol agrees with, and precedes (20), the hypothesis suggested by Peto et al (2) that β-carotene may be of greater significance in reducing lung cancer risk than retinol. Because the available dietary information was limited, only total vitamin A could be assessed and not the individual contribution of preformed vitamin A and β-carotene. Yet, with caution, one may speculate that the greater vitamin A intake in northern Louisiana may reflect the greater preponderance of fresh fruits and vegetables in the diet. Northern Louisiana is primarily agricultural, and one therefore would expect generous intakes of truck crops, such as many of the green and yellow vegetables that are rich in β-carotene. These suggestive findings strengthen the preliminary analysis of the case–control study carried out in the metropolitan New Orleans area.

Patients newly diagnosed as having primary lung cancer show that serum levels of retinol, β-carotene, and retinol-binding protein are significantly lower in affected persons than in matched controls. Furthermore, the difference between cases and controls seems to be greatest for serum β-carotene. This finding again supports the importance of the association of β-carotene with lung cancer when compared with the association of retinol. These findings agree with those of S. Atukorula et al (22), showing retinol and β-carotene to be lower in lung cancer patients than in the two control groups, although the difference for serum β-carotene in Atukorula's study is not statistically different.

The interpretation of our results on the relationship of serum levels with lung cancer incidence needs to be evaluated in the context of smoking habits and protein–calorie nutritional status. Cigarette smoking is known to be a major factor (23) in lung cancer development, and nutritional factors, such as retinol and/or β-carotene, may be modifying factors on the effect of cigarette smoke in lung cancer development. Also, it must be determined whether the lower levels of serum β-carotene are the result of a malnourished state caused by the malignant process or some other factor related to malnutrition. Preliminary evidence from our case–control study indicates that this is not the case, because the body mass index does not differ among lung cancer patients, hospital controls, and free-living subjects. Yet further analysis of more specific indexes of malnutrition, such as the concentration of somatic and visceral protein status, must be studied before malnutrition can be excluded as a contributing factor for the decrease in serum levels. An alternate approach for eliminating the potential contributory effect of malnutrition is to study serum values before the development of the lung cancer, as was done by Wald et al (24). In a prospective study of 16,000 men, they reported that serum retinol levels, independent of age and smoking habits, were lower in men who developed lung cancer than in persons who did not have lung cancer. Serum β-carotene levels were not reported.

In defining the role of β-carotene, retinol, or other nutritional factors in the development of lung cancer, an accurate and complete analysis of diet is essential. Early studies (7, 11) have failed in this area. In some studies, food frequency questionnaires were used to estimate grossly the vitamin A intake of persons who developed lung cancer as compared with persons serving as controls. For example, in a prospective study of 8278 men in Norway, Bjelke (7) reported that men with a high vitamin A index had a lower relative risk for lung cancer than did men with a low vitamin A index. The vitamin A index is derived from the frequency of consumption and the amount of vitamin A activity (IU) in an average serving size of that food.

This approach does not take into account the variability of serving sizes among different persons. Similarly, Mettlin (11) showed an inverse association of lung cancer incidence with a vitamin A index based on questionnaire-obtained information pertaining to the intake of 21 foods. Most of the 21 foods included were in the green and yellow vegetables category, foods that are rich in β-carotene. However, liver, one of the rich sources of retinol (preformed vitamin A) was not included in the evaluation. Because not all possible foods and vitamin supplements are included in such questionnaires, the index should only be used as a crude estimate of the relative consumption of vitamin A activity in foods. Furthermore, nutritional factors present in the same foods and having a procancer or anticancer effect, such as vitamin C, may be significant but not evaluated in the study. The net result of the algebraic sum of the procancer and anticancer effect in a food item may determine its final effect in promoting or preventing the development of cancer.

In our ongoing study, we will be better prepared to study the contribution of β-carotene, retinol, total vitamin A activity, and other related nutrients in absolute weight as well as a nutrient–calorie ratio. Our extensive interview on foods, including those specific for Louisiana, and our computerized nutrient analysis system enables us to quantify the nutrient under study as well as other vitamins and minerals. We will have a better overall picture of vitamin A, because information on dietary intake, serum levels, and body stores is being collected. Our laboratory also is studying retinol and β-carotene levels in liver specimens obtained at autopsies from persons who have died of lung cancer and other diseases. With the previously described information we will begin to help clarify the association of β-carotene and retinol with lung cancer incidence in Louisiana. Vitamin A nutritional status must be studied with the same intensity as information involving smoking and occupational exposures that has been analyzed in other studies.

This point is important if we are to show that nutritional differences contribute to the increased mortality for lung cancer in Louisiana.

Acknowledgments

Work reported here was supported by a grant from NCI, CA23205.

References

1. Mason TJ, McKay FW. U.S. cancer mortality by county 1950–1969. U.S. Department of Health, Education and Welfare (NIH) 74–615. Washington, DC: U.S. Government Printing Office, 1964.
2. Mason TJ, McKay FN, Hoover R, Blott WJ, Fraumeni JF. Atlas of cancer mortality for U.S. Counties: 1950–1969. Washington, DC: U.S. Government Printing Office, 1975.
3. Gottlieb MS, Pickle LW, Blott WJ, Fraumeni JF. Lung cancer in Louisiana: death certificate analysis. JNCI 1979;63:1131–7.
4. Rothschild H, Mulvey JJ. An increase risk for lung cancer mortality associated with sugarcane farming. JNCI 1982;755–60.
5. Blot WJ, Fraumeni JF. Geographic patterns of lung cancer: industrial correlations. Am J Epidemiol 1976;103:539–50.
6. Blot WJ, Brinton LA, Stone BJ, et al. Cancer mortality in U.S. counties with petroleum industries. Science 1977;198:51–3.
7. Bjelke E. Dietary vitamin A and human lung cancer. Int J Cancer 1975;15:561–5.
8. Basu TK, Donaldson D, Jenner M, Williams DC, Sakula A. Plasma vitamin A in patients with bronchial carcinoma. Br J Cancer 1976;33:119–21.
9. Suffiott U, Montesano R, Sellakumar AR, Borg SA. Experimental cancer of the lung. Inhibition by vitamin A of the induction of tracheobronchial squamous metaplasia and squamous cell tumors. Cancer 1967;20:857.
10. Sporn MB, Newton DL. Chemoprevention of cancer with retinoids. Fed Proc 1979;38:2528–33.
11. Mettlin C, Graham S, Swanson M. Vitamin A and lung cancer. JNCI 1979;62:1435–8.
12. Hirayama T. Diet and cancer. Nutr Cancer 1979;1:67–81.
13. Ten-State Nutrition Survey, 1968–70. U.S. Department of Health Education and Welfare Publ (HSM) 72-8129, 72-8130, 72-8131, 72-8132, 72-8133.
14. Neeld JB, Jr, Pearson WN. Macro and micromethods for the determination of serum vitamin A using trifluoracetic acid. J Nutr 1963;79:454–62.
15. Mancini G, Carbonara AO, Heremans JF. Immunochemical quantitation of antigens by single radial immunodiffusion. Immunochemistry 1965;2:35.
16. Moore MC, Judlin BC, Kennemur PM. Using graduated food models in taking dietary histories. J Am Diet Assoc 1967;51:447–50.
17. Moore MC, Moore EM, Beasley CD, Hawkins GJ, Judlin BC. Dietary atherosclerosis study on deceased persons. J Am Diet Assoc 1970; 56:14–22.
18. Key A, Fidanza F, Karvonen MJ, Kimura N, Taylor H. Indices of relative weight and obesity. J Chronic Dis 1972;25:329–43.
19. Underwood BA. The determination of vitamin A and some aspects of its distribution, mobilization and transport in health and disease. World Rev Nutr Diet 1974;19:123–72.
20. Lopez-S A, Yates B, Johnson WD, Nze R. The role of vitamin A and ascorbic acid in relation to respiratory system cancers. Am J Clin Nutr 1979;32:954.
21. Peto R, Doll R, Buckley JD, Sporn MB. Can dietary beta-carotene materially reduce human cancer rates? Nature 1981;2990:201–8.
22. Atukorala S, Basu TK, Dickerson JWT, Donaldson D, Sakula A. Vitamin A, zinc and lung cancer. Br J Cancer 1979;40:927–31.
23. Graham S, Levin ML. Smoking withdrawal in the reduction of risk for lung cancer. Cancer 1971;27:865–70.

24. Wald N, Idle M, Boreham L. Low serum vitamin A and subsequent risk of cancer. Lancet 1980;1:813-5.

CHAPTER **17**

Prevention of Smoking in Adolescents: Current Perspective on A Social-Behavioral Intervention

RICHARD I. EVANS

Social Psychology/Behavioral Medicine Research and Graduate Training Group, University of Houston, Houston, Texas 77004

ABSTRACT

The University of Houston Social Psychology/Behavioral Medicine Research Group has undertaken several investigations that evaluate the effectiveness of social-psychological strategies to deter the onset of frequent smoking in junior high school students. Smoking deterrence strategies were developed within a social-psychological framework consisting principally of a series of films and various student involvement techniques. In the films, in addition to information concerning effects of smoking, detailed techniques for coping with social influences (peers, parents, media) to smoke are depicted. Impact of the interventions are determined from measures of knowledge gained, intentions to smoke, and smoking behavior utilizing a specially designed saliva analysis procedure. Various junior high schools were assigned to experimental and control conditions. Seventh through ninth grade smoking deterrence interventions and evaluation measures were administered in the experimental schools, and the evaluation measures only were administered in the control schools. Analyses of the data revealed that the treatment group subjects smoked less frequently than did the control group subjects and that knowledge generated by the interventions was significantly related to smoking intention and behavior. Various short- and long-term followups (up to 3 years) appeared to confirm these findings. Various gender differences in susceptibility to social influences to smoke also were found. Discussion of the long-range implications of such programs, their strengths, and their weaknesses is presented.

Key Words: **Social psychology, behavioral medicine, social-psychological strategies, deterrence, adolescents**

Lung Cancer: Causes and Prevention.

It is obvious that an increasing focus of public policy in addressing cancer and other major diseases is in the area of primary prevention (1). It is apparent that because cigarette smoking has been linked both separately and synergistically to probably the greatest and most serious incidence of morbidity and mortality, a major thrust in a national program should be control of cigarette smoking. Although there has been a relative decline in incidence of smoking, smoking persists in about one-third of our adult population. This is partly true because smoking cessation efforts have a history of poor long-term effectiveness (2, 3). Influencing the cessation of smoking may, in fact, present a problem that is more clinical than social-psychological. So beginning in 1974, our Social Psychology/Behavioral Medicine Research Group began to focus on prevention. We decided to develop, implement, and evaluate social-behavioral strategies to prevent the onset of cigarette smoking in adolescents and were fortunate enough to be funded in these efforts by the National Heart, Lung, and Blood Institute and the National Cancer Institute.

The complex multidimensional nature of smoking, incorporating biologic, social-psychological, and behavioral variables, has now become even more specifically documented (2–6) than when we began this work. Identifying and coping with the factors involved in the initiation of smoking among adolescents is an endeavor that may require the utilization of diverse conceptualizations and strategies. Various conceptions in social and developmental psychology appear to be useful in generating hypotheses to account for the initiation of smoking and in providing conceptual bases for prevention programs.

In this chapter I first briefly review some of these general conceptions that have influenced the development of our intervention strategy, then describe the specific rationale for what may be described as our social inoculation approach, summarize some of our prospective investigations utilizing this intervention strategy, and finally consider some of the possible limitations of this approach.

Perspective From Earlier Research

The earlier research of the writer and his associates in the area of persuasive communications as it relates to disease prevention programs in schools (7, 8) yielded important insights that have proved to be particularly applicable to smoking investigations. These include: (a) the probability that reported health behavior may not be correlated with actual behavior; (b) that merely focusing on fear arousal in persuasion may not be the most effective means of influencing health enhancement behavior, and (c) that the school environment may be especially useful for systematic and controlled exposure to persuasive messages concerning disease prevention behavior. A fourth insight relates to the importance of tailoring both the content and the style of health-related messages to the particular audience. Therefore, a systematic process assessment of the knowledge, experiences, perceptions, beliefs, behaviors, and terminology of the target audience must form the basis on which persuasive communications are formulated. Results from our ongoing longitudinal smoking deterrence studies provide at least some support for the validity of these insights (9–11).

Theoretical and Empirical Foundations of Intervention Strategy

In order to apply any concept or rationale to the problem of smoking prevention, it should be noted that smoking begins reflecting an upward trend from elementary grades, and most significantly junior high school into high school (12–14). This trend has been reported consistently in the literature (4, 15, 16). So within this estimate of smoking frequency it was determined that the most effective way to attack the problem would be to influence entering junior high school students not to initiate smoking.

A survey of junior high school programs dealing with prevention of smoking (5) revealed that more traditional efforts (a) generally were focused perhaps too intensely on fear arousal; (b) largely emphasized the future consequences of smoking, such as heart disease or cancer, and failed to recognize that teenagers tend to care more about the present than the future; (c) in utilizing films and other media of communication, failed to utilize previous research on effective use of media; and (d) evoked responses that may even be counterproductive. In light of these findings, we decided to undertake a long-term study in the Houston Independent School District (10, 11, 17), among the largest school districts in the United States.

Interviews conducted before both a pilot study (17) and a 3-year study (10) with a large population of seventh graders, suggested that peer pressure, models of smoking parents, and smoking models or messages in the mass media, such as cigarette advertising, individually or collectively may outweigh the belief of adolescents that smoking is dangerous. By the time they had reached seventh grade, all the children believed smoking was dangerous. Some of them, between the ages of 4 and 11, had even spent time trying to persuade their parents to give up smoking. As they grew older, social pressures to smoke become superimposed on the fear of this behavior, and the fear and knowledge of the dangers of smoking became insufficient to prevent the onset of smoking.

From among the various available conceptions in psychology that generally might have related to our intervention strategy, Bandura's social learning theory (18, 19) offered particularly relevant insights. As applied to the initiation of smoking (20), this theory suggests that through observation children acquire expectations and learned behaviors with regard to smoking. For example, a child can learn vicariously that cigarette smoking relieves tension or anxiety. Thus, (s)he might come to expect that if (s)he feels tense, smoking will have a relaxing effect. In addition, when a model engages in an apparently enjoyable behavior that the observer expects to be socially prohibited, but negative consequences do not follow, disinhibition results. That is, the child's learned expectation of negative consequences is weakened, possibly to the point where the child engages in the same behavior as the model. Vicariously learned expectations, then, of the positive and

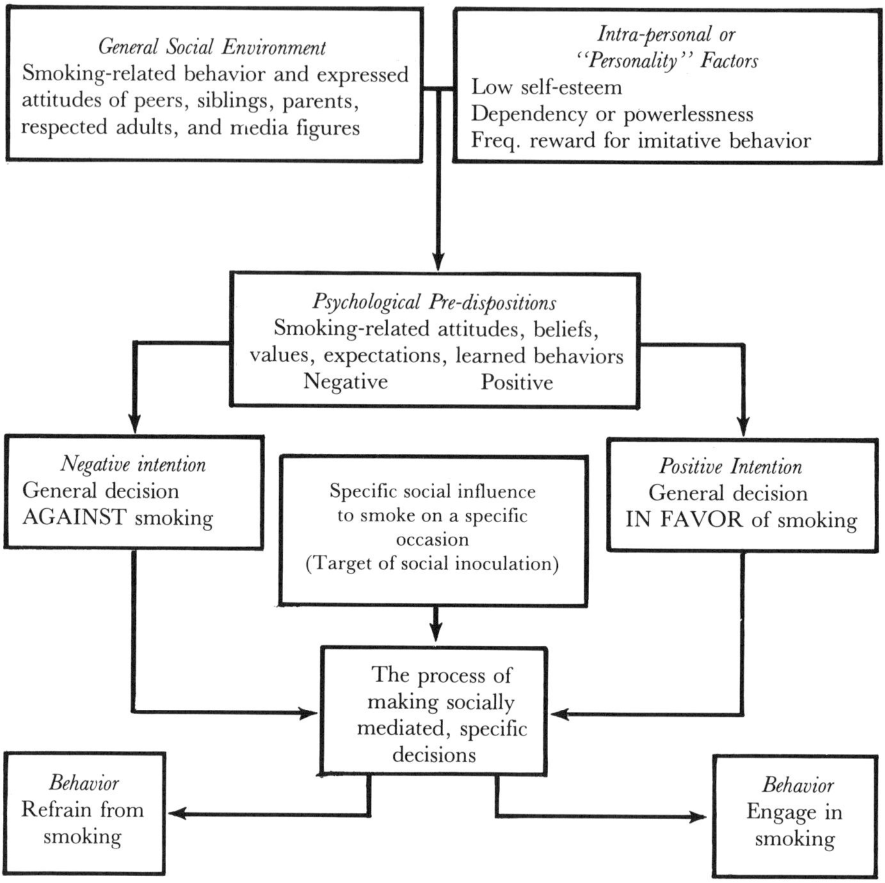

Figure 1. A model of smoking-related social-psychological processes impacting behavior

negative consequences of cigarette smoking appear to be important factors in the ultimate decision regarding smoking. As also first presented in an earlier publication (20), Figure 1 reflects the array of possible influences to smoke.

This model, which emerged from our investigations, postulates that both the social environmental and "personality" determinants contribute to the complex of psychological predispositions related to smoking. These psychological predispositions tend to produce an intention either to smoke or not to smoke. Nevertheless, the actual decision to smoke (or not to smoke) on a particular occasion may depend on the impact of situational social influences. Teaching adolescents to cope with such influences may decrease the probability of their initiating smoking. Also this approach logically could be incorporated within existing school health education programs. Examining the other components of smoking initiation as reflected in Figure 1, we felt that within the constraints in the school system with which we would be working we would not be able to design significant interventions modifying the social environment. Likewise, although other investigators (21, 22) subsequently developed interventions directed toward altering some of the intrapersonal determinants of smoking, we also felt that within the constraints of the institutions with which we would be working, such an alteration attempt would require too complex an array of commitments. So inoculation against social influences to smoke became the primary focus of our intervention.

To guide the development of our interventions, we found McGuire's (23) communication–persuasion model both relevant and provocative. It analyzes the impact of communications according to five components: attention, comprehension, yielding, retention, and action. Obviously, to be effective, a communication must hold the person's attention and be understandable to that person. In addition, the communication must elicit yielding (or agreement) on the part of the person exposed to the message. Induced agreement must be maintained (retention) over time in order for it to be translated into action in appropriate situations.

Various elements of the filmed messages we produced address problems of attention, comprehension, and yielding (20). First, instead of adults, adolescent narrators selected for their poise and appearance take the role of information brokers. Using language that is specifically geared to the audience's level of comprehension, the narrators present scientific information; however, in keeping with their role as information brokers, these student narrators make no claim to having a scientific expertise of their own. Thus, such phrases as "the researchers asked me to tell you. . ." and "the researchers found that. . ." are included at appropriate points.

Second, much of the content of the films and discussions dealing with psychosocial influences to smoke and with strategies for coping with these influences are based on data obtained from students who are similar to those in the audience. For example, most of the footage in the films shows students acting out situations which their peers have described to us in preintervention surveys and focused group interviews. Our process evaluations suggest that these scenes and situations are perceived by the student audience as being realistic.

Third, the messages in the films and discussions are presented in a manner directed toward reinforcing self-attributions or the ability of the members of the audience to self-determine the decision whether or not to smoke. The student narrators repeatedly tell the audience "you can decide for yourself " and "knowing these facts might help you to decide" and "here's something you might want to think about." Process evaluations have indicated that the student audiences are favorably impressed by this self-attributional aspect of the films and discussions.

In addition to tailoring our intervention to the model, as suggested earlier, we also employ a behavioral variation of McGuire's (24) "inoculation" approach to attitude change. McGuire suggests that existing attitudes may be strengthened by inoculating individuals against counterarguments to which they may be exposed. By explicating the nature of various social influences to smoke, our intervention program attempts to inoculate the audience against these influences. Further, we suggest to the students specific strategies that they can use to cope with these social influences when they encounter them.

To increase the probability of impact of the social inoculation interventions, information is presented that is intended to motivate the student to develop a negative smoking intention, an intention *not* to smoke. Information presented includes the immediate health effects of smoking, negative social consequences of smoking, and the cost of smoking. A film depicting immediate health effects includes statements of commonly held beliefs about smoking followed by demonstrations that either confirm or refute the accuracy of these beliefs. Another message attempts to increase student's awareness of the dangers of experimental smoking.

Prior to the presentation of the social inoculation messages, various messages familiarized the students with various social influences to smoke. Three social influences were defined in our pilot study (10)—modeling, peer pressure, and cigarette advertising—and scenes representing examples of each of these influences were presented. Our current investigation has incorporated adult nagging, because responses in a preintervention survey indicated this as a more frequently cited factor in smoking than had previously been apparent. In the case of cigarette advertising, content analyses of ads are used to reveal to students the techniques employed by advertisers. When a student subsequently encounters a situation in which a social influence to smoke is present, (s)he will be better able to consciously recognize that social influence and to understand how it operates. This recognition and understanding may well enable the student to make a specific decision that is based more on personal intention than on the demands of the particular situation. As indicated earlier, in the various filmed messages and group discussions, the student is encouraged to make a conscious decision about smoking, rather than to be influenced by external influences without being sufficiently vigilant concerning the effects of such external influences.

The social inoculation content consists of the presentation of strategies and skills for coping with social influences to smoke that they may encounter in the future. For example, various films depict specific strategies that the nonsmoking students themselves indicate they use for coping with peer pressure to smoke. During discussions following the films, students are given the opportunity to role play peer situations they may encounter, and to rehearse coping with them.

Evaluation

We concluded that school systems appeared to be the most promising agencies for the delivery of such smoking prevention programs to large groups of adolescents. There is no other agency in our culture that has the school's capability to reach adolescents from all racial, ethnic, religious, and socioeconomic groups. Within the context of the educational institution, however, an intervention program developer must consider the following constraints:

1. The amount of class time which the school is willing to allocate to smoking prevention
2. The amount of time required for school personnel to be trained adequately to implement the program

Guided by these considerations, it was decided to develop a system for delivering interventions that would require a minimum of class time, would not require prior training of school personnel or students, and would be relatively immune to the unique characteristics of the presenter. This delivery system involves four interrelated modes. First, a set of films or videotapes presents a number of messages. Second, discussions and role plays are used to reinforce, clarify, and personalize these messages. Third, posters assist students in retaining information. Fourth, feedback is provided concerning retention of knowledge and frequency of smoking as the intervention program progresses.

Time of each intervention session and frequency of intervention, of course, is negotiated with the school system officials. The central core of our intervention is designed to require one class period on each of four occasions. There appears to be a point of diminishing returns in terms of amount of classroom time devoted to the intervention because of possible habituation or "nag" effects.

Although in the pilot study, the sequence of presentation of the components of the intervention was more concentrated, the essence of the intervention procedure remained essentially the same. Films presented on the first day included information about the dangers of smoking to health and, most prominently, a section describing and illustrating peer pressure and its effect on smoking behavior. Other films recapped the first film and presented information about parental influence of smoking behavior, including a depiction of parental pressure to smoke and not to smoke, and children's modeling of parents' smoking behavior. Still other films recapped the first two films and presented information dealing with mass media pressures to smoke. These films included a pictorial analysis of such advertising techniques as artistically hiding the Surgeon General's warning on cigarette packages, and appeals based on implied sexual attractiveness and popularity. The final films were a general recap of earlier films. The various treatment films of the pilot were either presented in their entirety (all four films presented) or were absent (no treatment presented) in various experimental and control groups.

Following the films, students were asked for written and oral responses to questions. The experimenter distributed brief questionnaires for subjects' written responses. Four sets of questions were prepared and presented in conjunction with each film. The questions, which incorporated a quasi-role-playing device of allowing the respondent to make decisions concerning whether or not to respond to social pressure to smoke, were formulated in such a way as to attribute motivation to resist pressures to smoke to persons who have seen the film, and attribute ability to decide whether or not to smoke to persons subjected to smoking pressure.

Each film presentation is followed by a discussion that is designed to reinforce the messages in the films. Also to reinforce these messages, posters representing scenes from the films were displayed in the classrooms. These posters thus served as continuous reminders of the film messages.

The five dependent measures include smoking information, smoking attitudes, intention to smoke, and reported smoking behavior, as well as the nicotine in saliva analysis of Horning and his collaborators (25), which was used as an objective measure of the presence or absence of smoking. In the earlier investigations, the Horning test determined the amount of nicotine present in the saliva samples by a mass spectrometric analysis. In later investigations, thiocyanate analyses were employed. These analyses provided the basis for inferences about the degree of smoking behavior of the subjects. Cost of these chemical analyses precluded analysis for each subject on each occasion. So a sampling of saliva specimens from each group was analyzed both as an indicator of smoking frequency and as a part of a technique to increase the validity of self-reports of smoking. Earlier studies (26) found that when subjects learned from a short film that in some instances their saliva would be analyzed to determine smoking behavior and how this analysis was done, self-reports of smoking frequency increased.

In a 10-week pilot study (10), rates of onset of smoking in the treatment schools were significantly lower than the onset rates in the pretest single posttest control groups. More than 18% of the control groups had begun smoking, while less than 10% in the experimental groups had begun smoking. (The small number of subjects already smoking in the various experimental groups precluded a statistical comparison of onset rates among the experimental groups and the control group.) In a followup 3-year study (11) involving 13 junior high schools utilizing a complex multiple experimental–control group design, results indicate that those who gained information from films were smoking less than those who did not gain information. Using the criterion of smoking two cigarettes a day or more, 7% fewer in the treatment schools were smoking this frequently than were those in the control schools. Using the criterion of still not smoking at all, there were 8% fewer in the control schools than in the treatment schools; both these differences were statistically significant. Furthermore, significant interactions were found among information presented in the films and discussions, intention to smoke, and smoking. These results indicate that such interventions may prove more useful in deterring smoking among junior high school students than merely instructing them in more traditional health education programs. Perhaps of most importance is that these findings suggest that various kinds of interventions may be effective if they have a reasonable social psychological conceptual base framed in terms of data from the target audience about its perceptions of the influences to smoke and how to cope with them (2, 4, 5). Other investigators (22, 27), using variations of our conceptual and developmental approaches that also have reported promising results, appear to support this contention.

However, a word of caution may be introduced. Surely the results of this social-psychologically derived primary prevention program, this social inoculation–behavioral strategy, does demonstrate some promise. Yet, it must be remembered that the bottom line for prevention of smoking is not that which is demonstrated in a program's relatively short-termed effectiveness, that is, reduced smoking through the early adolescent years. Instead, as these adolescents move through high school, will such a strategy actually reduce the incidence of addictive smoking? This cannot be determined until individuals reach the end of their high school years, because very little cigarette smoking is initiated after the individual leaves high school and incidence of smoking addiction among high school seniors approaches the level of the general adult population (5). So it is important to continue to evaluate such interventions and their impact or to introduce additional interventions through later adolescent years. A similar caution must be considered in the evaluation of any program directed at the primary prevention of disease which involves children and/or adolescents, particularly when the endpoints of such programs involve not only influencing a behavior (as in the case of the social inoculation approach) but also ultimately influencing the incidence of morbidity and/or mortality.

References

1. U.S. Department of Health, Education and Welfare. Disease prevention and health promotion: Federal programs and prospects. Report of the department task force on prevention. U.S. DHEW (PHS) Publ 79-5507 IB. Washington, DC: U.S. Government Printing Office, 1979.
2. Evans RI, Henderson AH, Hill PC, Raines BE. Current psychological, social and educational programs in control and prevention of smoking: a critical methodological review. In: Gotto AM, Paoletti R, eds, Atherosclerosis review, Vol 6. New York: Raven Press, 1979:203–245
3. Leventhal H, Cleary PD. The smoking problem: a review of the research and theory in behavioral risk modification. Psychol Bull 1980; 88(2):370–405.
4. Evans RI, Henderson AH, Hill PC, Raines BE. Smoking in children and adolescents—psychosocial determinants and prevention strategies. In: Smoking and health: a report of the Surgeon General. U.S. Department of Health Education and Welfare Publ (PHS) 79-50066. Washington DC: U.S. Government Printing Office 1979.
5. Evans RI Raines BE. Control and prevention of smoking in adolescents: a psychosocial perspective. In: Coates T, Peterson A, Perry C, eds, Promoting adolescent health: a dialog on research and practice. New York: Academic Press, 1982:101–136
6. Reeder LG. Sociocultural factors in the etiology of smoking behavior: An assessment. In: Jarvik ME, Cullen JW, Gritz ER, Mogt TM, West LJ. eds, Research on smoking behavior. National Institute on Drug Abuse (NIDA) res monogr 17, U.S. DHEW, PHS, ADA/MHA, NIDA. U.S. Department of Health, Education and Welfare Publ (ADM) 78 – 581. Washington, DC: U.S. Government Printing Office, December 1977:186-201.
7. Evans RI, Rozelle RM, Lasater TM, Dembroski TM, Allen BP. Fear arousal, persuasion and actual versus implied behavioral change: new perspective utilizing a real-life dental hygiene program. J Pers Soc Psychol 1970;16(2):220–7.
8. Evans RI, Rozelle RM, Noblitt R, Williams DL. Explicit and implicit persuasive communications over time to initiate and maintain behavior change: new perspective utilizing a real-life dental situation. J Appli Soc Psychol 1975;5(2):150–6.
9. Evans RI. Modifying health lifestyles in children and adolescents: development and evaluation of a social psychological intervention. In: Baum A, Singer JE, eds. Handbook of psychology and health: issues in child health and adolescent health, Vol 2. Hillsdale, NJ: Lawrence Erlbaum Associates, 1982:231–245
10. Evans RI, Rozelle RM, Mittelmark MB, Hansen WB, Bane AL, Havis J. Deterring the onset of smoking in children: knowledge of immediate physiological effects and coping with peer pressures, media pressure, and parent modeling. J Appl Soc Psychol 1978;8:126–35.
11. Evans RI, Rozelle RM, Maxwell SE, et al. Social modeling films to deter smoking in adolescents: results of a three-year field investigation. J Appl Psychol 1981;66(4):399–414.
12. Johnson LD, Backman JG, O'Malley PM. Drugs and the class of '78. behaviors, attitudes and recent national trends. U.S. Department of Health, Education and Welfare Public Health Service Publ (ADM)79-877.1979.
13. Johnson LD, Bachman JG,O'Malley PM. 1979 highlights: Drugs and the nations' high school students, five-year national trends. U.S. Department of Health, Education and Welfare Public Health Service Publ (ADM) 80-930. Washington, DC: U.S. Government Printing Office, 1979.
14. National Institutes of Health. Teenage smoking: national patterns of cigarette smoking, ages 12 through 18, in 1972 and 1974. U.S. Department of Health, Education and Welfare Public Health Service Publ (NIH) 76-391. Washington, DC: U.S. Government Printing Office, 1976.
15. Creswell WH Jr, Huffman WJ, Stone DB. Youth smoking behavior characteristics and their educational implications. A report of the University of Illinois Anti-Smoking Education Study. Champaign, IL: University of Illinois Press, June 30, 1970.
16. Thompson EI. Smoking education programs 1960–1976. Am J Publ Health 1978;68:250–7.
17. Evans RI. Smoking in children: developing a social psychological strategy of deterrence. J Prevent Med 1976;5(I):122–7.

18. Bandura A. Social learning theory. Englewood Cliffs, NJ: Prentice-Hall, 1977.
19. Bandura A, Huston AC. Identification as a process of incidental learning. J Abnorm Soc Psychol 1961;63:311-8.
20. Evans RI, Smith CK, Raines BE. Deterring cigarette smoking in adolescents: a psycho-social-behavioral analysis of an intervention strategy. In: Baum A, Singer J, Taylor S, eds, Social psychological aspects of health. Hillsdale, NJ: Lawrence Erlbaum Associates, in press.
21. Botvin GJ, Eng A, Williams CL. Preventing the onset of cigarette smoking through life skills training. Perspect Med 1980;9(1):135-43.
22. Hurd PD, Johnson CA, Pechacek T, Bast LP, Jacobs DR, Leupker RV. Prevention of cigarette smoking in seventh grade students. J Behav Med 1980;3(1):15-28.
23. McGuire WJ. The nature of attitudes and attitude change. In: Lindzey G, Aronson E, eds, Handbook of social psychology, Vol 3. The individual in a social context. Reading, MA: Addison-Wesley, 1968.
24. McGuire WJ. The effectiveness or supportive refutational defenses in immunizing and restoring beliefs against persuasion. Sociometry 1961;24:184-97.
25. Horning EC, Horning MG, Carrol DI, Stillwell RN, Dzidic I. Nicotine in smokers, non-smokers and room air. Life Sci 1973;13(10):1331-46.
26. Evans RI, Hansen WE, Mittelmark MB. Increasing the validity of self-reports of smoking behavior in children. J Appl Psychol 1977;62(4):521-3.
27. McAlister AL, Perry C, Maccoby N. Adolescent smoking: onset and prevention. Pediatrics 1979;63:650-8.

CHAPTER 18

The Biology of Lung Cancer vis-à-vis the Emerging New Biotechnology

MERLE MIZELL

Laboratory of Tumor Cell Biology, Biology Department,
Tulane University, New Orleans, Louisiana 70118

ABSTRACT

The advent of recent biotechnology has changed our concept of the differentiated state. It is now unmistakably clear that morphologic criteria alone are inadequate to describe normal or neoplastic differentiation. Techniques that aid in revealing differential gene expression are now providing fundamental knowledge of tumor biology in natural tumors of outbred populations of animals, including man. This is especially true of lung cancer biology. New laboratory directions are evolving into useful clinical procedures. Indeed, small-cell lung cancer, with its unique chromosomal banding pattern, protein secretion, and cellular markers, provides powerful tools that hold promise of disclosing the critical events in tumorigenesis. The ability to uncover and/or activate latent genetic information has become routine with this new technology. These techniques provide insight into gene expression on a variety of levels, including (a) cellular and cell membrane, (b) nuclear and nuclear cloning, (c) chromosomal alterations and unique banding, and (d) DNA transfection and the level of the gene itself. The new directions that are evolving from these studies are discussed.
Key Words: **Small-cell lung cancer, natural tumors, tumor cell biology, emerging biotechnology, genetic reprogramming, nuclear transplantation, chromosomal rearrangement, cellular oncogenes, tumorigenesis**

The worldwide lung cancer epidemic continues unchecked. However, there is both good news and bad news concerning lung cancer. First the bad news. In our country the rate of lung cancer is rising in a predictable fashion: ever since the 1930s the slope of the lung cancer mortality rate per 100,000 males in the United

Lung Cancer: Causes and Prevention.

States has remained unchanged. And in the late 1970s more than 70 per 100,000 males died each year of lung cancer (Figure 1). With a notable increase in slope in the 1960s, the rate of female lung cancer mortality began to rise. The slope remains unchanged today, and lung cancer is predicted to become the number one cancer in United States women before the end of this century (Figure 2). (In early 1984 it was reported that lung cancer had already surpassed breast cancer in at least eight states and that this seemed to be a nationwide trend in the United States.)

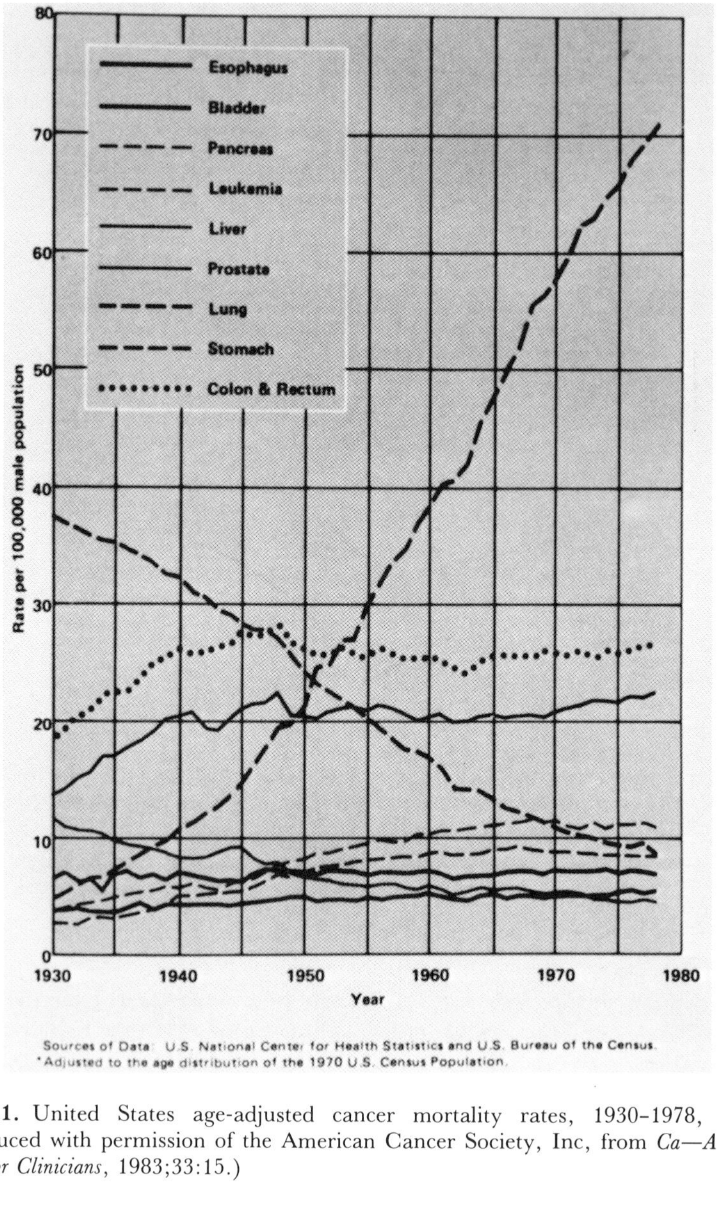

Figure 1. United States age-adjusted cancer mortality rates, 1930–1978, males. (Reproduced with permission of the American Cancer Society, Inc, from *Ca—A Cancer Journal for Clinicians*, 1983;33:15.)

These are horrendous rates, and appreciable changes are unlikely to occur soon, even with diligent application of the preventive measures discussed in this volume (see Chapter 1).

Now for the good news. Historically, high incidence of a number of diseases first occurred before inroads were made in understanding the disease conditions. For example, the fulfillment of Koch's Postulates and the ability to identify the causes of many diseases became possible only after elevated incidences of the disease or the advent of an epidemic. Also, in the past, crucial new insight often

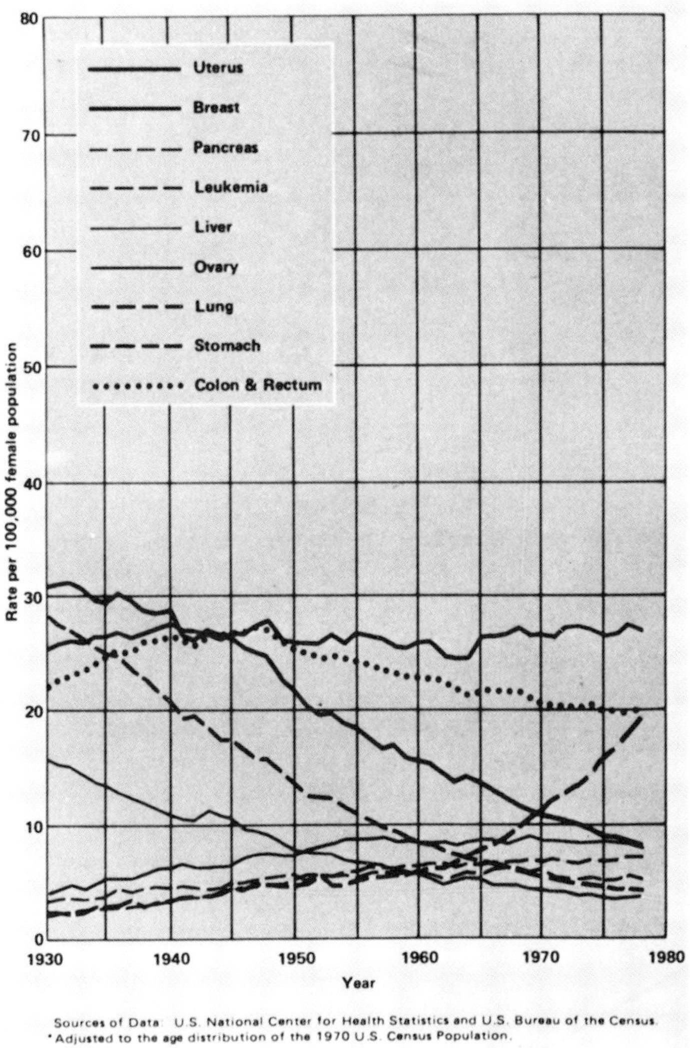

Figure 2. United States age-adjusted cancer mortality rates, 1930–1978, females. (Reproduced with permission of the American Cancer Society, Inc, from *Ca—A Cancer Journal for Clinicians*, 1983;33:14.)

went hand in hand with development of new techniques. The simultaneous existence of both factors invariably led to answers of fundamental questions. These factors, elevated incidence and the development of new techniques, currently exist for lung cancer investigations: more basic knowledge and understanding should soon be forthcoming.

This volume documents that smoking is one of the chief causes of lung cancer. However, it is not sufficient to know that smoking causes lung cancer—the ultimate question is *how?* What are the essential events in tumorigenesis?

Recent biotechnological advances already have provided answers to longstanding fundamental questions of molecular genetics. This emerging technology, in conjunction with the lung cancer epidemic, holds promise of disclosing the critical events in tumorigenesis. This is indeed good news. Small-cell lung carcinoma (SCLC) is a likely candidate to provide fundamental answers to "the" mechanism or steps involved in the development of natural cancers (see Chapters 19 and 20). Much of the work with inbred strains of mice and rats, although providing answers to important ancillary problems, ultimately cannot serve as accurate model in vivo systems for natural spontaneous tumors of man and other outbred animals.

Burkitt lymphoma (BL), a B-cell lymphoma of African children, and its association with an ubiquitous herpesvirus, the EB virus (Epstein-Barr virus), has provided important insight into the role of the immune system and tumor development (1). And although we still do not have definitive evidence to link the EB virus as the causative agent of BL, it has provided important immunologic data and has produced an understanding of the progression of malignancy in a natural tumor and its putative oncogenic virus (2).

It has been suggested that some cofactor(s) (perhaps, holoendemic malaria) interferes with the immune surveillance system of these African youngsters and results in BL (3). In any event, a prospective Ugandan seroepidemiologic study indicated that early contact and infection with EB virus was a prerequisite for the development of BL in this population (4).

At least two other natural tumors of outbred vertebrate animals exhibit the requirement of early viral infection if malignancy is to be transmitted: (1) transmission studies of leukemia and lymphoma in cats by the feline leukemia virus (FeLV) indicate that newborn kittens are susceptible to infection only prior to developing immunocompetence (5, 2). Similar results were obtained in our studies of the leopard frog renal adenocarcinoma (Lucké tumor) and its oncogenic herpesvirus, the Lucké tumor herpesvirus (LTHV) (6, 2). In a LTHV inoculation study of a series of developing embryo and larval stages, tumor induction occurred in a high percentage ($>50\%$) of these outbred animals. However, once the developing larvae reached immunocompetence, none of the inoculated animals gave rise to renal carcinomas (7). Therefore, in all three of these natural tumors of outbred vertebrates, an event associated with the attainment of immunocompetence thwarts tumor formation. Yet, the mechanism(s) of tumorigenesis remains unknown.

Nevertheless, it is now unmistakably clear that morphologic criteria alone are inadequate to describe normal or neoplastic differentiation. Techniques that aid in revealing differential gene expression are now providing fundamental knowledge of tumor biology in these natural tumors of outbred populations of animals. The ability to uncover and/or activate latent genetic information has become routine with this new technology. These techniques provide insight into gene expression on a variety of levels, including (a) cellular and cell membrane, (b) nuclear and nuclear cloning, (c) chromosomal alterations and unique banding, and (d) DNA transfection and the level of the gene itself.

Cellular and Cell Membrane

Viral infection results in many cellular and cell membrane changes. Epstein-Barr virus infection and the immune responses associated with BL tumor cells are manifold. Our knowledge of the viral-mediated changes in the tumor cell surface and the host cellular responses are continually evolving. However, the above-mentioned spontaneously arising natural tumors apparently are weakly immunogenic because they arise slowly in a graded tumor progression. These subtle changes nevertheless are reflected in cellular and cell membrane alterations, and most of these changes can be recognized immunologically. Certainly, future employment of monoclonal antibody techniques will permit precise detection of these important cell surface changes.

Nuclear Transplantation and Cloning

The procedure of nuclear transplantation has permitted the testing of nuclei from a variety of cells, including "differentiated cells." This technique of transferring the nucleus from a specialized somatic cell to an egg cell from which the nucleus has been removed has been used to test the latent ability of these "differentiated" nuclei and was first performed in 1952 in the leopard frog, *Rana pipiens*, by Briggs and King (8). Because the enucleated egg could follow normal developmental pathways after receiving nuclei from a variety of somatic cells, this landmark experiment and subsequent studies provided conclusive proof that "differentiated" cells have not lost the genes that govern a variety of activities (8–10).

The question then arises of whether the nucleus from a spontaneous tumor cell retains functional normal genes, and whether the tumor cell nucleus can be reprogrammed to provide the normal information required by egg cytoplasm to continue developmental processes. The frog renal adenocarcinoma and its oncogenic herpesvirus, LTHV, provided us with a unique opportunity to perform such a test (1, 2). It should be noted that LTHV is obtained directly from the carcinoma cells without intervening tissue culture. This is unique for oncogenic DNA tumor viruses to be harvested productively from tumor cells. By mere employment of a temperature shiftdown, the once nonpermissive tumor cells become permissive and produce large quantities of infectious herpesvirus in the tumor-bearing animal (6). Figure 3 diagrams the procedures involved in testing for functional normal developmental genes in these tumor cells. The experiment consists of two sequential genetic reprogramming operations: each step referred to in the following paragraphs is diagramed in Figure 3.

FIRST REPROGRAMMING: Reprogramming the Pronephric Cells To Form Tumor Cells

The eggs were fertilized (step 1) and subjected to hydrostatic pressure to produce triploid (3N) embryos (step 2). These were grown (steps 3 and 4) to a young embryonic stage, at which time they were inoculated with 0.2 μl of Lucké tumor herpesvirus (LTHV).

The upper right-hand corner of the diagram in Figure 3 depicts LTHV that has been recovered directly from an adult frog mesonephric tumor. Tumor-derived LTHV was then used to inoculate the pronephric region of the embryo (step 5). After inoculation, the first reprogramming took place: some of the left pronephric kidney cells were transformed into adenocarcinoma cells. Instead of atrophying as normally programmed, these transformed pronephric cells now continued to live. On the other hand, the right pronephric kidney cells died as originally programmed. The transformed left pronephric tumor cells continued to divide as the larva began to metamorphose into an adult frog (step 6). At this time the large 3N tumor was removed and dissociated (step 7), placed into monolayer culture at 26°C (step 8), and grown for several days while the tumor parenchymal cells attached, divided, and formed epithelial islands of tumor cells (step 9).

SECOND REPROGRAMMING: Testing for Functional Developmental Genes in the Tumor Nucleus

The monolayer was then dissociated, and 3N tumor nuclei were picked up by pipette (step 10) and transplanted into enucleated *Rana pipiens* eggs (step 11). The second reprogramming took place in the egg cytoplasm, and cleavage followed by normal (or near-normal) development proceeded (steps 12 and 13), producing a clone derived from tumor nuclei (tumor clone) (step 14). In one experimental series, partial blastulae that developed from a single tumor nucleus were used for serial retransfer (steps 15–18). A single tumor-derived blastula nucleus was removed (step 15) and transplanted to enucleated eggs (steps 16 and 17). The resultant developing embryos constitute a nuclear clone (step 18). (Note that the broken arrow lines in the Figure 3 diagram can be traced back to a single tumor nucleus, hence a nuclear clone). Also note the retention of the triploid marker throughout the experiment.

A total of 111 nuclear transplants were performed and an unusually high percentage of development ensued. Cleavage resulting in blastula formation occurred in 63 (74%) of the cases and development continued in most of these embryos; 15 of these blastulae continued development to postneurulae stages, three

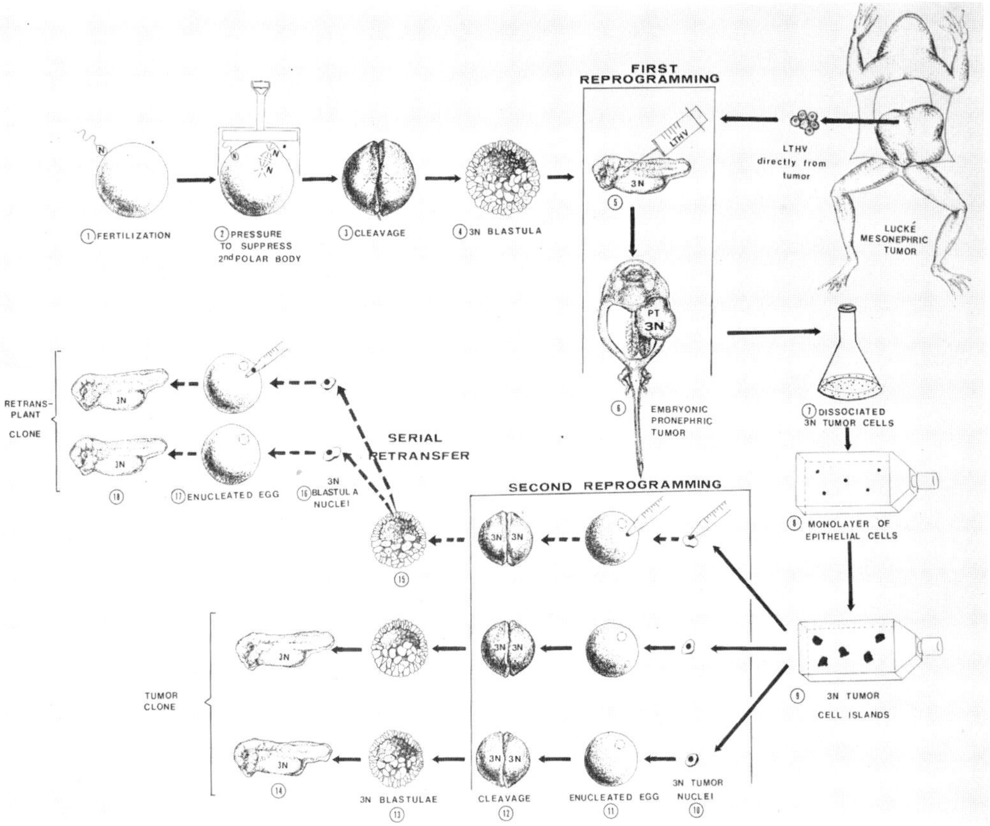

Figure 3. Diagram of experimental procedures: sequential genetic reprogramming in vivo, nuclear transplantation, and cloning. (See text for stepwise details.)

of which advanced to early larval stages containing the usual variety of differentiated tissues and organs: eg, brain, beating hearts, muscle, developing pronephric kidneys.

The animals were carefully examined histologically for tumors and none was found. This test for functional developmental genes in tumor cells, therefore, was positive and indicates that tumor cell nuclei do retain the genetic complement and ability to support the developmental program in egg cytoplasm (11, 12). Similar tests utilizing mouse teratocarcinoma cells placed into developing blastocysts also indicated an ability of mouse tumor cells to differentiate into a wide range of normal cell types (13). Lung cancer cells and/or nuclei have yet to be tested.

Chromosomal Alteration and Unique Banding

Modern cytogenetic banding techniques have made it possible to identify readily all human chromosomes and to recognize their alterations. This enhanced ability to recognize chromosomal rearrangements has revealed specific changes associated with specific cancers: eg, chronic myelocytic leukemia (CML) was recognized originally as possessing the "Philadelphia" chromosome, which was thought to represent a deletion of part of the long arm of chromosome 22 (14). The characteristic alteration is now known to consist of a translocation from chromosome 22 to chromosome 9 in the leukemic cells (15). Burkitt lymphoma lymphocytes also contain a reciprocal translocation, a translocation between chromosomes 8 and 14 (15, 16); and recently Whang-Peng et al (1982) have demonstrated a specific chromosomal defect associated with human small-cell lung cancer (SCLC): deletion 3p(14–23) (17). It shall be interesting to learn what genes are present in this chromosomal region. The full significance of this important marker in SCLC is yet to be realized but it already has provided important and useful knowledge (see Chapter 20).

DNA Transfection and the Level of the Gene Itself

The activity of purified cellular DNA and the transfection of cellular DNAs have shown that both normal and transformed cells contain genes that are capable of inducing oncogenic transformation of mouse cells. Cellular genes, capable of being activated and of thus becoming functional transforming genes, have now been identified and studied in a variety of animals, including man. Many of these DNA sequences present in normal uninfected cells are homologous to the transforming genes of acute retroviruses (18). Of special importance to the etiology of lung cancer is the fact that the retrovirus gene *ras*, a transforming gene of the Kirsten rat sarcoma virus (ras^k), has been found to be homologous to restriction fragments derived from human lung carcinoma DNA (19). Moreover, these human lung carcinoma DNA sequences are capable of transforming NIH3T3 cells (20). These or similar results have now been obtained from several laboratories, using different lung carcinomas; these results provide encouragement and suggest that the mechanism of human lung carcinoma may soon be more fully understood. In addition, it has been demonstrated that the transformation ability of the cellular homolog of the *ras* gene can be activated by adding a viral regulatory sequence upstream, which then results in enhanced formation of its protein product (20). This type of result leads one to reflect that the rearrangement of a segment of chromosome 3, an invariable chromosomal manifestation of small-cell lung carcinomas mentioned earlier (17), may indeed be a critical event in the activation of potential oncogenic DNA segments.

The results are clear: cellular *ras* genes lack transforming activity when associated with their normal cellular flanking regions. Moreover, potential transforming genes of normal cells can be activated as a consequence of DNA rearrangement.

Recently, another line of evidence has been developing to indicate that the active functioning of the immune system and/or another oncogene, *myc*, may be involved in the genesis of malignancy in BL. The reciprocal translocation of chromosome 8 and 14 in BL has been recognized since 1972, but the possible significance of the translocation remained unknown. However, it was disclosed recently that the immunoglobulin heavy-chain genes reside in this same region of chromosome 14.

Translocation of inactive gene sequences on chromosome 8 to an active site of transcription on 14 of this immunoglobulin-producing B-lymphocyte may be one of the critical events in BL oncogenesis (2). Furthermore, it was recently reported that the cellular *myc (c-myc)* oncogene is located on the region of chromosome 8 that is translocated, and that the crossover point between both chromosomes occurs in this region. Similarly, the cellular oncogene, *c-abl*, has been shown to be translocated from chromosome 22 to chromosome 9 in CML (see summary in Ref. 21). Whether malignancy is a result of activating a viral promotor or insertion of an oncogene downstream from a normal cellular promoter, pathogenesis may be the result of qualititative or quantitative (dosage) changes in the product of a normal cellular "proto-oncogene". Therefore, the provocative questions raised in 1975 as to the possible cellular origin of oncogenes, and that these same genes "might perform a necessary function during normal embryonic development" (22) are now accepted as fact. It therefore becomes especially desirable to obtain animal models in which proto-oncogenes can be analyzed: (a) first as they regulate the orderly growth of embryonic cells, and then, (b) to be followed during tumor initiation and growth (23). Less than two dozen different oncogenes have so far been found in retroviruses. Moreover, although the proteins encoded by these oncogenes illustrate remarkable diversity (eg, many are tyrosine-specific protein kinases located on the plasma membrane, some are nuclear proteins that bind to chromatin DNA), the emerging results represent our best insight into the biochemical events that lead to neoplastic growth (24).

The specific 3p deletion reported last year in small-cell lung cancers (17, see also Chapter 11) requires closer examination to see whether the observed rearrangement indeed activates oncogenic sequences in a manner analogous to that in B-cell lymphomas and CML. However, the ability to precisely locate these unique alterations indicates the clarity and explicit nature of our newly acquired biotechnology.

Gene splicing and recombinant DNA techniques in conjunction with procedures to rapidly determine the sequence of nucleotides in a genome have now become routine. Unique monoclonal antibodies are being prepared for both diagnostic and therapeutic purposes in a variety of tumors. However, the inherent antigenic features of small-cell lung cancer make this tumor especially amenable to analysis and investigation by this technique. Besides providing useful clinical procedures of both diagnostic and therapeutic value, this methodology is undoubtedly to play an important role in disclosing the critical events in the pathogenesis of lung cancer.

These techniques already have extended our knowledge of lung cancer biology and will continue to provide insight into gene expression on a variety of levels. The new biotechnology therefore has moved us into an era where we can now study natural tumors of outbred animals such as man and, in doing so, expect to obtain answers to fundamental questions of tumorigenesis.

Acknowledgments

The author's work reported here was supported by grants from the National Institute of Health, American Cancer Society, and the Cancer Association of Greater New Orleans.

References

1. Epstein MA, Achong BG. The relationship of the virus to Burkitt's lymphoma. In: Epstein MA, Achong BG, eds, The Epstein-Barr virus. New York: Springer-Verlag, 1979:321–37.
2. Klein, G. Mini review: specific chromosomal translocations and the genesis of B-cell-derived tumors of mice and man. Cell 1983;32:311–5.
3. Burkitt DP. Etiology of Burkitt's lymphoma—an alternative hypothesis to a vectored virus. J Natl. Cancer Inst 1969;42:19–28.
4. de The G, et al. Epidemiological evidence for causal relationship between Epstein-Barr virus and Burkitt's lymphoma from Ugandan prospective study. Nature 1978;274:756–61.
5. Essex M. Horizontally and vertically transmitted oncornaviruses of cats. Adv Cancer Res 1975;21:175–248.
6. Mizell M. State of the art: Lucké renal adenocarcinoma. In: Mizell M, ed, Biology of amphibian tumors. New York: Springer-Verlag, 1969:1–25.
7. Mizell M, McCue R, Charbonnet L. "Neonatal" tumor induction: the emerging immune surveillance mechanism and amphibian embryo tumorigenesis. In: de The G, Henle W, Rapp F, eds, Oncogenesis and herpesviruses III. Lyon: International Agency for Research on Cancer Scientific Publications, 1978:835–44.
8. Briggs R, King TJ. Transplantation of living nuclei from blastula cells into enucleated frogs' eggs. Proc Natl Acad Sci USA 1952;38:455–63.
9. Laskey RA, Gurdon JB. Genetic content of adult somatic cells tested by nuclear transplantation from cultured cells. Nature 1970;228:1332–4.
10. Gurdon JB. Nuclear transplantation and regulation of cell processes. Br Med Bull 1973; 29:259–63.
11. Mizell M, DiBerardino MA, Friesendorf DG, Hoffner NJ. Normal development programmed by the Lucké tumor cell nucleus. Am Zool 1980; 20:737.
12. DiBerardino MA, Mizell M, Hoffner NJ, Friesendorf DG. Frog larvae cloned from nuclei of pronephric adenocarcinoma. Differentiation 1983;23:213–7.
13. Mintz B, Fleischman RA. Teratocarcinomas and other neoplasms as developmental defects in gene expression. Adv Cancer Res 1981; 34:211–78.
14. Nowell PC, Hungerford DA. Chromosome studies on normal and leukemic human leukocytes. J Natl Cancer Inst 1960;25:85–109.
15. Rowley JD. A new consistent chromosomal abnormality in chronic myelogenous leukemia identified by quinacrine fluorescence and Giemsa-staining. Nature 1973;243:290–3.
16. Zech L, Hagland V, Nilsson K, Klein G. Characteristic chromosomal abnormalities in biopsies and lympoid cell lines from patients with Burkitt's and non-Burkitt lymphomas. Int J Cancer 1976;17:47–56.
17. Whang-Peng J, et al. Specific chromosome defect associated with human small-cell lung cancer: deletion 3p (14–23). Science 1982;215:181–2.
18. Bishop JM. Enemies within: the genesis of retrovirus oncogenes. Cell 1981;23:5–6.
19. Der CJ, Krontiris TG, Cooper GM. Transforming genes of human bladder and lung carcinoma cell lines are homologous to the *ras* genes of Harvey and Kirsten sarcoma viruses. Proc Natl Acad Sci USA 1982;79:3637–40.
20. Cooper GM. Cellular transforming genes. Science 1982;217:801–6.
21. Rowley JD. Human oncogene locations and chromosome aberrations. Nature 1983;301:290–1.
22. Mizell M. The biology of cancer. Science 1975;190:373–4.
23. Mizell, M. The Lucké frog carcinoma virus. In: Klein G, ed, Advances in viral oncology. New York: Raven Press, 1984; Vol 5, In press.
24. Bishop JM. Cancer genes come of age. Cell 1983;32:1018–20.

CHAPTER **19**

Transforming Genes of Human Lung Carcinomas

GEOFFREY M. COOPER

Dana-Farber Cancer Institute and Department of Pathology, Harvard Medical School, Boston, Massachusetts 02115

ABSTRACT

The DNAs of a variety of neoplasms, including human lung carcinomas, contain activated transforming genes that efficiently induce transformation of NIH 3T3 mouse cells on transfection. The transforming gene activated in human lung and colon carcinomas has been identified as a cellular homolog of the transforming gene (ras^K) of Kirsten sarcoma virus. Analysis of the expression of the ras^K-encoded gene product in normal human epithelial cells and a variety of carcinomas has indicated that activation of the transforming activity of this gene in carcinomas is a consequence of mutations that alter the structure of its gene product.
Key Words: **Transforming genes, DNA, transfection, gene, ras^K gene, virus.**

Activation of Transforming Genes in Neoplasms

The DNAs of a variety of neoplasms induce oncogenic transformation when introduced into NIH 3T3 cells by transfection. These neoplasms include carcinomas, sarcomas, and lymphoid neoplasms of chicken, mouse, and human origin (1). In contrast, DNAs of normal cells lack efficient transforming activity, including DNAs of homologous normal tissues of the same individual animals and/or inbred strains of mice whose neoplasms have yielded transforming DNA (2–4). These findings indicate that dominant genetic alterations occur during the development of some neoplasms and result in the activation of cellular transforming genes, which then can be detected by their biologic activity in transfection assays.

The cells used as recipients in transfection of tumor DNAs have been an established line of mouse cells, NIH 3T3 cells. These cells have been used as recipients because they display unusually high efficiences of uptake and stable integra-

Lung Cancer: Causes and Prevention.

tion of exogenous DNA. It should be noted, however, that NIH 3T3 cells are not normal primary fibroblasts. Instead they are an established cell line with the capacity for continuous proliferation in cell culture. Therefore, if neoplasia is considered a multistage process involving a series of preneoplastic and neoplastic alterations, it is likely that NIH 3T3 cells already have undergone some of these events and may be more properly considered preneoplastic rather than normal cells. If this is the case, activation of the transforming genes detected by transfection NIH 3T3 cells may represent only one event in the process of carcinogenesis, probably occurring late in the progression of preneoplastic cells to the full neoplastic phenotype. In mammary carcinomas and lymphoid neoplasms, this concept is supported by identification of other potential transforming genes that do not induce transformation of NIH 3T3 cells and that may function in earlier stages of oncogenesis (2, 3, 5, 6).

NIH cells transformed by neoplasm DNAs acquire, in vitro, characteristics of neoplastic cells, such as growth to high saturation densities and anchorage- independence, as well as in vivo tumorigenicity. In addition, they contain active transforming genes, derived from the original neoplasm DNAs, that can be transmitted efficiently to new recipient cells in serial transfection assays (1).

Activated transforming genes have been detected in a wide variety of neoplasms of different cell types and different species (1). These tumors include virally induced, chemically induced, and spontaneously occurring neoplasms. In addition, DNAs from primary neoplasms of either human or animal origin, as well as from tumor-derived cell lines, efficiently induce transformation, indicating that activation of transforming genes occurs in primary neoplasms and is not an artifact of in vitro culture of tumor cell lines.

Overall, approximately 50% of the neoplasm DNAs investigated possess transforming activity (1). However, the fraction of positive neoplasms differs among different types of tumors. In the case of lymphoid neoplasms, greater than 90% of the individual primary tumors and tumor cell lines that have been tested contain active transforming genes (2, 4). Activation of transforming genes in these neoplasms, therefore, appears to be a highly frequent event in oncogenesis, supporting the hypothesis that these genes play a role in induction of neoplasia. In mammary, colon, and lung carcinomas, transforming genes also are activated in many neoplasms. In these cases about 50% of those examined. In other tumor types, however, activation of cellular transforming genes is a less regular event in oncogenesis. The first transforming gene reported in a human neoplasm was identified originally in two bladder carcinoma cell lines (8, 9) and subsequently in a third (10). However, later analysis indicated that all three of these bladder carcinoma cell lines were cross contaminated (11). Activation of this transforming gene has not been detected in any other bladder carcinomas studied, so it has, in fact, been found in only a single tumor, making its role in bladder oncogenesis less compelling.

Further supporting the role of the more frequently detected neoplasm transforming genes in tumor development are results indicating that the same transforming gene is activated repeatedly in independent neoplasms of the same cell type. For example, restriction endonuclease analysis of human and mouse lymphoid neoplasm transforming genes indicated that the same transforming gene was activated in multiple neoplasms representing the same stage of normal B or T lymphocyte differentiation but different transforming genes were activated in neoplasms representing different stages of cell differentiation (pre B, intermediate B, mature B, intermediate T, and mature T), (4). Additional specific transforming genes have been observed in human and mouse mammary carcinomas (3), and human sarcomas (12). A single transforming gene has been reported in six independent human lung carcinomas, all of which are probably of the adenocarcinoma type (7, 10, 13). This gene is also activated in colon carcinomas (7, 10, 13).

Identification of the Transforming Gene of Lung and Colon Carcinomas

Analysis of the transforming gene activated in human lung carcinomas was facilitated greatly by experiments that identified this gene as a cellular homolog of the transforming gene of Kirsten sarcoma virus, an acute transforming retrovirus. The acute transforming retroviruses are laboratory isolates that are highly oncogenic in vivo and efficiently induce cellular transformation in vitro (1). All of the viruses of this class contain specific transforming genes responsible for their oncogenicity. In all cases, these viral transforming genes are related closely to cellular genes that are found in all vertebrate species, including man. Because the cellular homologs of these retroviral transforming genes represent one class of potential transforming genes in the cellular genome, it was of interest to investigate the possibility of relationships between them and the transforming genes detected by transfection of tumor DNAs.

Molecular clones of the viral transforming genes designated *src, myc, myb, mos, fes*, ras^H, ras^K, *erb*, and *sis* (1) were used as probes for blot-hybridization analysis of DNAs of NIH cells transformed by a variety of different human neoplasm DNAs. NIH cells transformed by DNAs of human lymphoid neoplasms, Wilm tumor, mammary carcinoma, and a pancreatic carcinoma did not contain exogenous DNA sequences homologous to any of these retroviral transforming gene probes, indicating that the transforming genes activated in these neoplasms were not related to the retroviral transforming genes studied (13, 14). In contrast, the transforming gene activated in a human bladder carcinoma was identified as a cellular homolog of the transforming gene of Harvey sarcoma virus (ras^H) (13, 15, 16) and the transforming gene of a lung carcinoma was identified as a cellular homolog of the ras^K transforming gene of Kirsten sarcoma virus (13). Activation of the same cellular ras^K homolog has now been reported in a total of six independent human lung carcinomas (7, 13, 14), three colon carcinomas (7, 14), a bladder carcinoma (7), a gall bladder carcinoma (7), a pancreatic carcinoma (7) and a rhabdomyosarcoma (7). These neoplasms include primary carcinomas of the lung and pancreas as well as cell lines (7).

These findings have provided a link between the transforming genes of viruses and the transforming genes activated in non-virus-induced human tumors. The frequent activation of a cellular homolog of *ras*^{K} further indicates that this gene may be involved in oncogenesis in a variety of carcinomas occurring at different anatomic sites, including the lung.

Organization of ras^K Genes in Normal Cells and Carcinomas

The same *ras*^{K} DNA sequences were detected in DNAs of both normal human cells and carcinomas, indicating that activation of the transforming activity of *ras*^{K} in tumors was a consequence of alteration of a normal cellular gene (13). Further comparisons of normal and tumor DNAs by blot-hybridization analysis did not reveal either significant amplification or rearrangement of *ras*^{K} sequences in neoplasms (13, 14). Therefore, activation of this gene appeared to be a consequence of more subtle mutational events, eg, point mutations, which were not detectable by overall structural comparisons. Such mutations could be envisioned a priori to affect either (1) the level of *ras*^{K} expression or (2) the structure and function of the *ras*^{K}-encoded gene product.

Mechanism of Activation of ras^K in Lung and Colon Carcinomas

A major advantage of identifying the transforming gene of lung and colon carcinomas as a homolog of *ras*^{K} was that previous studies of this viral transforming gene could be applied to analysis of the transforming genes activated in carcinomas. Both *ras*^{H} and *ras*^{K} are members of a multigene family and encode related proteins of 21,000 daltons (17). Antisera against these proteins have been used to demonstrate that they are expressed at high levels in virus-transformed cells and that similar proteins are expressed at low levels in normal cells (18). Since a monoclonal antibody was available that was highly cross-reactive with both viral and cellular *ras*^{K}-encoded proteins (p21s) (19), we were able to investigate p21 expression in a variety of human carcinomas and normal human cells.

Immunoprecipitation assays indicated that p21 proteins were expressed in both normal human epithelial cells and human carcinoma cells (14). The levels of p21 expression in carcinomas were approximately five-fold higher than in normal epithelial cells. Levels of p21 expressed in lung, colon, and bladder carcinomas that contained activated *ras*^{K} or *ras*^{H} transforming genes were similar to those in carcinomas of the same types whose DNAs lacked transforming activity (14). Therefore, changes in p21 expression did not appear to be correlated with activation of the transforming activity of *ras*^{K} or *ras*^{H} in neoplasms.

In contrast, however, structural alterations in p21 were associated with activation of transforming activity of *ras*^{K} in lung and colon carcinomas (14). The p21 proteins expressed in normal human cells migrated in sodium dodecyl sulfate (SDS)-polyacrylamide gel electrophoresis as a closely spaced doublet. The same p21 species were detected in four human carcinomas (bladder, mammary, pancreatic, and Wilm tumors) that contained transforming genes other than *ras*^{K} and in nine human carcinomas (bladder, lung, colon, prostate, cervical, and adrenal cortical) the DNAs of which lacked transforming activity. In contrast, two lung and two colon carcinomas that contained activated *ras*^{K} genes all expressed abnormal species of p21, electrophoretically distinguishable from the normal p21 doublet. These results indicated that expression of abnormal species of p21 was specifically associated with activation of *ras*^{K} transforming activity.

Interestingly, the abnormal p21 proteins of one lung and two colon carcinomas comigrated with an electrophoretic mobility corresponding to an apparent molecular weight increase of 1.5–2 kdaltons compared to normal p21 proteins. However, a different abnormal p21 protein was expressed in a second lung carcinoma that contained the same activated *ras*^{K} gene. The electrophoretic mobility of this abnormal protein was slower than that of normal p21 proteins but faster than the abnormal p21 proteins of the other three carcinoma cell lines.

The p21 proteins expressed in NIH cells transformed by DNAs of these lung and colon carcinomas were investigated to determine whether the abnormal p21 species detected in the carcinomas were encoded by the *ras*^{K} genes responsible for transforming activity of the carcinoma DNAs. NIH 3T3 cells and NIH cells transformed by DNAs of neoplasms containing transforming genes other than *ras*^{K} expressed p21 proteins of similar electrophoretic mobility. In contrast, NIH cells transformed by DNAs of the lung and colon carcinomas, which contained active *ras*^{K} transforming genes, expressed abnormal species of p21 that comigrated with the abnormal p21 proteins detected in the donor human carcinoma cells. Therefore, these abnormal p21 proteins were encoded by the activated human *ras*^{K} genes.

These results indicate that activation of *ras*^{K} in four different human lung and colon carcinomas is a consequence of mutations that alter the structure of the *ras*^{K}-encoded gene product rather than the level of gene expression. In addition, because different abnormal p21 proteins are encoded by the same *ras*^{K} gene activated in different carcinomas, it appears that different mutations can activate the transforming activity of this gene in different individual neoplasms.

Implications

The identification of *ras*^{K} as the transforming gene activated in human lung carcinomas and the finding that its activation is a consequence of detectable changes in the structure of its gene product, have implications both for increased understanding of the mechanism of oncogenesis and for potential therapeutic applications. Studies of viral *ras* gene products have provided some foundation for consideration of the cellular *ras*^{K} proteins in carcinomas and, therefore, are summarized here.

Cellular localization of p21 in virus-transformed cells has indicated that the protein is present on the inner side of the cytoplasmic membrane and does not appear to be expressed on the cell surface (20). Some viral p21 proteins are phosphorylated in vivo and display autokinase activity in vitro (21). However, p21s encoded by other transforming viruses and by cellular genes in either normal cells or carcinomas are not phosphorylated and do not exhibit autokinase activity (14, 21). All forms of p21 bind guanine nucleotides (21) and a portion of the sequence of p21 is homologous to that of other nucleotide metabolizing enzymes (22). It is possible that cellular, as well as viral, p21 proteins function as kinases, but that some of these proteins have a more restricted substrate specificity than those which display autokinase activity. Finally, viral p21 proteins are modified by covalent attachment of lipid, which may contribute to their membrane localization (23). Whether modification of this type also occurs in the cellular p21 proteins of either normal cells or carcinomas is currently unknown. Further comparative studies of p21 proteins encoded by normal and activated cellular transforming genes may elucidate the biochemical activities of p21 that are important in oncogenesis.

The qualitative differences in the p21 proteins encoded by normal and activated cellular *ras*^{K} genes may suggest eventual clinical application. For example, it may be possible to generate monoclonal antibodies with specificity for the activated carcinoma proteins. Because p21 is located on the inside of the cell, such antibodies are unlikely to be useful as therapeutic agents, although they may have potential application in histologic diagnosis. However, at least two obvious problems need to be considered: (1) only about 50% of the lung carcinomas investigated have activated *ras*^{K} genes and (2) the active *ras*^{K}-encoded p21s present in different individual carcinomas may differ from each other. Clinical application of these findings at present, therefore, appears uncertain, although further understanding of the role of these proteins in both normal and malignant cells may make such applications possible.

References

1. Cooper GM. Cellular transforming genes. Science 1982;217:801–6.
2. Cooper GM, Neiman PE. Transforming genes of neoplasms induced by avian lymphoid leukosis viruses. Nature 1980;287:656–9.
3. Lane M-A, Sainten A, Cooper GM. Activation of related transforming genes in mouse and human mammary carcinomas. Proc Natl Acad Sci USA 1981;78:5185–9.
4. Lane M-A, Sainten A, Cooper GM. Stage-specific transforming genes of human and mouse B- and T-lymphocyte neoplasms. Cell 1982;28:873–80.
5. Cooper GM, Neiman PE. Two distinct candidate transforming genes of lymphoid leukosis virus-induced neoplasms. Nature 1981;292:857–8.
6. Lane M-A, Neary D, Cooper GM. Activation of a cellular transforming gene in tumours induced by Abelson murine leukemia virus. Nature 1982;300:659–61.
7. Pulciani S, Santos E, Lauver AV, Long LK, Aaronson SA, Barbacid M. Oncogenes in solid human tumours. Nature 1982;300:539–42.
8. Krontiris TG, Cooper GM. Transforming activity of human tumor DNAs. Proc Natl Acad Sci USA 1981;78:1181–4.
9. Shih C, Padhy LC, Murray M, Weinberg RA. Transforming genes of carcinomas and neuroblastomas introduced into mouse fibroblasts. Nature 1981;290:261–4.

10. Perucho M, Goldfarb M, Shimizu K, Lama C, Fogh J, Wigler M. Human-tumor derived cell lines contain common and different transforming genes. Cell 1981;27:467-76.
11. O'Toole CM, Povey S, Hepburn P, Franks LM. Identity of some human bladder carcinoma cell lines. Nature 1983;301:429-30.
12. Marshall CJ, Hall A, Weiss RA. A transforming gene present in human sarcoma cell lines. Nature 1982;299:171-3.
13. Der CJ, Krontiris TG, Cooper GM. Transforming genes of human bladder and lung carcinoma cell lines are homologous to the *ras* genes of Harvey and Kirsten sarcoma viruses. Proc Natl Acad Sci USA 1982;79:3637-40.
14. Der CJ, Cooper GM. Altered gene products are associated with activation of cellular ras^K genes in human lung and colon carcinomas. Cell 1983;32:201-8.
15. Parada LF, Tabin CJ, Shih C, Weinberg RA. Human EJ bladder carcinoma oncogene is homologue of Harvey sarcoma virus *ras* gene. Nature 1982;297:474-8.
16. Santos E, Tronick GR, Aaronson SA, Pulciani S, Barbacid M. T24 human bladder carcinoma oncogene is an activated form of the normal human homologue of BALB- and Harvey-MSV transforming genes. Nature 1982;298:343-7.
17. Ellis RW, DeFeo D, Shih TY, et al. The p21 *src* genes of Harvey and Kirsten sarcoma viruses originate from divergent members of a family of normal vertebrate genes. Nature 1981; 292:506-11.
18. Langbeheim H, Shih TY, Scolnick EM. Identification of a normal vertebrate cell protein related to the p21 *src* of Harvey murine sarcoma virus. Virology 1980;106:292-300.
19. Furth ME, Davis LJ, Fleurdelys B, Scolnick EM. Monoclonal antibodies to the p21 products of the transforming gene of Harvey murine sarcoma virus and of the cellular *ras* gene family. J Virol 1982;43:294-304.
20. Willingham MC, Pastan I, Shih TY, Scolnick EM. Localization of the *src* gene product of the Harvey strain of MSV to plasma membrane of transformed cells by electron microscopic immunocytochemistry. Cell 1980;19:1005-14.
21. Papageorge A, Lowy D, Scolnick EM. Comparative biochemical properties of p21 *ras* molecules coded for by viral and cellular *ras* genes. J Virol 1982;44:509-19.
22. Gay NJ, Walker JE. Homology between human bladder carcinoma oncogene product and mitochondrial APT-synthase. Nature 1983;301:262-4.
23. Sefton BM, Trowbridge IS, Cooper JA. The transforming proteins of Rous sarcoma virus, Harvey sarcoma virus and Abelson virus contain tightly bound lipid. Cell 1982;31;465-74.

CHAPTER **20**

In Vitro Studies of the Biology of Lung Cancer

DESMOND N. CARNEY, ADI F. GAZDAR, FRANCIS CUTTITTA, and JOHN D. MINNA

NCI-Navy Medical Oncology Branch, (DCT, NU/NIH) Naval Hospital, Bethesda, Maryland 20814

ABSTRACT

The establishment of multiple continuous cell lines of lung cancer has permitted important new biologic studies of lung cancer. Small-cell lung cancer (SCLC) cell lines, unlike non-SCLC cell lines, express a variety of biochemical markers including L-dopa decarboxylase, neuron-specific enolase, creatine kinase-BB, and bombesin. In patients with SCLC, serum determinations of these biomarkers have demonstrated clinical value in staging patients and in monitoring responses to therapy. A specific cytogenetic abnormality (del 3p–, 14–23) has been observed in all cell lines and fresh specimens of SCLC but is absent in non-SCLC cells. Using a soft agarose clonogenic assay, in vitro chemosensitivity and radiation studies of fresh specimens and cell lines of lung cancer have demonstrated an excellent correlation with the observed clinical responses of these tumors to cytotoxic therapy. These cell lines also have permitted the identification of the specific serum-free growth requirements of lung cancer cells and have been used to develop monoclonal antibodies to different histologic types of lung cancer, and may be useful in the identification of transforming genes associated with these tumors.
Key Words: **Small-cell lung cancer, SCLC, continuous culture, SCLC "conversion," agarose cloning, clonogenic assay, DNA, HITES, medium**

Introduction

Lung cancer accounted for more than 100,000 deaths in the United States in 1983 (1). Although considerable advances have been made in the treatment of this disease, most patients will die from their tumor. Whereas there are four major forms of primary lung cancer — epidermoid (or squamous cell), adenocarcinoma, large-cell carcinoma, and small-cell lung cancer — a number of important biologic differences distinguish small-cell lung cancer (SCLC) from the other forms of lung cancer (the so-called non-SCLC lung cancers) (2). Small-cell lung cancer is associated with a propensity to early, widespread dissemination, such that the diagnosis of this histologic type of lung cancer usually precludes surgical intervention, in contrast to the other forms of lung cancer in which the hope for cure or long-term survival is directly related to the resectability of the tumor. Small-cell lung cancer also is associated with a marked sensitivity to a variety of chemotherapeutic agents and to radiation therapy, such that the vast majority of patients achieve a remission with combination therapy, and a small percentage of patients achieve long-term (greater than 2 years), disease-free survival (3).

Our understanding of the biology and the cell of origin of different forms of lung cancer has been greatly facilitated by the recent development of techniques that support the long-term continual in vitro culture of cell lines of most forms of lung cancer, in particular, SCLC (4–7). These cell lines have permitted the identification of specific biomarkers associated with these tumors and of specific growth requirements of lung cancer. In the case of SCLC, these cell lines have permitted the identification of a specific cytogenetic abnormality that has been identified consistently in continuous cell lines and fresh biopsy specimens of SCLC.

Growth and Characterization of Continuous Cell Lines of Lung Cancer

Whereas several laboratories have reported on the continuous growth of single cell lines of lung cancer, two laboratories (4–7) recently have reported considerable success on the in vitro growth of specimens of SCLC. In general, two culture conditions have been used to isolate and culture SCLC. These include growth in serum-supplemented medium (SSM), usually either RPMI 1640 medium supplemented with 10–20% fetal bovine serum, or Waymouths medium supplemented with serum; and more recently, growth in a serum-free chemically defined hormone-supplemented medium (SFM) (7) (vide infra). Using either technique, continuous cell lines of SCLC retain common characteristics (Table 1).

Cell lines have been established from both primary lung cancer biopsy specimens and from a variety of metastatic sites, including bone marrow aspirates, pleural effusions, lymph node aspirates and biopsies, and other less common sites, such as liver and brain. In addition to the successful culture of tumor cells from fresh biopsies, some groups have reported success on culture of SCLC from autopsy specimens (5, 6). No significant differences on the biologic behavior of SCLC cell lines cultured from these different sites have been observed.

In continuous culture, SCLC cell lines usually grow as floating cell aggregates of tightly packed cells, in contrast to non-SCLC cell lines, which demonstrate substrate adherence. In a few instances, adherent cell lines of SCLC have been observed (5, 6). Small-cell lung cancer cell lines have doubling times of 48–96 hours and colony-forming efficiencies in soft agarose ranging from 1 to 5%. They form classic SCLC tumors in athymic nude mice when inoculated either in-

Table 1. In vitro biologic properties of small-cell lung cancer and non-small-cell lung cancer cell lines

Characteristic	Small cell	Non-small cell
Morphology	Floating aggregates	Adherent monolayer
Tumorigenicity	Yes	Yes
Cloning efficiency	1–5%	5–20%
Doubling time	24–96 h	20–48 h
L-Dopa decarboxylase	Elevated	Low/absent
Neuron-specific enolase	Elevated	Low/absent
Bombesin	Elevated	Absent
Creatine kinase BB	Elevated	Low/absent
Hormone production	Common	Uncommon
Epidermal growth factor Receptors	Absent	Present
Chromosome Deletion (3p, 14–23)	Present	Absent

tracranially or subcutaneously (8, 9). Non-SCLC cell lines also form colonies in soft agarose with an efficiency of 5–10% and form tumors in athymic nude mice. Metastatic lesions of lung cancer have not been observed in these nude mice.

Continuous cell lines of SCLC express a variety of amine precursor uptake and decarboxylation (APUD) properties. These include high levels of the key APUD enzyme L-dopa decarboxylase (E.C.4.1.1. 28) (DDC), neuron-specific enolase (NSE), and the brain neuropeptide bombesin. These three markers have been found in the majority of cell lines established from patients with SCLC and either are present in very low amounts or are absent in continuous cell lines of other forms of lung cancer (10–13). In addition, elevated levels of DDC have been demonstrated in fresh biopsy specimens of SCLC, whereas DDC usually is absent in fresh biopsies of non-SCLC lung cancer (11). These data suggest that measurement of DDC levels and other APUD markers in fresh biopsies may be of value in determining the histologic type of lung cancers with anaplastic morphology. Because of the differences in the treatment of SCLC and non-SCLC, confirming the origin of the tumor may have considerable importance in the prognosis of the patient.

In addition to DDC, NSE, and bombesin, SCLC cell lines express high levels of the BB isozyme of creatine kinase (CK-BB) whereas non-SCLC cell lines have low levels of this enzyme (11). Similarly to DDC, high levels of CK-BB also have been demonstrated in fresh specimens of SCLC but not in non-SCLC fresh specimens. The role of CK-BB in the metabolic behavior of SCLC has not been determined, but the association of high levels of CK-BB with SCLC and its absence in non-SCLC suggests that these tumor groups have different pathways in their energy requirements.

Because in most patients with lung cancer tumor dissemination has occurred at the time of diagnosis, a number of investigators have evaluated the usefulness of serum markers in evaluating extent of disease and response to therapy in these patients. Both in vitro and in vivo production of a number of hormones by SCLC has been demonstrated; these include calcitonin, adenocorticotropic hormone

(ACTH), antidiuretic hormone (ADH), and neurophysins (8, 9, 14–17). Although elevated serum levels of these hormones have been found in patients with a variety of lung cancers, none of these hormones has been sensitive or selective enough to achieve widespread application in the management of patients with lung cancer. The presence of high levels of CK-BB and NSE in cell lines of SCLC prompted us to evaluate the usefulness of these markers in the serum of patients with SCLC (18, 19).

Among 94 newly diagnosed and extensively staged patients with SCLC, elevated serum NSE levels (>12.0 ng/ml) were present in 69% of all patients and in 87% of patients with extensive-stage disease (mean 52.35 ± 11.56, range 4.1–850 ng/ml) (18). Extensive-stage patients had a significantly higher serum NSE level (58 ng/ml) compared to patients with limited stage (13.8 ng/ml). Additionally, in patients with three or more metastatic sites, elevated serum NSE was osberved in all cases. Sequential serum NSE determinations in 23 patients demonstrated an excellent correlation between response to therapy and NSE levels. In a study of serum CK-BB determinations in 105 patients with SCLC, a similar correlation between tumor extent and response to therapy was observed, whereas elevated levels were observed in only 2% of patients with limited-stage disease compared to elevated serum NSE in 39% of patients with limited-stage disease. Serum CK-BB was elevated in 44% of patients with extensive-stage disease. As for serum NSE levels, an excellent correlation between tumor burden (ie, number of metastatic sites detected) and the presence of an elevated serum CK-BB was observed. These data suggest that both serum NSE and CK-BB determination may be of value in the staging and management of patients with SCLC. However, as with other markers, because their detection in the serum is correlated with tumor burden, the usefulness of these and other markers in the early detection of lung cancer, both at diagnosis and at early relapse, remains to be determined. The demonstration of NSE in all cell cultures of SCLC suggests that immunohistochemical staining of lung cancer for NSE, especially those with anaplastic histology, may differentiate clearly those of SCLC lineage from other varieties of lung cancer. Such distinction clearly would have a major impact on selection of therapy.

In Vitro Soft Agarose Cloning of Human Lung Cancer Clinical Specimens

Although soft agarose cloning has been used for a long time to assess the "tumorigenic" potential of established cell lines, the recent work of Salmon et al (20, 21) suggests that this technique can be used to culture tumor cells selectively from fresh biopsy specimens. In addition, several investigators have shown that this cloning assay can be used to select, in a specific manner, chemotherapy for individual patients (22–24). At the present time, most patients are treated with chemotherapeutic agents that have been shown in previous studies to benefit the majority of patients with a tumor of a given histology. This mode of chemotherapy selection suggests that many patients receive drugs that are not active against "their" tumor or do not receive agents that are of benefit. Therefore, the development of in vitro assay systems, comparable to in vitro microbiologic assay systems, for the selection of specific cytotoxic agents for individual patients would be of major benefit to medical oncology.

Following the initial reports of successful soft agarose cloning of fresh tumor specimens by Salmon and Hamburger (21), we and others have tested the ability of clinical specimens of both SCLC and non-SCLC to form tumor cell colonies when plated in agarose (24–27). Methods for the collection, processing and plating of tumor cells from clinical specimens have been described previously (25–26). Briefly, a single-cell suspension of cells, obtained by mechanical dissociation and pipetting and mixed in culture medium and 0.3% (v/v) agarose, are plated over a base layer of culture medium and agarose (0.5% v/v) which has hardened. After 2–3 weeks, culture plates are observed for colony formation (cell aggregates of more than 50 cells), and the number of colonies is scored using an inverted phase microscope.

So far, we have evaluated the in vitro soft agarose cloning of 318 specimens obtained from patients with SCLC. Specimens were obtained from a variety of metastatic sites and from both newly diagnosed, untreated patients and from patients who had relapsed from prior intensive multiple drug combination chemotherapy. Although no tumor cell colony formation was observed in 238 specimens that were histocytopathologically negative for SCLC tumor cells, SCLC tumor colony formation was observed in 86% of the 80 specimens containing pathologically identifiable SCLC tumor cells. The number of colonies per 10^5 viable mononuclear cells plated ranged from 3 to 350 (mean 66; median 22), with no significant differences in colony-forming efficiency between specimens obtained from different metastatic sites.

Although no tumor colony formation was observed in cytologically negative specimens, suggesting the tumor cell origin of colonies in positive specimens, in a small number of bone marrow specimens, and in the absence of specific growth factors, typical hematopoietic stem cell colony growth was observed.

The nature of the colonies cultured in SCLC-positive specimens was confirmed by gross morphology, by cytology examination, by DNA content analysis using flow cytometry (FCM), and by the inoculation of colonies into athymic nude mice. (27). Typical SCLC colonies consisted of tight aggregates of 50 to several hundred cells, which attained peak size and viability approximately 14 days after plating. Cytology examination revealed cells with the typical morphology of SCLC: scanty cytoplasm, inconspicuous nucleoli, and nuclear molding (26). The DNA content analysis confirmed that the colonies cultured were aneuploid and also demonstrated that no change in DNA content was observed with culture of these cells. Finally, the "stem" cell origin of colonies was confirmed by the ability of colonies (as few as two colonies per mouse) to form typical SCLC tumors when inoculated intracranially into nude mice. (27). Continuous cell lines with the typical characteristics of SCLC could be established readily from these tumors. For a small number of specimens of non-SCLC lung cancer, colony formation in soft agarose was observed in 66% of specimens, with a colony-forming efficiency of 0.17% (27).

Whereas these data confirm the usefulness of the soft agarose clonogenic assay to culture tumor cells selectively from fresh clinical specimens of lung cancer, as has been described for a number of other tumors, in these conditions, the colony-forming efficiency is low (usually less than 0.1%) with most plates containing less than 30 colonies per 10^5 viable cells plated (28). Whether this low cloning efficiency is a reflection of the inherent biology of the tumors, the methods used to obtain single-cell suspensions, or the culture conditions remains to be determined. It is likely that, whereas all these factors may contribute, improvements in cloning efficiency will come with the characterization of the specific growth requirements of individual tumor types.

Because of the poor CFE observed with fresh SCLC specimens, of the 86% of positive tumor specimens which formed colonies in agarose, in vitro drug sensitivity testing was possible in only 18 (22%) of these specimens. In a retrospective correlation of in vitro drug sensitivity and patient responses to these drugs, the in vitro soft agarose assay accurately predicted sensitivity in 73% of the tests, and resistance in 100% of the cases, confirming the potential value of this assay in chemotherapy selection (29). It should be stressed, however, that most patients were treated with combination multiple drug therapy, whereas in vitro drug assays were performed using single agents. These data are similar to data reported by others for the clonogenic assay where, for a large number of tumor specimens, successful in vitro drug sensitivity data could be obtained only in 30% of specimens (24, 28). The in vitro assay appears most useful in predicting which drug *not* to give a patient, rather than in predicting the agent most likely to obtain a clinical remission in that patient. If the soft agarose clonogenic assay is to achieve widespread use in the management of patients with cancer, including lung cancer, then growth conditions must be identified that support the cloning of the majority of tumor specimens at a much higher efficiency. Because of the low cloning efficiency of clinical specimens in soft agarose, we have evaluated the in vitro sensitivity of established cell lines to a large number of cytotoxic agents clinically useful in the treatment of lung cancer (29). As was observed for fresh clinical specimens, drug sensitivity data obtained with established cell lines, in continuous culture for periods ranging from 4 months to 3 years, accurately predicted the clinical responses observed in the patients from whom the lines were established. Cell lines established from untreated patients were sensitive to most drugs in vitro, whereas cell lines established from patients who had relapsed from multiple drug combination therapy retained reistance in vitro to these agents. Although these data suggest that drug testing may be determined successfully using established cell lines, they also suggest that established cell lines may be a useful model for understanding mechanisms of drug resistance in human cells and for screening new agents with potential clinical usefulness in the treatment of lung cancer.

Recently, we observed that a cell line (NCI H249p), established from a patient with SCLC who had relapsed from multiple courses of high-dose methotrexate as a single agent, had, after several months in continuous culture, become sensitive in vitro to methotrexate, although the fresh biopsy specimen and the early passage of the cell line were resistant to this drug (30). Further studies of this cell line revealed that the early-passage cell line displayed amplification of the gene coding for dihydrofolate reductase and a large number of double minute chromosomes. With serial passage in culture, the loss of drug resistance was associated with loss of the double minute chromosomes and a decline in dihydrofolate reductase levels. These results suggest that, in some cell lines of SCLC, instability of drug resistance may occur and may be related to gene amplification on double minute chromosomes.

Cytogenetic and DNA Content Analysis of Human Lung Cancer

Although considerable data are available on the cytogenetic analysis of hematopoietic malignancies, there is a paucity of data concerning the cytogenetic analysis of fresh specimens of human solid tumors. The major reasons are (1) the low number of metaphase spreads observed in fresh biopsy specimens, and (2) the uncertainty in these fresh specimens whether what is observed represents tumor cells or the frequently admixed nonmalignant cells. There are, however, several studies in which the DNA content of lung cancer cells has been determined by flow cytometry (FCM) (31–33). A DNA content analysis of FCM allows rapid determination of the DNA content of tumor cells independently of the proliferative state of the cells. In severral studies of human SCLC clinical specimens, in 65–75% of patients in whom tumor cells were identified, an aneuploid population of cells was identified with a DNA content of 1.1–2.3 times the diploid. Multiple aneuploid cell lines were identified in 10–20% of all clinical specimens, confirming the heterogeneous nature of these tumors. The failure to detect tumor cells by FCM in up to 35% of specimens containing tumor cells may be explained by the fact that in many instances, the number of tumor cells present in clinical samples is too small to be detected by FCM. In addition, as has been confirmed by DNA content analysis of continuous cell lines, in several instances both SCLC and non-SCLC lung cancer cell lines have near-diploid DNA contents.

Although a considerable range in total DNA content was observed among both SCLC and non-SCLC clinical specimens, the survival of patients was similar for patients with near-diploid and aneuploid DNA content. In addition, in several patients in whom tumor DNA content was analyzed prior to and after relapse from intensive combination chemotherapy, no significant changes in the DNA content were observed.

Of considerable interest is the recognition that with continuous cell culture in the majority of cases examined, a significant change in DNA content does not occur (33). This finding suggests that frequent measurement of the total DNA content of cell lines may be a useful method to screen for cross-contamination of cell lines in laboratory research.

Recently, using established cell lines of SCLC and fresh specimens of SCLC, we have demonstrated the presence in tumor cells of a specific cytogenetic defect associated with this tumor (34). Among established cell lines, although a wide range of chromosomal abnormalities was observed, all of the cell lines and the fresh specimens evaluated had a common deletion on a short arm of chromosome three. Use of the shortest region of overlap analysis showed that the common deletion was of the short arm in the regions p (14–23). This abnormality has been demonstrated in tumor cells of SCLC derived from a variety of metastatic sites and from primary lung specimens, and has been demonstrated in newly diagnosed, untreated and heavily pretreated patient specimens. This abnormality has not been identified in cell lines of non-SCLC lung cancer (in which no specific defects have been observed) and has not been observed in B lymphoblastoid autologous cell lines derived from patients with SCLC.

Although this abnormality was first identified in established cell lines of SCLC (35), the use of a serum-free defined medium selective for the growth of SCLC (vide infra) permitted the cytogenetic analysis of fresh specimens of SCLC after 2–3 days culture. This analysis is similar to PHA stimulation of bone marrow specimens prior to cytogenetic analysis. The presence of the 3p deletion in fresh specimens suggests that this defect is not an artifact of cell culture but a specific defect of SCLC. Whether the deletion is directly related to the malignant behavior of SCLC, or merely an association, remains to be determined. If confirmed by other investigators, the presence of 3p deletion in lung cancer will be of major biologic and diagnostic importance.

Serum-Free Defined Culture Media for Lung Cancer

At present, the growth of human tumor specimens in culture requires the use of serum-supplemented medium. Although the use of serum supplementation has facilitated the growth of cell lines, there are several problems associated with its use (36, 37). In addition to the fact that serum contains a variety of proteins, both known and unknown, that may have both stimulatory and inhibitory effects on the growth of the cells, serum supports the growth of both normal, nonmalignant cells and tumor cells. Because serum is nonselective, in many instances the growth of the normal cells occurs at a much faster rate such that overgrowth of the tumor cells occurs and the cells are lost.

Recently Sato and co-workers demonstrated for several continuous cell lines that the serum requirements could be replaced by the addition of hormones and growth factors (36, 37). Of interest was the observation that the growth-factor requirements were different for tumors of different histologies, suggesting that the identification of the specific growth factors of individual tumors might provide a means of regulating its growth both in vivo and in vitro.

Using established cell lines of SCLC that had been cultured continuously in serum-supplemented medium (SSM), the influence of a wide variety of growth factors and hormones on the proliferation of these cells was evalauted (38). A serum-free medium consisting of hydrocortisone, insulin, transferrin, estradiol, and selenium (HITES medium) added to RPMI 1640 medium was shown to support the continuous growth of the established cell lines. When transferred from SSM into HITES medium, after an initial lag phase, cell proliferation was at a rate similar to that observed in SSM.

To evaluate the specificity and selectivity of the HITES medium for the growth of SCLC tumor cells, a study comparing the growth of tumor cells from fresh biopsy specimens in both SSM and in HITES medium was carried out (7). At the present time, more than 60 tumor specimens of SCLC have been plated in SSM and in HITES medium. In the SSM, growth and proliferation of SCLC cells was observed in only 49% of all specimens. In contrast, in HITES medium, growth of tumor cells was observed in 74% of all specimens. Of major importance was the observation that in HITES medium, growth of SCLC tumor cells was selective. In SSM, growth of both normal admixed stromal cells and tumor cells was observed, whereas in the HITES medium growth of only SCLC tumor cells occurred, with death and lysis of other cells 7–14 days after plating. Thus, a pure population of rapidly dividing SCLC tumor cells was observed in the HITES medium. With the HITES medium, successful growth of tumor cells was obtained with specimens obtained from a wide variety of metastatic sites and with equal efficiency in specimens obtained from newly diagnosed, previously untreated patient specimens, and from specimens obtained from heavily pretreated patients.

The origin of the cells cultured in the HITES medium was confirmed by cytologic examination; by DNA content analysis, which confirmed the selective growth of tumor cells in the HITES medium (using aneuploid DNA as a marker for tumor cells); and by nude mouse tumorigenicity studies.

Although most specimens demonstrated a rapid initial proliferation in HITES medium, for approximately 50% of these specimens a growth crisis was observed after 12–24 weeks culture (6–12 passages). At this time, growth rate slowed and occasionally ceased. For these specimens, the addition of a small volume of fetal bovine serum (2.5% v/v) was sufficient to support the continuous growth of the tumor cells. This suggests that the HITES medium is not yet a complete medium for the growth of all specimens of SCLC. For 17 clinical specimens of SCLC, continuous cell lines have been established in HITES medium alone. These cell lines express the typical morphologic and biochemical properties of cell lines established using SSM and form typical SCLC tumors in athymic nude mice. For cell lines cultured in parallel in SSM and in HITES medium, no differences in the expression of biomarkers, etc, has been observed.

The failure of the HITES medium to support the continuous growth of all clinical specimens of SCLC and the failure of most specimens to form colonies in soft agarose in HITES medium alone without serum (7, 39, 40) suggests that this medium is not yet complete. Recently, we have evaluated the influence of a number of hormones produced by SCLC on the growth of SCLC in vitro. Two hormones, bombesin and arginine vasopressin (AVP), have been demonstrated in most cell lines of SCLC (5, 6, 13, 41). In addition, AVP excess has been demonstrated in the sera of the majority of patients with SCLC. Using a clonogenic assay with serum-free medium, we have shown that both bombesin and AVP stimulate the cloning of SCLC in agarose. We also have demonstrated that bombesin-like peptide receptors are present in cell lines of SCLC, but not in other lung cancer cell lines (41). The presence of these receptors on SCLC cells, the recognition that the majority of SCLC cell lines express high amounts of bombesin, and the demonstration in vitro that bombesin can influence the growth of these cells suggests that bombesin may be an important "autocrine" growth regulatory peptide in SCLC. The characterization of the receptor and the generation of monoclonal antibodies to both bombesin and its receptors may provide a novel approach to regulating the growth of this tumor in vivo. The data also suggest that the screening of tumor cells for hormone receptors may aid in the rapid identification of hormones and growth factors essential for the growth in vivo and in vitro.

In addition to defining the serum-free growth requirements for SCLC, considerable success has now been achieved in defining the growth requirements for other types of lung cancers (36, 37, 42). However, in contrast to SCLC, where the essential growth requirements are selenium, insulin, and transferrin (hydrocortisone and estradiol are stimulatory but not essential), the growth of non-SCLC cell lines in serum-free medium requires the addition of several other factors (Table 2). Although the defined media for non-SCLC have been shown to support the growth of established cell lines of non-SCLC, data are not yet available to show whether these defined media are superior to serum-supplemented media for the growth and establishment of continuous cell lines from fresh clinical specimens. Of interest is the requirement by non-SCLC cell lines for epidermal growth factor (EGF) which is nonstimulatory to SCLC cell lines (38). It has been demonstrated previously that cell lines of non-SCLC, but not SCLC, have EGF receptors. These data suggest that the recognition of cell surface receptors for growth factors and hormones may be a means for identifying agents essential for the growth of specific cell lines. In addition, they may provide a means for regulating the growth of these cells both in vivo and in vitro.

Table 2. Serum-free growth factor and hormone requirements of small-cell and non-small-cell lung cancer cell lines[a]

Growth factor	Cell type[b] Small cell	Adenocarcinoma	Squamous cell
Basal medium	RPMI-1640	F12/DMEM	F12/DMEM
Hydrocortisone	+	+	+
Insulin	+	+	+
Transferrin	+	+	−
Estradiol	+	−	−
Selenium	+	+	+
T3	−	−	+
Glucagon	−	−	+
Epidermal growth factor	−	+	−
Albumin	(+)	+	−

[a]Data from Refs. 7, 36–38, and 42.
[b]+, essential requirement; −, not required; (+), stimulatory but not essential.

"Conversion" of Small-Cell Lung Cancer to Large-Cell Morphologic Variants

Among the histologic types of SCLC a number of histologic variants have been recognized, including the classic lymphocyte or oat cell type, the fusiform, polygonal, and other cell types (43–45). In several clinical studies, a comparison of the clinical presentation, response to therapy, and survival have not shown significant differences in the biologic behavior of these histologic subtypes (43). However, in addition to these subtypes of SCLC, in approximately 6% of patients with SCLC at diagnosis, a mixture of SCLC with another histologic type of lung cancer, most frequently large cell (LC), is observed. In contrast to SCLC, the presence of this SCLC/LC mixture is associated with a poor prognosis, including an overall lower response rate to combination chemotherapy than "pure" SCLC, and a significantly shorter median survival (44, 45). Whether the presence of two cell types means the presence of two different tumors or the "conversion" of one to the other has not yet been determined. Although this mixture of SCLC/LC is observed in only 6% of previously untreated patients with SCLC at autopsy (usually following intensive cytotoxic therapy), it has been seen in up to 35% of all patients, including those who initially present with "pure" SCLC in their biopsy specimen (44, 46). Of interest is the observation that when patients with SCLC relapse from initial induction therapy, further responses to cytotoxic therapy, including radiation therapy, are much less than those observed in newly diagnosed patients.

We and others have observed in continuous cell lines of SCLC that a small percentage undergoes "conversion" from SCLC to large-cell morphology (46–49). This change is uncommon but is associated with a number of important biologic changes in the cell. In addition to altered morphology, the LC cancer "variant" cell lines grow in much looser aggregates than SCLC, form colonies in agarose at a much higher efficiency (18–25% compared to 1–5% for SCLC), and have a much shorter latent period to tumor formation when inoculated into athymic nude mice. These observations suggest that the change to LC is associated with a more "malignant" behavior in the cell.

In addition to the biologic changes, when cells convert from SCLC to a LC variant, there is a loss in the expression of the classic APUD cell markers, including L-dopa decarboxylase and bombesin. However, these cells do retain the 3p cytogenetic deletion, confirming their SCLC lineage.

To determine whether the "conversion" of SCLC to LC with changes in biologic behavior and with the loss of APUD cell properties is related to a decrease in sensitivity of cells to cytotoxic therapy, we evaluated the in vitro radiation "sensitivity" of classic SCLC cell lines and LC variant cell lines using a soft agarose clonogenic assay (50).

The radiation survival curves of the SCLC cell lines were characterized by D_0s ranging from 51 to 140 rads and extrapolation values (n) ranging from 1.0 to 3.3 While the D_0s of the radiation survival curves of the LC variant cell lines were similar (91 and 80 rads) the extrapolation values of 5.6 and 11.1 were significantly greater than the classic SCLC cell lines. In addition, at a 200-rad dose, there was a two-to fivefold increase in survival of the LC variant lines compared to the SCLC cell lines. This suggests that the transformation of SCLC to LC with loss of APUD characteristics is associated with a marked increase in radiation resistance (n) in vitro. The observation of increased survival at 200 rads of the LC suggests that in patients with this histology the use of larger daily fraction of radiation may lead to a greater clinical response in these patients.

Surface Membrane Protein Phenotypes of Lung Cancer Cell Lines

Although monoclonal antibodies may be used to identify and isolate membrane determinants of human tumor cells, another approach in membrane characterization is to identify surface proteins by two-dimensional gel electrophoresis. Recently Baylin et al (51), using iodinated cell membranes followed by isoelectric focusing in the horizontal axis and then isoelectric focusing in the vertical axis, showed that SCLC cells have a similar phenotype with 12 protein spots distinguishing SCLC fron non-SCLC. The non-SCLC lung cancer cells had a very similar protein phenotype compared to each other, but one very distinct from the SCLC phenotype. Three of these 12 proteins identified in SCLC appear to be unique as they were not present in non-SCLC cells of human fibroblasts. Thus, this two-dimensional system may provide a means for biochemically typing different forms of lung cancer. The characterization of the different protein phenotypes of the tumors also may aid in our understanding of the differences in the biologic behavior of the varying histologic forms of lung cancer.

Summary

With improved techniques—most notably the use of chemically defined serum-free culture conditions—cell lines now can be established from the majority of clinical specimens of lung cancers, in particular, SCLC. These cell lines have facilitated greatly our knowledge of the biology of lung cancer and the identification of biomarkers associated with these tumors. Data generated from cell lines have been confirmed both by studies on fresh clinical specimens and by examining serum for the presence of markers identified in continuous cell lines. All of these data confirm our belief that cell lines of human tumors are excellent models for studying the biology of human tumors. In addition to the identification of biomarkers, these cell lines of lung cancer have permitted the identification of a specific cytogenetic marker associated with SCLC, the characterization of specific growth factor requirements for both SCLC and non-SCLC cell lines, and the characterization of membrane protein phenotypes of lung cancer cells.

All of these have important application in both our understanding of the biology of these tumors and the management of patients with these diseases.

References

1. American Cancer Society. Cancer statistics 1980 Ca—A Cancer Journal for Clinicians 1981; 31:13-28.
2. Minna JD, Higgins GA, Glatstein EJ. Cancer of the lung. In: DeVita VT, Hellman S, Rosenberg SA, eds, Cancer principles and practice of oncology. Philadelphia: J.B. Lippincott, 1982;396-475.
3. Carney DN, Minna JD. Small cell lung cancer. Clin Chest Med 1982;3:389–98.
4. Gazdar AF, Carney DN, Russel E, et al. Establishment of continuous clonable tumorigenic cell lines of small cell carcinoma of the lung having amine precursor uptake and decarboxylation properties. Cancer Res 1980;40:3502–7.
5. Sorenson GD, Pettengill OS, Brink-Johnson T, et al. Hormone production by cultures of small cell carcinoma of the lung. Cancer 1981;47:1289–96.
6. Pettengill OS, Sorenson GD. Tissue culture and in vitro characteristics of small cell lung cancer. In: Greco FA, Bunn PA, Oldham RK, Small cell lung cancer. New York: Grune and Stratton, 1981;51–79.
7. Carney DN, Bunn PA, Gazdar AF, Pagan JA, Minna JD. Selective growth in serum-free hormone supplemented medium of tumor cells obtained by biopsy from patients with small cell carcinoma of the lung. Proc Natl Acad Sci USA 1981;78:3185–9.
8. Chamber WF, Pettengill OS, Sorenson GD. Intercranial growth of pulmonary small cell carcinoma cells in nude athymic mice. Exp Cell Biol 1981;49:90–7.
9. Gazdar AF, Carney DN, Sims HL, Simmons A. Heterotransplantation of small cell carcinoma of the lung into nude mice. I. Comparison of intracranial and subcutaneous routes. Int J Cancer 1981;28:773–83.
10. Baylin SB, Sbeloff MD, Goodwin G, Carney DN, Gazdar AF. Activities of *L*-dopa decarboxylase and diamine oxidase (histaminase) in human lung cancers: the decarboxylase as a marker for small (oat) cell cancer in tissue culture. Cancer Res 1980;40:1990–6.
11. Gazdar AF, Zweig MH, Carney DN, Van Stierteghen AC, Baylin SB, Minna JD. Levels of creatine kinase and its isozyme in lung cancer tumors and cultures. Cancer Res 1981;41:2773–7.
12. Marangos PJ, Gazdar AF, Carney DN. Neuron specific enolase in human small cell carcinoma cultures. Cancer Lett 1982;15:67–71.
13. Moody TW, Pert CB, Gazdar AF, Carney DN, Minna JD. High levels of intracellular bombesin characterize human small cell lung cancer. Science 1981;214:1246–8.
14. Richardson RL, Greco FA, Oldham RC, Liddle GW. Tumor products and potential markers in small cell lung cancer. Semin Oncol 1978;5:253–62.
15. North WG, Maurer H, Valtin H, O'Donnel JF. Human neurophysins as potential markers for small cell carcinoma of the lung: applications of specific radioimmunoassay. J Endocrinol Metab 1980;51:892–6.
16. Gropp C, Havemann K, Scheurer A. Ectopic hormones in lung cancer patients at diagnosis and drug therapy. Cancer 1980;46:347–54.
17. Hansen M, Hammer M, Hummer L. ACTH, ADH, and calcitonin concentrations as markers for response and relapse in small cell carcinoma of the lung. Cancer 1980;46:2062–7.
18. Carney DN, Zweig MH, Minna JD, et al. Creatine-kinase BB: A clinical marker for tumor burden in patients with small cell carcinoma of the lung. AFCR, 1981;433A.
19. Carney DN, Marangos PJ, Ihde DC, Cohen MH, Minna JD, Gazdar AF. Neuron specific enolase: A marker for disease extent and response to therapy in patients with small cell lung cancer. Lancet 1982;1:583–5.
20. Hamburger AW. Use of in vitro tests in predictive cancer chemotherapy. JNCI 1981;66:981–8.
21. Hamburger AW, Salmon SE. Primary bioassay of human tumor stem cells. Science 1977:197: 461–3.
22. Salmon SE, Hamburger AW, Soehnlen BJ, Durie BGM, Alberts DS, Moon TC. Quantitation of differential sensitivities of human tumor stem cells to anticancer drugs. N Engl J Med 1978;298: 1321–7.

23. Alberts DS, Chem HSG, Soehnlen B, et al. In vitro clonogenic assay for predicting response of ovarian cancer to chemotherapy. Lancet 1980;2:340–2.
24. Von Hoff DD, Casper J, Bradley E, Sandbach J, Jones D, Makuch R. Association between human tumor colony-forming assay results and response of an individual patient's tumor to chemotherapy. Am J Med 1981;70:1027–32.
25. Carney D, Gazdar AF, Minna JD. Positive correlation between histologic tumor involvement and generation of tumor cell colonies in agarose in specimens taken directly from patients with small cell carcinoma of the lung. Cancer Res 1980;40:1820–3.
26. Carney DN, Bunn PA, Gazdar, AF, Minna JD. In vitro cloning of small cell carcinoma of the lung. In: Greco, FA, Bunn PA, Oldham RK, eds, Small cell lung cancer. New York: Grune and Stratton, 1981;79–94.
27. Carney DN, Gazdar AF, Bunn PA, Guccion JG. Demonstration of the stem cell nature of clonogenic cells in lung cancer specimens. Stem Cells 1981;1:149–64.
28. Selby P, Buick RN, Tannock I. A critical appraisal of the human tumor stem-cell assay. N Engl J Med 1983;308:129–34.
29. Carney DN, Gazdar AF, Minna JD. In vitro chemosensitivity of clinical specimens and cell lines of small cell lung cancer. Proc ASCO 1982;1:C-37.
30. Curt G, Carney DN, Cowan K, et al. Unstable methotrexate resistance in human small cell carcinoma associated with double minute chromosomes. N Engl J Med 1983;4:199–203.
31. Barlogie B, Drewinko B, Schuman T, et al. Cellular DNA content as a marker of neoplasia in man. Am J Med 1980;69:195–203.
32. Vindeløv LL, Hansen HH, Christensen IJ, et al. Clonal heterogeneity of small cell anaplastic carcinoma of the lung demonstrated by flow-cytometric DNA analysis. Cancer Res 1980; 40:4295–300.
33. Bunn PA Jr, Carney DN, Gazdar AF, Whang-Peng JW, Matthews MJ. Flow cytometric DNA content analysis in lung cancer; diagnostic and biologic implications. Cancer Res 1983; 43:5026–32.
34. Whang-Peng J, Kao-Shum CS, Lee EC, et al. A specific chromosome defect associated with human small cell lung cancer. Deletion 3p (14–23). Science 1982;215:181–3.
35. Whang-Peng JW, Bunn PA, Kao-Shum CS, et al. A non-randomal chromosomal abnormality, del 3p (14–23) in human small cell lung cancer. Cancer Genet Cytogen 1982;G:119–34.
36. Barnes DW, Sato GW. Serum-free cell culture: A unifying approach. Cell 1980;22:649–55.
37. Barnes D, Sato G. Methods for growth of cultured cells in serum-free medium. Anal Biochem 1980;102:255–70.
38. Simms E, Gazdar AF, Abrams PG, Minna JD. Growth of human small cell (oat cell) carcinoma of the lung in serum-free growth factor supplemented medium. Cancer Res 1980;40:4356–63.
39. Minna JD, Carney DN, Oie, H, Bunn PA, Gazdar AF. Growth of small cell lung cancer in defined medium. In: Pardee J, Sato GW, eds, Growth of cells in defined medium, Vol 6. New York: Cold Spring Harbor Press, 1982;627–39.
40. Sorensen GD, Bloom SR, Ghatei MA. Bombesin production by human small cell carcinoma of the lung. Regul Pept 1982; 4:59–66.
41. Moody TW, Bertness V, Carney DN. Bombesin-like peptides and receptors in human tumor cell lines. Peptides 1983;4:683–6.
42. Brower M, Carney DN, Oie H, et al. Growth of human adenocarcinoma of the lung cell lines and clinical specimens in serum-free defined medium. Proc ASCO 1982;C:543.
43. Carney DN, Matthews MD, Ihde DC, et al. Influence of histologic subtype of small cell carcinoma of the lung on clinical presentation, response to therapy and survival. JNCI 1980; 65:1225–9.
44. Mathews MJ, Gazdar AF. Pathology of small cell carcinoma of the lung and its subtypes. A clinico-pathologic correlation. In: Livingston RB, ed, Lung cancer I. Boston: Martinus Nijhoff, 1981:283–306.
45. Radice PA, Matthews MJ, Ihde DC, et al. The clinical behavior of mixed small cell/large cell bronchogenic carcinoma compared to pure small cell subtypes. Cancer 1982;50:2894–2902.
46. Abeloff MD, Eggleston JC, Mendelsohn G, Ettinger DS, Baylin SB. Changes in morphologic and biochemical characteristics of small cell carcinoma of the lung: A clinicopathologic study. Am J Med 1979;66:757–62.
47. Gazdar AF, Carney DN, Guccion JG, Baylin SB. Small cell carcinoma of the lung; Cellular origin and relationship to other pulmonary tumors. In: Greco FA, Oldham RK, Bunn PA, eds, Small cell carcinoma of the lung. New York: Grune and Stratton 1981;145–75.

48. Brereton HD, Matthews MJ, Costa J, Kent CH, Johnson RE. Mixed anaplastic small cell and squamous cell carcinoma of the lung. Ann Int Med 1978;88:805-6.
49. Goodwin G, Baylin SB. Relationships between neuroendocrine differentiation and sensitivity to radiation in culture line OH-1 of human small cell lung carcinoma. Cancer Res 1982;42:1361-7.
50. Carney DN, Mitchell JB, Kinsella TK. In vitro radiation and chemotherapy sensitivity of established cell lines of human small cell lung cancer and its large cell morphologic variants. Cancer Res 1983;43:2806-11.
51. Baylin SB, Gazdar AF, Minna JD, et al. A unique cell surface protein phenotype distinguish human small cell from non-small cell lung cancer. Proc Natl Acad Sci U.S. 1982;9:4650-4.

CHAPTER **21**

Radioactivity and Cigarette Smoke

THOMAS H. WINTERS and JOSEPH R. DIFRANZA

Department of General Internal Medicine
Department of Family and Community Medicine
University of Massachusetts Medical Center, 55 Lake Avenue, North Worcester, Massachusetts 01605

ABSTRACT

Alpha radiation from tobacco smoke is a significant factor in the induction of lung cancer. The smoker receives α radiation at bronchial bifurcations from three sources: from ^{214}Po in mainstream smoke and particles; from ^{210} Po that grows up into ^{210} Pb-enriched particles, which persist at bifurcations; and both from atmospheric and soil (phosphate fertilizer) radon progeny as well as from indoor radon decay products. A cumulative α dose at the bifurcation of smokers dying of lung cancer is 1600 rems, enough radiation to induce malignant transformation of basal epithelial cells.

We have found when educating smokers that more are encouraged to quit as they learn of the presence of radioactivity in cigarette smoke.

Acquisition of Radioisotopes by Tobacco

It has been known for 20 years that all varieties of tobacco contain the α emitting radioisotope polonium (−210) (^{210}Po) and its β-emitting precursor, lead − 210 (^{210}Pb). However, the mechanism by which the tobacco plant acquires these isotopes has been the subject of some debate.

One mechanism is the uptake of radioisotopes through the roots (Figure 1). In support of this mechanism Tso demonstrated that tobacco plants are capable of absorbing ^{210}Pb and ^{210}Po added to their potting mixture (1). All soils contain radium and its breakdown products ^{210}Pb and ^{210}Po. In addition, the phosphate ore that is the substrate for the phosphate fertilizers used on tobacco fields also contains these isotopes.

A second mechanism involves the airborne deposition of these isotopes on leaf surfaces (Figure 1). Tobacco leaves are coated with tiny leaf hairs called trichomes. Trichomes have glandular heads that are coated with a sticky organic

Lung Cancer: Causes and Prevention.

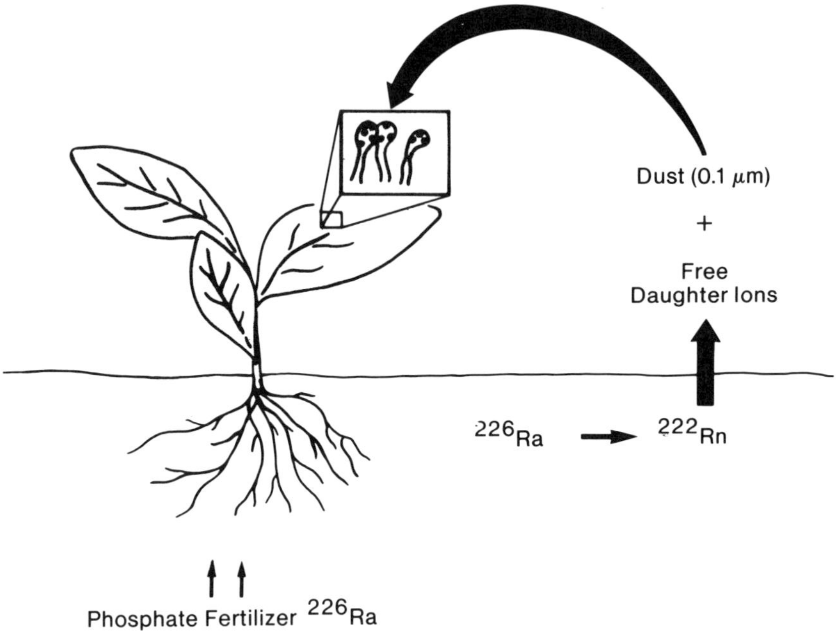

Figure 1. Radon daughter migration to trichomes of tobacco plant.

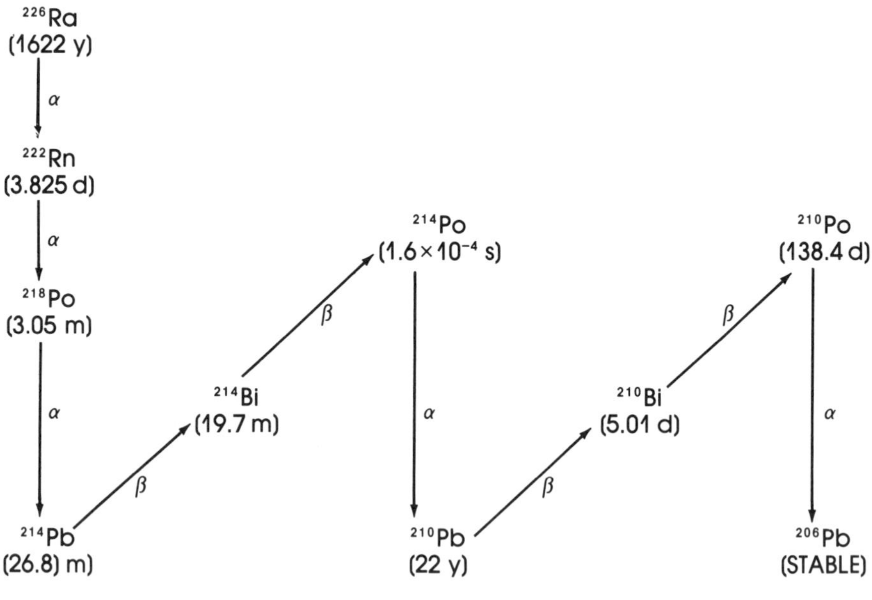

Figure 2. Radium-226 (uranium-238) decay series with half-lives.

exudate. Martell was able to demonstrate that the radioisotopes are found on the trichome heads in concentrations about 10,000 times that of the bulk leaf (2).

The source of the isotopes is the soil and phosphate fertilizers. When radium -226 decays, it gives rise to radon -222, an inert gas that emanates from the soil into surface air. There it decays into a series of radon daughters. The electrically charged radon daughters have a high affinity for suspended particulates and become attached to dust particles $< 0.1\ \mu m$ in diameter (2). These particles bearing radon daughters in turn become attached to the sticky trichome heads (Figure 2). Tso demonstrated that radon daughters ^{210}Pb and ^{210}Po, when applied to the surface of tobacco leaves, did not migrate but remained where applied (3). Which of these mechanisms represents the major route of acquisition? Certain grasses share tobacco's property of acquiring radioisotopes on their surfaces. Hill studied the ratio of ^{210}Pb to stable ^{206}Pb in soils and grasses (4). Both lead isotopes should be absorbed with equal avidity by the roots. However, Hill found the ratio of ^{210}Pb to ^{206}Pb in the plants to be 20 times greater than that for the soil, eliminating root uptake as a major mechanism of acquisition.

Smoking and Lung Clearance Mechanisms

In healthy lungs inhaled particulates would be phagocytized by pulmonary macrophages and transported via the mucocilliary clearance mechanism out of the lungs.

Smoking impairs the efficiency of the mucocilliary clearance mechanism by slowing ciliary action. The average time required to clear 50% of inhaled particles is 172 min for smokers compared to 90 min for nonsmokers (5). In addition, smoking causes metaplasia whereby the normal ciliated columnar bronchial epithelium is replaced by nonciliated squamous epithelium. Auerbach et al (6) demonstrated such areas of metaplasia in 100% of the lungs of smokers he examined. The most common site for metaplastic changes to occur is at the bifurcations of bronchi (6). Even in healthy lungs, the bronchial bifurcations are areas of inefficient mucus transport because the mucus stream must split and change directions in order to continue its upward journey. At bifurcations, where metaplasia has occurred, the mucus transport is impaired severely.

Polonium-210 in Tobacco Smoke

Once deposited on the trichome heads, radon daughters continue to decay according to the scheme in Figure 2. Because of the long time between harvesting and consumption of the tobacco, ^{210}Pb and ^{210}Po are found in physical equilibrium (7). When the cigarette is burned, the ^{210}Po on the trichomes is completely volatilized, entering the smoke in gaseous form. The volatilized polonium rapidly absorbs onto particulates in the smoke.

Polonium-210 inhaled in gaseous form deposits on the alveolar membranes, whereas that attached to particulates mostly deposits along the tracheobronchial tree with preferential deposition at bronchial bifurcations. In either case, the ^{210}Po is soluble and dissolves in the surrounding fluid. It is removed from the lung by the lymphatics, the blood stream, and the mucociliary clearance mechanism. Once dissolved in the body water, polonium has a biologic half-life of 25 days (8). Because the intake of polonium is constant and the interval between doses (cigarettes) is short compared to the half-life, smokers maintain a steady-state level of polonium in their tissues. Smokers have significantly higher levels of ^{210}Po in lungs, bone, blood, and urine (7, 9, 10). Higher levels of ^{210}Po have been consistently found in smokers in the liver, kidneys, spleen, pancreas, gonads, and semen (11-13).

Eventual elimination is by radioactive decay or renal clearance. Active smokers (two packs a day) excrete 0.065 pc/24° of ^{210}Po whereas those who do not actively smoke excrete 0.011 pc/24° (7).

Radford and Hunt demonstrated that 50% of the ^{210}Po in cigarette smoke appears in the sidestream smoke. Hill, using a different smoking technique, found 70% of the ^{210}Po in the sidestream smoke. Polonium-210 in the sidestream smoke is inhaled by passive smokers.

Radford and Hunt derived a minimum dose estimate for the α dose to the bronchial epithelium from soluble ^{210}Po alone (7). It is based on measurements of ^{210}Po in tobacco smoke and the assumption (incorrect) that soluble ^{210}Po is deposited (99%) on the alveolar epithelium. Their minimum estimate for a two pack a day smoker is 36 rem over 25 years. The fact that soluble ^{210}Po deposits preferentially at bifurcations would lower the overall dose estimate but increase the proportion delivered to the bifurcations. This estimate would have to be adjusted upward to take into account prolonged clearance times resulting from the ciliary slowing effect of smoke and the mucus stagnation at metaplastic bronchial bifurcations.

Insoluble ^{210}Pb

As mentioned above, fresh trichomes contain ^{210}Pb and ^{210}Po in physical equilibrium (7). Martell has demonstrated combustion of the trichomes results in insoluble particles 1 μm in diameter (14). The ^{210}Po on the trichomes is stripped off by the 600–800 °C temperature of the cigarette, leaving behind the ^{210}Pb encased in the insoluble particles. When inhaled, these insoluble particles deposit preferentially at the bifurcations of the segmental bronchi (Figure 3).

At bifurcations where metaplasia has occurred and the mucus is stagnant, these insoluble particles remain where deposited for several months (Figure 4). The insoluble ^{210}Pb encased within these particles decays to ^{210}Po which also is trapped in an insoluble form. By measuring the ratio of ^{210}Pb to ^{210}Po in the insoluble particles found at the bronchial bifurcations of smokers, Radford and Martell were able to demonstrate a mean residence time of 3–5 months for these particles (15). Although the physical half-life of ^{210}Pb is long, 22 years, the quantity of ^{210}Pb present is large enough to produce a quantity of ^{210}Po sufficient to

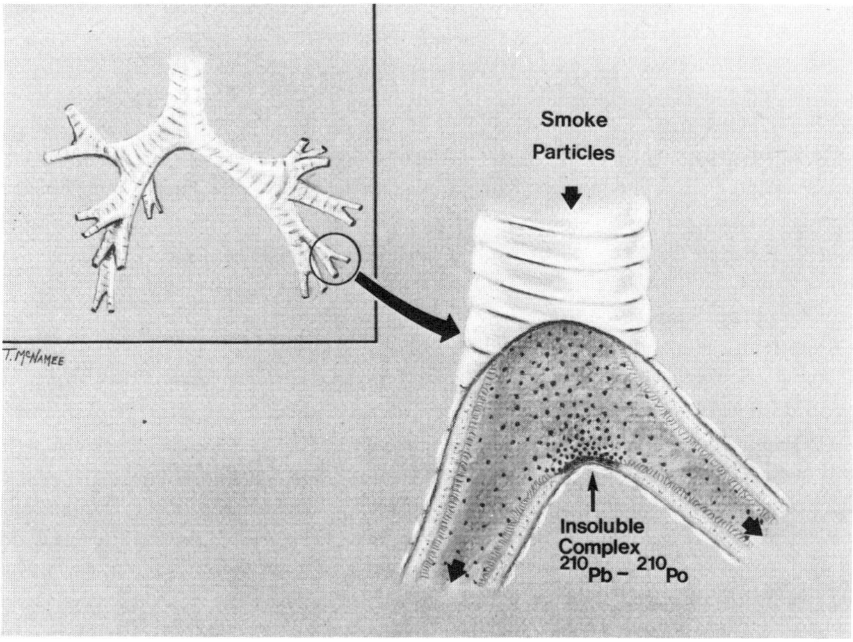

Figure 3. Tracheal tree with ^{210}Pb-^{210}Po complex deposition at bronchial bifurcations.

deliver a substantial dose of α radiation to the already metaplastic epithelium.

Little et al measured ^{210}Po in epithelial samples from 40 subjects. The highest concentrations were found in smokers at the bifurcations of segmental bronchi (9). They calculated the ^{210}Po α dose at these locations to be 200 rems over 25 years for a 1½ pack a day smoker. This is equal to the skin dose from 8000 chest x-rays.

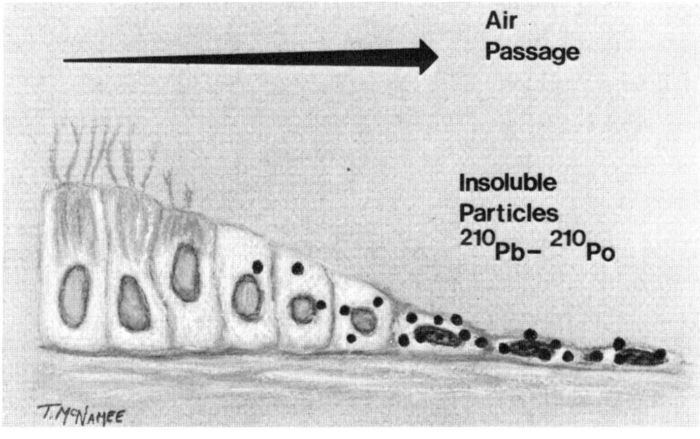

Figure 4. Deposition of insoluble complex in metaplastic bronchial epithelial cells.

Indoor Radon Daughters

Radium-226 is found in all soils. There it decays to radon-222, an inert gas that emanates from the soil into the surface air. Radon enters buildings through porous construction materials and is found in indoor air at levels tenfold higher than in outdoor air. Levels in some buildings are such that the U.S. Surgeon General has recommended that remedial action be taken to reduce the exposure of occupants to indoor radon.

Electrically charged radon daughters have a high affinity for surfaces. When the level of suspended particulates in indoor air is low (10^3 particles/cm^3) the radon daughters predominantly become attached to room surfaces (16). Martell and Sweder have demonstrated that when cigarette smoke is present (10^6 particulates/cm^3) the radon daughters rapidly attach to smoke particles 0.5–1.0 μm average diameter (16).

By increasing the level of respirable radon daughters, indoor air pollution from cigarettes increases the exposure of both active and passive smokers to radiation from radon daughters.

When smoking indoors, the smoker draws the suspended smoke particles bearing radon daughters in through the cigarette (Figure 5). This results in the radon daughters becoming associated with the 1–2 μm particles in the mainstream smoke. Martell and Sweder have demonstrated that the radon daughter ^{218}Po is in a soluble form and thus it decays before clearance because of its very short, 3.5 min half-life. It "contributes significantly to the alpha irradiation of the bronchial epithelium" (16).

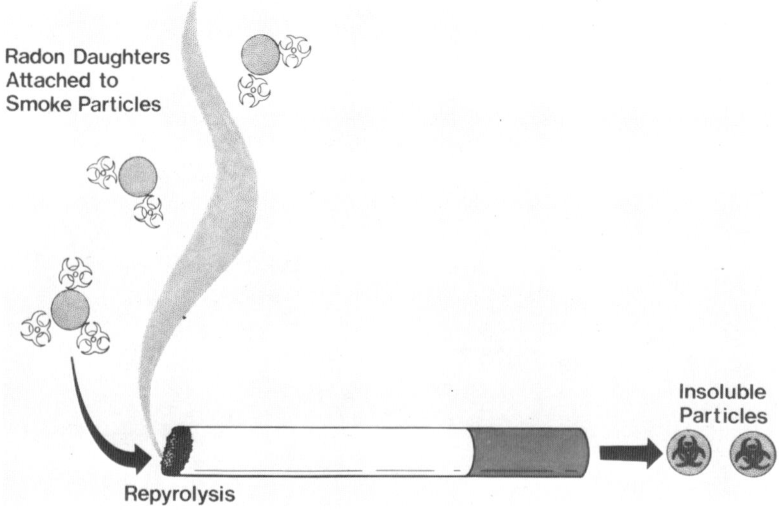

Figure 5. Indoor radon progeny attachment to smoke particles: insoluble ^{210}Pb formation.

After being drawn through the burning cigarette, the radon daugher ^{214}Pb is found in association with insoluble particulates (smoke tar) and would be preferentially deposited at bronchial bifurcations. Its decay product ^{214}Po contributes to the α irradiation of the epithelium at these sites.

Martell estimates the 40-year α-radiation dose for a smoker, which includes the ^{210}Po radiation from tobacco, indoor radon daughters, and the same inhaled through cigarettes, to be 80–100 rads—equivalent to 1600–2000 rems (17).

Extrapolating from the incidence of bronchial cancer in underground miners exposed to radon daughters, Radford and Hunt estimated that a radiation dose of 1300 rems would be necessary to account for the observed incidence of lung cancer in two pack a day smokers (7).

Tumor Induction

It is a common practice to assume that the exposure received from a radiation source is distributed throughout a tissue. In this way a high level of exposure in a localized region, eg, bronchial epithelium, is averaged out over the entire lung mass. However, α particles travel only a short distance in tissue (40 μm for ^{210}Po). A cell nucleus 5–6 μm in diameter, traversed by a single α particle, receives a dose of 1000 rems. Therefore, although the total tissue dose may be thought to be negligible, cells close to an α source receive very high doses. The α particles traveling through tissue leave a dense track of ionization. When such a track intersects a chromosome closely spaced chromosomal breaks are likely to occur, with a possible result being permanent mutation of the genetic material and carcinogenesis.

The α radiation associated with smoking is delivered in highest concentrations to the metaplastic epithelium at bronchial bifurcations. Metaplastic tissue is fertile ground for neoplasia. Auerbach's results indicate that the highest frequency of premalignant lesions in the bronchi of smokers occurred at the bifurcations (6). It has been demonstrated that α-particle doses greater than 80 rads are very effective in producing malignant transformations in cultured mammalian cells (18). Little et al demonstrated lung cancer in 94% of Syrian golden hamsters after intratracheal instillation of ^{210}Po (19).

Whether radiation, chemicals, or physical factors associated with smoking cause the metaplasia found in all smokers is not clear. However, the fact that these high doses of radiation are delivered to vulnerable tissue at the location where malignancy is most frequently observed argues strongly for α radiation playing the major role in the etiology of lung cancer.

Passive Smoking

In a 14-year prospective study involving 91,540 subjects, Hirayama demonstrated that passive smokers are at increased risk of developing lung cancer (20). His results have been confirmed by a case control study by Trichopoulos et al (21). Radiation may play a role in the induction of cancer in passive smokers as well.

The passive smoker is exposed to the same radioelements in the tobacco as the smoker; moreover, 50–70% of the ^{210}Po appears in sidestream smoke (7, 21).

In addition, the exposure of the passive smoker to naturally occurring radon daughters is increased in a smoky environment (16). Extrapolating from uranium miner experience, Harley and Pasternack estimate that radon daughter exposure accounts for 20–100% of lung cancers seen in nonsmokers (22). Increased exposure to radon daughters through passive smoking would be expected to increase the risk of lung cancer in passive smokers. There has been no study comparing isotope levels in passive smokers and nonsmokers (23). When Little et al did their autopsy study, passive smoking was not a medical issue (9). In Little's study, four out of eight "nonsmokers" had significant ^{210}Po at the bifurcations, demonstrating exposure to airborne ^{210}Po or ^{210}Pb. The fact that in the remaining four "nonsmokers" no ^{210}Po activity was found in any epithelial sample makes it very unlikely that the ^{210}Po in the lungs of the others was from natural atmospheric sources. It is more likely that those "nonsmokers" with significant ^{210}Po levels were actually passive smokers. Further research is needed to evaluate the magnitude of the dose to passive smokers (23, 24).

In conclusion, passive smoking is associated with an increased exposure to several isotopes; α radiation should be considered as an etiology of the increased incidence of lung cancer seen in passive smokers.

Comment

After our first publication on this subject, we received hundreds of phone calls from smokers who quit smoking upon learning of the radioactive content of cigarette smoke. In addition to its contribution to solving the mysteries of lung cancer etiology, knowledge of the presence of radioactivity in cigarette smoke (in the setting of increased public concern about radiation) may play a vital role in motivating people to quit smoking.

References

1. Tso TC, Harley N, Alexander LT. Source of lead-210 and polonium-210 in tobacco. Science 1966;153:880–2.
2. Martell EA. Radioactivity of tobacco trichomes and insoluble cigarette smoke particles. Nature 1974;249:215–7.
3. Tso TC, Fisenne I. Translocation and distribution of lead-210 and polonium-210 supplied to tobacco leaves. Radiat Bot 1968;8:457–62.
4. Hill CR. Lead-210 and polonium-210 in grass. Nature 1960;187:211–2.
5. Albert RE, Lippmann M, Briscoe, W. The characteristics of bronchial clearance in humans and the effects of cigarette smoking. Arch Environ Health 1969;18:738–55.
6. Auerbach O, Stout AP, Hammond EC, Garfinkel L. Changes in bronchial epithelium in relation to cigarette smoking and in relation to lung cancer. N Engl J Med 1961;265:253–67.

7. Radford EP Jr, Hunt VR. Polonium-210: a volatile radioelement in cigarettes. Science 1964;143:247-9.
8. International Committee on Radiation Protection (1959) Committee II. Health Physics 1960;3:1.
9. Little JB, Radford EP Jr, McCombs HL, Hunt VR. Distribution of polonium-210 in pulmonary tissues of cigarette smokers. N Engl J Med 1965;273:1343-51.
10. Holtzman RB, Icewicz FH. Lead 210 and polonium 210 in tissues of cigarette smokers. Science 1966; 153:1259-60.
11. Blanchard RL. Concentrations of ^{210}Pb and ^{210}Po in human soft tissues. Health Physics 1967;13:625-32.
12. Hill CR. Polonium 210 in man. Nature 1965;208:423-8.
13. Hunt V. Penn State University. Personal Communication, 1983.
14. Martell EA. Radioactivity of tobacco trichomes and insoluble cigarette smoke particles. Nature 1974;249:215-7.
15. Radford EP, Martel EA. Polonium 210: lead 210 ratios as an index of residence times of insoluble particles from cigarette smoke in bronchial epithelium. In: Walton WH, ed, Inhaled particles, IV. Oxford: Pergamon Press, 1977:567-80.
16. Martell EA, Sweder KS. The roles of polonium isotopes in the etiology of lung cancer in cigarette smokers and uranium miners. In: Gomez M ed. Proceedings, radiation hazards in mining. New York: American Institution of Mining Engineers, 1981:383-9.
17. Martell EA. Alpha radiation dose at bronchial bifurcations of smokers from indoor radon progeny exposure. Proc Natl Acad Sci USA 1983;80:1285-9.
18. Lloyd EL, Gemmell MA, Henming CB, Gemmell DS, Zabransky BJ. Transformation of mammalian cells by alpha particles. Int J Radiat Biol 1979;36:467-78.
19. Little JB, O'Toole WF. Respiratory tract tumors in hamsters induced by benzo [a] pyrene and ^{210}Po radiation. Cancer Res 1974;34:3026-39.
20. Hirayama T. Non-smoking wives of heavy smokers have a higher risk of lung cancer: a study from Japan. Br Med J 1981;282:183-5.
21. Trichopoulos D, Kalandidi A, Sparros L, MacMahon B. Lung cancer and passive smoking. J Cancer 1981;27:1-4.
22. Harley NH, Pasternack BS. A model for predicting lung cancer risks induced by environmental levels of radon daughters. Health Physics 1981;40:307-16.
23. Winters TH, DiFranza JR. Radioactivity in cigarette smoke. N Engl J Med 1982;306:364-5.
24. DiFranza JF, Winters TH. Radioactivity in cigarette smoke. N Engl J Med 1982; 307:310-3.

CHAPTER **22**

Lung Cancer Incidence and Type of Cigarette Smoked[1]

PETER N. LEE

Independent Consultant in Statistics and Epidemiology, 25 Cedar Road, Sutton SM2 5DG, United Kingdom

ABSTRACT

During the last 30 years smokers in many countries have switched from plain cigarettes to filter cigarettes with a reduced yield of tar and nicotine. Although smokers do not appear to compensate for the reduced nicotine yield by increasing their cigarette consumption, they do achieve some compensation by altering the way in which they smoke their cigarettes. This compensation is only partial, so that tar intake is reduced on average in smokers of low tar cigarettes. A number of epidemiologic studies has shown that filter cigarette smokers have a lower risk of lung cancer than plain cigarette smokers, although more evidence is still needed on the risk of lung cancer in smokers of low-tar cigarettes. That a benefit of tar reduction has occurred is strongly suggested by the sharply reducing lung cancer rates in younger men and women in the United Kingdom. Claims that tar reduction has resulted in an increased risk of lung cancer in the United States are unsoundly based.
***Key Words:* Lung cancer, cigarette smoking, epidemiology, filter/plain, high tar/low tar**

Trends in the Type of Cigarette Smoked

Evidence relating cigarette smoking to lung cancer first started to emerge clearly some 30 years ago. At that time the great majority smoked were untipped plain cigarettes. Although no data on sales-weighted tar yields were available at that

[1]Any views expressed in this chapter are those of the author and not of any other person or company.

Lung Cancer: Causes and Prevention.

Table 1. Changes in type of cigarette sold, United Kingdom, 1955–1981[a]

Year	Market share (%)			Mean tar (mg/cigarette)		
	Plain	Filter	Low tar	Plain	Filter	All brands
1955	98.1	1.9	—	No data	No data	No data
1965	47.0	53.0	—	35.0	29.3	31.4
1972	18.3	81.7	—	27.8	18.9	20.5
1981	6.4	93.6	15.5	18.5	15.6	15.8

[a]Data from Lee (9); data for low tar (0–10 mg/cigarette) market share supplied by the tobacco industry.

time, it is fairly clear from a number of sources of evidence (1–3) that these cigarettes were "high tar," yielding perhaps 35–40 mg per cigarette. Since that time a three-stage change has occurred in the type of cigarette smoked.

Taking the United Kingdom data by way of illustration (Table 1) the first change, mainly between 1955 and 1965, was from high-tar plain to high-tar filter cigarettes, early filters being inefficient and reducing tar yields only slightly. Although, by 1965, filter cigarettes formed over half of the United Kingdom market, their average tar delivery, 29.3 mg, fell within the Department of Health and Social Security league tables high-tar classification of 29+ mg.

Between 1965 and 1972, the market share of filter cigarettes continued to rise and the second change, the switch from high-tar filter to middle-tar (17–22 mg) filter cigarettes occurred. Middle-tar filter cigarettes formed some 75% of the United Kingdom market in 1972.

Since then the third change, the switch to low-tar (0–10 mg) filter cigarettes, has started to occur, so that by 1981, some 15% of cigarettes smoked were low tar and 19% low to middle tar (11–16 mg). Currently only about 0.2% of the United Kingdom market are of middle to high (23–28 mg) or high-tar cigarettes, partly because the tar yield of plain cigarettes also has fallen considerably in recent years.

This general pattern also has occurred in many other countries, tending to occur rather earlier in the United States of America, Germany, and Switzerland and later in France (4). The majority of developed countries now has sales-weighted average tar yields in the middle- to low-tar group (Table 2). More recently, a dramatic fall in tar levels has been seen also in many developing countries and now virtually all have average tar levels in the low- to middle-tar or middle-tar group (Table 3). It is

Table 2. Sales-weighted average tar deliveries in 14 developed countries, 1982[a]

Tar group (mg per cigarette)	Countries			
Low tar (0–10 mg)	None			
Low to middle tar (11–16 mg)	Australia	Belgium	Canada	Finland
	Holland	New Zealand	Sweden	Switzerland
	United States	United Kingdom	West Germany	
Middle tar (17–22 mg)	France	Italy		
Middle to high tar (23–28 mg)	Denmark			
High tar (29+ mg)	None			

[a]Data supplied by the tobacco industry.

Table 3. Sales-weighted average deliveries in 33 developing countries, 1982[a]

Tar group (mg per cigarette)	Countries				
Low tar (0–10 mg)	None				
Low to middle tar (11–16 mg)	Chile	El Salvador	Fiji	Guatemala	Kenya
	Mauritius	Nicaragua	Panama	Papua-New Guinea	Trinidad
	Venezuela				
Middle tar (17–22 mg)	Argentina	Bangladesh	Barbados	Brazil	Costa Rica
	Cyprus	Hong Kong	India	Malawi	Malaysia
	Malta	Mexico	Nigeria	Sierra Leone	Singapore
	South Africa	Sri Lanka	Suriname	Zimbabwe	
Middle to high tar (23–28 mg)	Indonesia	Pakistan	Zaire		
High tar (29+ mg)	None				

[a]Data supplied by the tobacco industry.

notable that none of the countries listed in either Table 2 or Table 3 falls in the high-tar group.

What Benefits Do We Expect from Tar Reduction?

That the general tar reductions of over 50% that have occurred in most countries are likely to result in a substantial reduction in risk of lung cancer seems apparent a priori from the clear epidemiologic evidence that risk is strongly related to number of cigarettes smoked and the often repeated demonstration that application of tar to the skin of mice results in tumor development. There are, however, four salient points to be borne in mind.

First, there is abundant evidence that lung cancer risk is strongly dependent on duration of smoking (5), implying that past exposure to cigarettes is relevant. This being so, early evidence in which smokers have smoked reduced-tar cigarettes for only a relatively small proportion of their smoking life may not indicate the full extent of the reductions in risk obtained by lifelong smoking of lower tar cigarettes. In any event the expected reduction in risk from switching to lower tar cigarettes hardly can exceed that related to giving up smoking. Even after 10 years cessation the lung cancer risk of ex-smokers is five times that of lifelong nonsmokers (6).

Second, the extent of reduction in risk associated with smoking the same number of cigarettes but with a fraction of the tar yield need not necessarily be the same as that associated with a fraction of the number of cigarettes but with the same tar yield. It is only the latter dose–response relationship for which one has good evidence (7).

Third, there may have been qualitative changes in the tar to which the smoker is exposed because of modification of the cigarette design. In fact such evidence as there is suggests that the mouse skin carcinogenicity per unit dose of tar has been steadily reducing (8).

Fourth, there is the problem of "compensation." For most of the period over which tar reductions have occurred (although not over the last 7 or 8 years in the United Kingdom) there have been concomitant reductions in the nicotine yield of cigarettes (9) and there is a strong correlation between tar and nicotine deliveries of brands on the market (10). As it is widely believed that a substantial proportion of smokers smoke for nicotine, it has been suggested that a smoker switching to a brand with a lower machine yield of nicotine will alter his smoking characteristics so as to attain a required "dose" of nicotine (11). This compensation can occur in two ways, either by smoking more cigarettes or by altering the manner of smoking so as to "get more out of" a cigarette, or both.

Compensation by Increased Consumption

Stepney (12), reviewing evidence from 16 published experiments in which smokers switched to brands of lower yield for up to 6 weeks, concluded that there was some evidence of a modest increase in consumption in relation to a decrease in nicotine yield (Table 4). In view of the short-term nature of these studies it is not clear that this small degree of compensation is anything but a transitory effect. More relevant seems the analysis of Garfinkel (13) (Table 5), based on the American Cancer Society million-person study that changes in consumption were essentially independent of whether or not men changed the tar/nicotine yield of the brand they smoked. Wald et al (14) came to a similar conclusion in an analysis of data from the British United Provident Association (BUPA) study sample, although this was based on smaller numbers of smokers and relied on memory for past smoking habits. Based on the observation in some countries of long-term increases in cigarette consumption per smoker in conjunction with long-term decreases in sales-weighted tar yields, one might suggest that compensation by increased consumption is important. However, such correlations are potentially misleading as changes in cigarette consumption also depend on a number of other important factors that must be taken into account. Among these are: changes in relative price, available money, degree of Westernization, and liberation of women. Two observations from national statistics in fact argue against this form of

Table 4. Estimated increase in cigarette consumption in relation to reductions in nicotine delivery[a]

	Percentage change				
Reduction in nicotine delivery	10	30	50	70	90
Increase in cigarette consumption	1	5	9	13	18

[a]Based on linear regression fitted by Stepney (12) to results from 16 short-term switching studies.

Table 5. Lack of relationship between tar reduction and cigarette consumption[a]

		Change in cigarette consumption (%)		
Change in tar/nicotine level	**Men studied**	**Increase**	**No change**	**Decrease**
None	8,190	31.7	34.7	33.6
Decrease	16,991	31.5	34.1	34.4

[a]From Garfinkel's (13) analysis of the American Cancer Society million person study data.

Table 6. Average annual consumption of cigarettes per smoker, United Kingdom, 1981[a]

Usual brand	Men	Women
Low tar	6700	5300
Low to middle tar	7300	6050
Middle tar	7500	6150

[a]Research Services (unpublished data).

compensation. One is that in the United Kingdom consumption of cigarettes per smoker is 10–15% less for low-tar smokers than for middle-tar smokers (Table 6). Although this does not necessarily prove negative compensation, as those who reduced tar may have been smokers with below average consumption, it certainly does not support the thesis of positive compensation. The second is that an analysis carried out by the tobacco industry of data from a number of Third World countries, where very rapid reductions in tar yield have occurred, failed to show any discernible effect on sales trends.

Compensation by Altered Manner of Smoking

Compensation in terms of manner of smoking may occur by altering the puffing characteristics in order to increase the amount of smoke presented to the smoker, changing the proportion blown out of the mouth before inhalation, altering the pattern of inhalation so that the relative uptake from a given amount of smoke is increased, or even, on occasion, by tampering with the cigarette itself by removing the filter or by placing fingers over some of the air holes on cigarettes with ventilated filters. A number of studies (14–17) have investigated the relationship between machine nicotine yield and nicotine uptake, either as measured directly by blood or urinary nicotine or cotinine, or as estimated indirectly via an "inhaling index" based on blood carboxyhemoglobin values. In some studies the same smoker has smoked different types of cigarettes, whereas in others the comparison has been between smokers. The first type of study suffers from the objections that it is usually small scale, it measures short-term effects, and the subjects are not representative of those who freely choose to switch. The second type of study suffers from the alternative objection that there may be systematic differences between different smokers of different types of cigarette in innate "desire to smoke". Table 7 summarizes the evidence from some of these studies and indicates that, although compensation in terms of altered manner of smoking exists, it is by no means complete.

In all the studies cited the smoker took in less nicotine when switching to a product with a lower machine nicotine yield, although the percentage reduction in intake was less than the percentage reduction in yield. Overall, although there is considerable variation in the data, it may not be unreasonable to state that for a given proportional reduction in nicotine yield, the average smoker reduces nicotine intake by about half as much. One study by Russell et al (11), which purported to demonstrate blood nicotine levels were virtually invariant of machine nicotine yields, has been widely quoted as support for the conflicting viewpoint of complete

Table 7. Reduction in nicotine intake in relation to reduction in machine nicotine delivery

Study	Type of study	Comparison	Percentage reduction: Nicotine delivery	Percentage reduction: Nicotine intake[a]
Ashton et al (15)	Within smoker	Middle nicotine vs high nicotine	24	23
		Low nicotine vs middle nicotine	57	6
Russell et al (16)	Within smoker	Low tar/nicotine vs middle tar/nicotine	46	35
Stepney et al (17)	Within smoker	Low tar/nicotine vs. middle tar/nicotine	55	33
Wald et al (14)	Between smoker	Unventilated filter vs plain	32	19
		Ventilated filter vs plain	58	30

[a]24- urinary nicotine for Ashton and Stepney studies; plasma nicotine for Russell study; estimated nicotine intake via inhaling index from COHb data for Wald study.

Table 8. Percentage of unventilated filter cigarette smokers with plasma nicotine levels above 200 mole/liter[a]

Nicotine delivery of cigarette	Percentage
>1.5 mg	67
1.1–1.5 mg	49
<1.0 mg	21

[a]From an analysis by Kozlowski et al (18) of data collected by Russell et al (11).

compensation; however, a reanalysis of their data (18) (Table 8) shows that there was in fact a clear trend for blood nicotine levels to be reduced in those smoking lower nicotine cigarettes.

Evidence from Epidemiologic Studies

Lee and Garfinkel (19) summarized the evidence then available from three prospective (20–22) and four retrospective (23–26) studies of lung cancer and type of cigarette smoked. These data are brought up to date in Tables 9 and 10 by the addition of information from a recently published study by Rimington (27). It is notable that the results consistently show a reduced risk of lung cancer in smokers of filter or lower tar/nicotine cigarettes than in smokers of plain or higher tar/nicotine cigarettes. Most relevant are the results from the American Cancer Society million-person study because of its prospective nature and the large numbers of deaths involved. The only relative mortality estimate out of the 18 figures cited that shows an increased mortality in filter cigarette smokers is based on a small sample and is not statistically significant.

That smokers of lower tar cigarettes have a reduced risk is probably supported also by a study by Kunze and Vutuc (28), who found that the risk of lung cancer was almost four times lower in those with a tar exposure score of less than 500 than in those with a score of 5000 or more. However this result is not clear because the

Table 9. Relative lung cancer mortality[a] by type of cigarette smoked: evidence from four prospective studies

Study	Comparison	Men: Deaths/ cases	Men: Relative mortality	Women: Deaths/ cases	Women: Relative mortality
Hammond et al (20) 1960–1966	Low vs high tar/nicotine	229	0.82	76	0.57
	Middle vs high tar/nicotine	843	0.95	119	0.88
Hammond et al (20) 1966–72	Low vs high tar/nicotine	162	0.80	94	0.63
	Middle vs high tar/nicotine	784	0.94	150	0.74
Hawthorne and Fry (21)	Filter vs plain	80	0.84	—	—
Migrants (22)	Filter vs plain	99	1.12	21	0.98
Rimington (27)	Filter vs plain	104	0.65	—	—

[a]Lung cancer incidence for Rimington (27) study.

Table 10. Relative lung cancer mortality by type of cigarette smoked: Evidence from four retrospective studies

Study	Comparison	Men: Deaths/ cases	Men: Relative/ mortality	Women: Deaths/ cases	Women: Relative/ mortality
Dean et al (23)	Filter vs plain	332	0.54	101	0.68
Bross and Gibson (24)	Filter vs plain	265	0.59	—	—
Wynder et al 1970 (25)	Filter vs plain	157	0.55	—	—
Wynder and Stellman 1979 (26)	Filter vs plain	293	0.76	63	0.75

Table 11. Frequency of lung changes seen in men dying in 1955–1960 and 1970–1977[a]

	1955–1960	1970–1977
Percentage with basal cell hyperplasia and 50% + cells with atypical nuclei		
Never smoked regularly	0.0	0.1
1–19 cigarettes a day	56.7	9.6
20–39 cigarettes a day	84.1	26.3
40+ cigarettes a day	98.6	56.1
Percentage with lesions with cilia absent and 50% + cells with atypical nuclei		
Never smoked regularly	0.0	0.0
1–19 cigarettes a day	10.0	2.2
20–39 cigarettes a day	21.9	6.0
40+ cigarettes a day	30.3	9.3

[a]Data from Auerbach et al (29).

score used fails to dissociate clearly between effects of tar level, duration of smoking, and number of cigarettes smoked per day.

Auerbach's pathology study (29) comparing the degree of changes seen in subjects dying in 1955-1960 with those seen in subjects dying in 1970-1977 (Table

11) is also important to note. If the lesions studied by Auerbach have a direct relationship to lung cancer, one old cigarette would seem to be equivalent to perhaps three or four modern cigarettes and lifetime exposure to lower tar cigarettes may involve markedly less risk than lifetime exposure to higher tar cigarettes.

Although the epidemiologic evidence is promising, it should be realized that it all refers to the first and second changes in cigarettes that have occurred. The switch to low-tar cigarettes, the third change, has occurred only fairly recently and its effects have not yet been reliably documented in an epidemiologic study. It is of obvious importance that further mortality studies be carried out to monitor this continuing trend.

Trends in National Mortality Figures

In any interpretation of national mortality trends for lung cancer it is of importance first to exclude artifacts caused by changes in diagnostic standards, which in the United Kingdom and United States accounted for something like a tenfold rise in observed death rates between 1900 and 1950 (30, 31), and second to take into account the crucial role played by duration of smoking. Doll and Peto (7) have shown that, whereas lung cancer risk is related only to the first or second power of daily "dose" of cigarettes, it is related to the fourth or fifth power of number of years smoked. The importance of this is indicated by considering the hypothetical example of a population, all of whom took up smoking at the same level in 1915 or at age 15 if they were born after 1900.

If risk is taken to be proportional to the fourth power of duration of smoking and to be independent of non-smoking-related factors then Table 12 gives the relative risk of lung cancer by age and year assuming no changes in the type of cigarette smoked. It is apparent that in this population, which in some ways is not dissimilar from United Kingdom males, any effect of changing type of cigarette would be virtually impossible to pick up clearly in the oldest age groups. In the younger age groups an effect should be discernible and, as Table 13 shows, it clearly is, with

Table 12. Trends in relative lung cancer risk for a hypothetical population all of whom took up smoking in 1915, or at age 15 if born after 1900[a]

	Year						
Age at year stated	**1930**	**1940**	**1950**	**1960**	**1970**	**1980**	**Risk increases up to year**
40	1	8	8	8	8	8	1940
50	1	8	30	30	30	30	1950
60	1	8	30	81	81	81	1960
70	1	8	30	81	181	181	1970
80	1	8	30	81	181	353	1980
90	1	8	30	81	181	353	1990

[a]Assumptions: (1) Risk is proportional to fourth power of duration of smoking, (2) no change in cigarettes, (3) non-smoking-related factors ignored.

quite a striking decrease seen in the youngest age groups over the last years. For United Kingdom females, where smoking started considerably later, it is to be expected that any reductions in lung cancer risk will be seen only over a smaller age range and Table 14 supports this prediction.

Although the trends in the United Kingdom are consistent with a strong effect of tar reduction a word of caution is necessary. One must bear in mind that there also have been concomitant reductions in air pollution and in occupational exposures. Even if it seems unlikely from other data that these can have played a great part in the reduction, one requires a satisfactory explanation of the fact that reductions in lung cancer rates in young men and women were seen before 1965 when, according to Todd (3), little or no reductions in tar levels occurred. Doll and Peto invoke Wald's 1981 study (2) of old packets of cigarettes, which showed higher tar levels in brands manufactured before 1962 than in those manufactured in 1962–1968, as suggesting that substantial earlier tar reductions did occur. This is not convincing, because most of the filter cigarettes Wald tested for the critical period 1962–1968 were made in 1967–1968, a time by which large tar reductions were already known to have occurred. Despite these doubts, it seems that tar reductions are likely to have had a marked effect in reducing lung cancer rates in the United Kingdom.

In some ways the situation in the United Kingdom, especially for males, is easier to analyze than it is in other countries, as there was a long period between about 1940 and 1975 when cigarette consumption per adult remained similar. In the United States, as Doll and Peto (5) show in their detailed analysis, there was a

Table 13. Trends in England and Wales male lung cancer rates relative to 1956–60

Age	1956–1960	1966–1970	1976–1979
30–34	100	68	46
35–39	100	81	59
40–44	100	86	54
45–49	100	90	67
50–54	100	93	81
55–59	100	95	81
60–64	100	111	100
65–69	100	134	126
70–74	100	159	171
75–79	100	177	240

Table 14. Trends in England and Wales female lung cancer rates relative to 1956–60

Age	1956–1960	1966–1970	1976–1979
30–34	100	80	53
35–39	100	97	70
40–44	100	133	98
45–49	100	149	151
50–54	100	166	205
55–59	100	165	222
60–64	100	154	244
65–69	100	170	251
70–74	100	159	230
75–79	100	150	226

Table 15. Trends in United States respiratory cancer deaths per billion packs smoked

Age	1955	1960	1965	1970	1975
35–39	12	14	19	20	19
40–44	23	28	34	46	45
45–49	52	52	61	73	85
50–54	90	97	102	118	130
55–59	139	152	160	183	186
60–64	201	220	225	249	270

[a]Data from Gerstein and Levison (32).

sharp postwar increase in consumption, which makes it more difficult to assess precisely what trends in lung cancer would have been expected in the absence of any changes in tar level per cigarette smoked. Nevertheless Doll and Peto (5) were able to show, fairly convincingly in my view, that the trends in lung cancer rates that have been seen in recent years are consistent with a benefit of tar reduction. This view recently has been challenged by a report from the United States National Research Council (32). In this report they present a table giving male trends in respiratory cancer rates divided by estimated number of lifetime packs smoked (Table 15) and observe that this adjusted rate has been increasing at all ages above 45 and has only started to level off in the youngest age groups.

Unfortunately, the analysis is seriously unsound for two reasons. First, duration of smoking only comes linearly into the correction, when it should enter as a fourth or fifth power. As noted before, in the absence of any changes in cigarettes, one would have expected to see a substantial increase in lung cancer death rate in the older age groups. In the youngest age groups this is not so serious a criticism because durations of smoking are similar in successive cohorts, but here the second objection is important, namely that the cigarette consumption data on which the estimates have been based are known not only to be inaccurate but also to have different inaccuracy in different years. Todd (33), in a study of national estimates of cigarette consumption from various countries, noted that for the 1955 and 1966 surveys it was necessary to multiply the reported cigarette consumption by 32% and 28%, respectively, to bring the figures into line with known sales totals, and noted that "errors of between 20% and 40% suggest some fundamental defect in this survey." For the 1970 and 1975 surveys, he noted that the correction factors needed were even higher, 52% and 56%, repectively, and indeed represented the largest understatements in any of the surveys he had studied in any country. He suggested that this was caused by asking for views on health questions before asking for questions on smoking habits. It is clear that adjustment for this differential bias would have reduced 1970 and 1975 data relatively to earlier years and suggested that an advantage of tar reduction really did exist.

Conclusion

Although it is of obvious importance to carry out further studies, both of epidemiology and of national trends, the data reviewed here suggest very strongly indeed that the switch to lower tar yield cigarettes has resulted in lower average tar intake by the smoker and consequently to substantially lower death rates from lung cancer. The reduction in death rates indicated so far may be considerably less than that which ultimately will occur with ever-reducing tar levels and with lower tar cigarettes having been smoked for an ever-increasing fraction of a smoker's lifetime.

References

1. U.S. Public Health Service. Smoking and health. A report of the Surgeon General of the Public Health Service. U.S. Department of Health and Human Services, Office on Smoking and Health. Washington, DC: U.S. Government Printing Office, 1979.
2. Wald N, Doll R, Copeland G. Trends in tar, nicotine and carbon monoxide yields of U.K. cigarettes manufactured since 1934. Br Med J 1981;282:763-5.
3. Todd GF. Changes in smoking patterns in the U.K. Tobacco Research Council Occasional Paper 1. London: Tobacco Research Council 1975.
4. Weber KH. Recent changes in tobacco products and their acceptance by the consumer. Proceedings of the Sixth International Tobacco Scientific Congress. Paris: Coresta 1976:15-30.
5. Doll R, Peto R. The causes of cancer: quantitative estimates of avoidable risks of cancer in the United States today. JNCI 1981;66:1193-308.
6. Doll R, Peto R. Mortality in relation to smoking: 20 years' observations on male British doctors. Br Med J 1976;2:1525-36.
7. Doll R, Peto R. Cigarette smoking and bronchial carcinoma: dose and time relationships among regular smokers and lifelong non-smokers. J Epidemiol Community Health 1978;32:86-96.
8. Wynder EL, Hoffman D. Tobacco and health: a societal challenge. New Engl J Med 1979;300:854-903.
9. Lee PN. Statistics of smoking in the United Kingdom. Tobacco Research Council Research Paper I, 7th ed. London: Tobacco Research Council 1976 and annual supplements.
10. Fairweather FA, Carmichael IA, Phillips GF. Changes in the tar, nicotine and carbon monoxide yields of cigarettes sold in the United Kingdom. Health Trends 1981;13:77-81.
11. Russell MAH, Jarvis M, Iyer R, Feyerabend C. Relation of nicotine yield of cigarettes in blood nicotine level of smokers. Br Med J 1980;280:972-6.
12. Stepney R. Consumption of cigarettes of reduced tar and nicotine delivery. Br J. Addiction 1980;75:81-8.
13. Garfinkel L. Changes in the cigarette consumption of smokers in relation to changes in tar/nicotine content of cigaretes smoked. Am J Public Health 1979;69:1274-6.
14. Wald NJ, Idle M, Boreham J, Bailey A. Inhaling habits among smokers of different types of cigarette. Thorax 1980;35:925-8.
15. Ashton M, Stepney R, Thompson JW. Self-titration by cigarette smokers. Br Med J 1979; 2:357-60.
16. Russell MAH, Sutton SR, Iyer R, Feyerabend C, Vesey CJ. Long term switching to low-tar lownicotine cigarettes. Br J Addiction 1982;77:145-8.
17. Stepney R. Would a medium-nicotine, low-tar cigarette be less hazardous to health? Br Med J. 1981;283:1292-6.
18. Kozlowski LT, Frecker RC, Lei H. Nicotine yields of cigarettes, plasma nicotine in smokers and public health. Prevent Med 1982;11:240-4.
19. Lee PN, Garfinkel L. Mortality and type of cigarette smoked. J Epidemiol Community Health 1981;35:16-22.
20. Hammond EC, Garfinkel L, Seidman H, Lew EA. 'Tar' and nicotine content of cigarette smoke in relation to death rates. Environ Res 1976;12:263-74.
21. Hawthorne VM, Fry JS. Smoking and health; cardiorespiratory disease, mortality and smoking behaviour in West Central Scotland. J Epidemiol Community Health 1978;32:260-6.
22. Reid DD. Studies of disease among migrants and native populations in Great Britain, Norway, and the United States. I. Background and Design. National Cancer Institute Monogr 19. Bethesda, MD: National Institutes of Health, 1966:287-99.
23. Dean G, Lee PN, Todd GF, Wicken AJ. Report on a second retrospective mortality study in North-East England. Part I: Factors related to mortality from lung cancer, bronchitis, heart

disease and stroke in Cleveland County, with particular emphasis on the relative risks associated with smoking filter and plain cigarettes. Tobacco Research Council Research Paper 14, Part I. London: Tobacco Research Council, 1977.

24. Bross IDJ, Gibson R. Risk of lung cancer in smokers who switch to filter cigarettes. Am J Public Health 1968;58:1396–1403.
25. Wynder EL, Mabuchi K, Beattie EJ. The epidemiology of lung cancer. Recent trends. JAMA 1970;213:2221–8.
26. Wynder EL, Stellman SD. The impact of long-term filter cigarette usage in lung and larynx cancer risk: a case-control study. JNCI 1979;62:471–7.
27. Rimington J. The effect of filters on the incidence of lung cancer in cigarette smokers. Environ Res 1981;24:162–6.
28. Kunze M, Vutuc C. Threshold of tar exposure: analysis of smoking history of male lung cancer cases and controls. In: Gori G, Bock F, eds. A safe cigarette? Banbury report 3. New York: Cold Spring Harbor Laboratory, 1980:29–6.
29. Auerbach O, Hammond EC, Garfinkel L. Changes in bronchial epithelium in relation to cigarette smoking 1955–1960 vs. 1970–1977. N Engl J Med 1979; 300:381–6.
30. Rigdon RH, Kirchoff H. Cancer of the lung from 1900 to 1930. Surg Gyn Obstet 1958;107:115–8.
31. Royal College of Physicians of London. Smoking *or* Health. Third Report. London: Pitman, 1977.
32. Gerstein DR, Levison PK, eds. Reduced tar and nicotine cigarettes: smoking behaviour and health. Committee on Substance Abuse and Habitual Behavior, Commission on Behavioral and Social Sciences and Education, National Research Council. Washington DC: National Academy Press 1982.
33. Todd GF. Cigarette consumption per adult of each sex in various countries. J Epidemiol Community Health 1978;32:289–93.

CHAPTER **23**

Smoking Cessation Programs and Lung Cancer Prevention

ELLEN R. GRITZ

Macomber-Murphy Cancer Prevention Program, Division of Cancer Control, Jonsson Comprehensive Cancer Center, University of California, Los Angeles, California 90024

ABSTRACT

For those who smoke cigarettes, cessation of smoking is the most important lifestyle change that can be made to prevent the incidence of lung cancer. A variety of modalities—including pharmacotherapy, behavior modification, education, and psychotherapy, alone or in combination—have been utilized in smoking cessation programs, with long-term success rates averaging 25–50%. Recent trends in smoking cessation research have focused upon (1) targeting high-risk populations, (2) techniques to ensure long-term maintenance of abstinence and prevention of relapse, (3) the development of self-help and mass media interventions to reach large audiences, and (4) the involvement of health care professionals (primarily physicians) in minimal smoking cessation interventions. The components of a successful smoking cessation program are reviewed and new developments in research and smoking control highlighted.
Key Words: **Smoking, lung cancer prevention, smoking cessation programs**

Introduction and Overview

The statistic that 85% of lung cancer cases are attributable to cigarette smoking provides a powerful challenge to those who work in cancer control (1). Indeed, the definition of primary cancer prevention as the "identification and control by appropriate interventions of those environmental and host factors that influence the occurrence of cancer and its progression to clinical disease" (2) finds its most outstanding application in this instance. For no other cancer site can the behavioral scientist or health professional produce such a potential impact on cancer incidence. My goal today is to offer a practical as well as theoretical overview of the state of the art in smoking cessation programs.

Smoking Prevalence

The public health movement has made a measurable and substantial impact on smoking prevalence in the United States, although 52.3 million adult Americans (32.6%) continue to use cigarettes. Adult male smoking has fallen from a prevalence of 51.1% in 1965 to 36.7% in 1980, and adult female smoking has changed from a prevalence of 33.3% in 1965 to 28.9% in 1980 (3, 4). While the decline in women's smoking may seem small, it is historically relevant that women only began to smoke in significant proportions after World War II, almost 30 years later than men. Their smoking prevalence has never equaled that of men, and the trends reflect a mix of changing patterns of initiation as well as cessation. For example, smoking among adolescent females now exceeds that of adolescent males, averaging 12.7% vs 10.7% across the age group 12–18 (5). However, there is cause for optimism regarding women's smoking cessation trends. Adult men and women smokers are now indistinguishable with respect to the probability of attempting to quit smoking and the likelihood of success, according to the 1980 U.S. Surgeon General's Report (3). Between 1978 and 1980, 1.8 million adults quit smoking, 60% of whom were women (4). A variety of interpersonal forces are aiding the public health movement in breaking down the earlier resistances of women to smoking cessation (3).

As a whole, 33 million adults have quit smoking, an estimated 95% of these by their own efforts. Approximately one-third of current smokers make a fairly serious attempt to quit smoking each year, and one-fifth of those who try report success, resulting in an annual temporary quit rate of about 6% (3). I say temporary because recidivism is not accounted for in that statistic, and recidivism takes a heavy toll on smokers. Some 41–47% of (more permanent) ex-smokers report having succeeded on their first try; only 25–30% report having made three or more unsuccessful attempts before the winning try (6, 7).

Smoking: A Complex Behavior

It is natural at this point to ask why people have so much trouble giving up smoking and abstaining permanently. The answer lies in the complex reinforcement system underlying tobacco use. Whereas teenagers take up smoking for a set of socially determined reasons (discussed in Chapter 17) the maintenance of the behavior has a strong pharmacologic component. Of the more than 3600 compounds present in tobacco smoke, nicotine is the most important alkaloid, comprising almost 95% of the total alkaloid content (1, 8, 9). Nicotine is carried on particles of tar (condensate) into the alveoli of the lungs and reaches the brain in less than 7.5 s via the arterial circulation (10). Many excellent reviews of the actions of nicotine summarize its organ system effects, including the autonomic nervous system, endocrine glands, voluntary musculature, gastrointestinal tract, cardiovascular system, and brain (10–13). The potential reinforcing effects of nicotine lie in its alteration of central nervous system arousal processes, both as stimulating and sedative-like changes, as well as various organ system effects such as the release of catecholamines from the adrenal medulla, the inhibition of gastric hunger contractions, and musculoskeletal relaxation (10, 14).

Regular use of tobacco leads to a dependence syndrome that has been described in the psychiatric nomenclature and in the behavioral literature (15–17). Tobacco dependence is characterized by compulsive use, tolerance to certain pharmacologic effects of nicotine, and, upon discontinuation, the occurrence of a withdrawal syndrome with both physiologic and psychological components (16, 17).

There are also complex social and habitual (conditioned) components of tobacco use that further contribute to difficulty in abandoning its use. Doses of nicotine delivered approximately 10 times per cigarette, 20 times a day, 365 days a year provide 73,000 opportunities for association with almost every cognitive, behavioral, and social act in the human repertoire. Some of the more important social and coping functions with which smoking commonly is associated are illustrated in Tables 1 and 2. The elements of conditioning embedded in these associations may be derived partially from the pharmacologic actions of nicotine temporally associated with given behaviors or from the sociocultural "benefits" attributed to smoking. The latter result from clever marketing by the tobacco industry and/or from long-held beliefs stemming from adolescent adulation of valued role models.

Table 1. Smoking as a coping mechanism

Stimulant for:	Fatigue, lethargy
	Depression
	Lack of concentration
Sedative for:	Anxiety, tension
	Anger
	Hostility
Time marker:	After meals
	As a "break"
Food related:	Depress appetite
	Substitute for eating

Table 2. Social factors in smoking

Peers	Shared habit
Media	Image of attractiveness
	Sexuality
	Slenderness
	Beauty
	Popularity
	Happiness
	Image of liberation, sophistication
	Image of social conformity
	Ignores:
	Wrinkles
	Osteoporosis, early menopause, etc
	Tobacco stains on teeth, fingers, clothes
	Extra cost
Family	Spouse smokes
Common situations	Legal drugs
	Coffee
	Alcohol
	Socializing
	Meals
	Parties

Smoking Cessation

Promoting permanent cessation of smoking often has been viewed with great pessimism, sometimes akin to despair, when recidivism curves depicting 70% relapse to smoking within 6 months after quitting are cited (18). These figures, derived from the treatment literature (and paralleled by results from studies in alcoholism and heroin addiction), present only one aspect of a complex scenario. The most important facet upon which to fix our gaze is the 33 million adults who have quit smoking, who represent 38% of those who have ever smoked. I consider that a remarkable proportion. The treatment literature data reflect only a single cross-sectional view of what is essentially a longitudinal process in a smoker's history. This process is understood in greater perspective from the consideration of national survey data cited earlier.

The determinants of relapse are complex and likely represent a combination of factors in any given case. First, dysphoric withdrawal symptoms and craving may play an especially prominent role in the period immediately following cessation. Second, certain environmental situations have been identified as high-risk triggers for relapse (19, 20). These precursors of relapse include social models and pressures to smoke, negative affect (feelings of frustration, anxiety, depression, anger), or stress in over 70% of cases. Such situations represent almost archetypal associations for smokers and are further linked to pharmacologic actions of nicotine [eg, the facilitation of smoking by alcohol, see Ref (21)]. Third, a "slip" or relapse may occur at almost any time when an especially strong stimulus formerly associated with smoking, such as a period of intense negative affect or powerful peer pressure, supercedes coping mechanisms developed to replace the alleged mood-modulating effects of cigarettes. At such times, a complex cognition known as the abstinence violation effect (AVE) may prompt a return to smoking (20). The AVE is a reaction to initial relapse consisting of self-attribution of insufficient skill to remain abstinent, feelings of depression or failure, and anticipated positive benefit from smoking. Studies of near and actual relapse also have revealed naturalistic cognitive and behavioral coping mechanisms used by smokers with and without success, suggesting leads for treatment strategies to prolong abstinence (19).

Smoking Cessation Programs

With this foundation I will now discuss critical advances in our concepts of smoking cessation programs: what they must evolve toward to meet the challenges of new research findings, how we must wisely allocate scarce resources, and how we may capitalize upon technological progress.

Components of Smoking Cessation Programs

Practitioners in smoking cessation have concentrated primarily on the techniques to achieve cessation and, more recently, to maintain abstinence. Yet models of smoking behavior have long taken into account a succession of stages through which a smoker must pass in the transition from confirmed smoker to confirmed quitter (22). Recently, the cyclical nature of such stages—immotive smoking (precontemplation), contemplation, decision, activity, and relapse—has been emphasized (23). Smoking cessation programs may have an important (and unmeasured) preliminary function of affecting motivation, thus moving the smoker from a preaction to an action phase. Special events such as the Great American Smokeout, sponsored annually by the American Cancer Society and accompanied by much print and viewing media publicity, seem to serve such trigger functions and even result in a small gain in permanent quitting (24). Other examples are provided by the release of the 1964 (and subsequent) U.S. Surgeon General's Reports, a strong personalized warning by a physician, or the death of a loved one from a smoking-related disease. The general persistence of the public health movement and growing antismoking societal attitude has had such a facilitatory effect in preventing the rise in smoking prevalence that might otherwise have occurred (25).

Once motivation has reached the level critical to action, effective smoking cessation programs usually have included a selection of techniques to assist quitting that have been discussed at length in many review articles (1, 3, 9, 26). These include: self-monitoring of smoking behaviors and urges, aversive methods of smoking meant to decrease the pleasurable sensory (reinforcing) component of smoking, a structure for quitting (cold turkey or gradual reduction), cognitive and behavioral techniques for dealing with urges to smoke and substitutions for smoking, positive reinforcement for not smoking, some form of social support from significant others or formally assigned buddies, stress management techniques, weight control, and preparation for withdrawal. The higher rates of success (approximately 50% abstinence) achieved by several formal treatment programs have been attributed to heavy doses of coping techniques aimed at preventing relapse, including such strategies as building reinforcement into the natural environment, the use of contingency contracts (tangible rewards for abstinence and punishments for recidivism), workplace-based programs, and self-reward (27–31). The Multiple Risk Factor Intervention Trial (MRFIT) utilized a particularly good example of a broadly based, multiple-technique smoking cessation program with a strong social support component that resulted in very high rates of abstinence (over 40%) at the 4-year evaluation (32).

I would like point out that no given set of elements has been identified as optimal, either for attaining cessation or for maintaining it, and we toss such packages at smokers with the general intent that they self-select the components that prove most efficacious for them as individuals. Such selection of techniques may even vary for a given individual from one quit attempt to another.

Delivery of Smoking Cessation Programs

The term "smoking cessation program" need not imply a single format. There is a continuum of program delivery ranging from the complete lack of direct involvement by any external figure (self-help manuals, audiovisual materials, broadcast media programs, informal personal groupings) to some minimal leadership involvement (simple advice to quit from a health professional) to intense direction (large or small group clinics, individual treatment). In our search for cost-effective delivery of programming, increasingly greater emphasis is being placed on the development of effective interventions requiring minimal or no leadership, and on taking advantage of naturally occurring opportunities to promote cessation, such as routine visits to health care professionals. More will be said about this in the section entitled *The Role of The Physician.*

Modalities: The Promise of the Future

Instead of reviewing existing modalities of smoking cessation programs I am going to intrigue you with what appear to be the most exciting possibilities for advances and applications.

Targeting High-Risk Populations

Certain smokers are at elevated risk of premature mortality and excess morbidity. Because it clearly is impossible to reach all smokers with intensive programs, one strategy is to concentrate resources on reaching those persons who we know to be at greatest risk for adverse health consequences (of which lung cancer is only one). At the November 1981 National Conference on Smoking *OR* Health, three important subgroups of high-risk smokers were identified, and a number of recommendations were set forth, several of which I will cite (33). The first subgroup consists of smokers with coexisting medical conditions that either are exacerbated by smoking, interact with cigarette smoking to raise mortality and morbidity rates, or pose special risks to smokers. In this category are pulmonary diseases, coronary heart disease, peripheral arterial disease, peptic ulcer, cancers considered related to smoking, alcoholism-associated diseases, and familial history of smoking-related diseases. Pregnancy also is included in this list because of the increased risk of serious complications to the fetus among women who smoke.

Smokers with environmental exposure to certain substances fall into the second category of high risk. Certain occupational exposures discussed at length in this volume pose known hazards. With regard to lung cancer, asbestos has received the greatest attention in the past few years.

Finally, certain lifestyle factors may predispose to high risk. Smokers who have a higher cumulative smoke dose (determined by age of initiation, number of years smoked, T/N content of cigarette, number of cigarettes smoked daily, and intensity of puffing) are at greater risk of developing smoking-related diseases. Those who work in occupations where smoking is prevalent as well as those with certain substance abuse disorders (opiate addiction, alcoholism, polydrug use) are also less likely to give up smoking. Smoking is also relatively more prevalent among blue collar workers, certain segments of minority populations, and persons in the lower socioeconomic strata.

Recommendations were made to formulate and encourage the adoption of standards of practice for dealing with smokers at high risk in the first two subgroups. Such standards of practice would be distributed to health professionals and relevant industrial professionals with emphasis on the duty to inform, as well as on the duty to understand and act on the part of targeted individuals. Consonant with the latter responsibility was a third goal to develop procedures for self-assessment of high-risk smoking that would be widely distributed. Educating health professionals, patients, and other persons at high risk, as well as providing the resources for assisting in permanent smoking cessation are, of course, concomitant and critical activities. A substantial amount of work already has occurred on turning these conceptual goals into concrete realities.

Reaching Large Audiences

The continual evaluation of scarcity of financial and human resources and the emphasis on needing to reach populations, not clinic-sized groups, with our smoking cessation aids has led to serious attempts to utilize our communications technology effectively. This is especially salient in view of the evidence that most smokers express a preference for quitting on their own, without formal aid (1). Experimentation with televised smoking cessation programs (34–38), manuals published by voluntary health organizations such as the American Cancer Society and the American Lung Association (39, 40), and manuals published by behavioral experts in smoking cessation (41, 42) have been most promising. Evaluations of written materials show 5–20% abstinence at long-term followup. Evaluations of televised programs yield highly variable outcome estimates, which is not unexpected because of the heterogeneity of sampled participants, and the lack of standardization of format, geographic locale, materials, and airing time. However, as previously pointed out, these community- and nation-wide programs may serve a motivational function impelling smokers into a greater readiness to quit, which is much more difficult to assess than how many actually quit after viewing. Intriguing interventions that combine school-based prevention curricula with network television programming aimed at smoking parents of participating children represent other avenues of facilitating intentional or behavior change (43). We have only begun to explore the power of the mass media in this aspect of health promotion.

The Role of the Physician

In our attempts to mobilize powerful segments of our health care professions to promote attitudinal and behavioral change in smokers, new light has been focused on physicians. For many years, the physician's role in this task was unguided and largely thankless. Griffiths has commented that the discouragement of physicians with their rate of success in helping patients stop smoking rather should be compared favorably to their rate of success in curing lung cancer, which is much lower (44). Moreover, I would add, the latter cure is at much greater cost to patient, society, and perhaps even physician. Reviews of the literature on physician advice to quit smoking in the areas of general practice, obstetrics, pulmonary, and cardiovascular disease generally show a positive relationship between severity of disease and likelihood of quitting smoking (3, 25, 45, 46). This finding may be attributable to greater physician involvement with the more severely ill patient and greater salience of message (46), but the power of such a "teachable moment" should not be undervalued.

The efforts of general practice physicians to provide minimal interventions to all smoking patients in the course of routine care is now receiving greater attention.

For example, a study conducted in England involving 28 physicians and over 2000 patients reported a 3–5% abstinence rate at 1-year followup among patients given a 1–2 min message (some with other materials), compared to 0.3% in nonintervention controls (47). The major effect of the physician advice in this study was to increase motivation in terms of the percentage of patients attempting to quit, and to reduce relapse. The variability in obtained success rates among participating physicians has led investigators in this country to develp protocols to guide physicians in their efforts (48). Communication skills generally not taught in our medical schools do need to be improved among physicians practicing health education with patients (44). A five-stage model of helping roles offers separable or unified guidance for the physician: (1) serving as a nonsmoking, healthy lifestyle role model; (2) providing information on smoking risks and the health benefits of cessation; (3) suggesting quitting by direct advice; (4) offering a referral network for smoking cessation resources; and (5) prescribing and following up on the use of specific cessation and maintenance strategies (45).

Although pharmacologic aids to smoking cessation have been discouragingly unsuccessful in placebo-controlled trials in the past (49), promising results have emerged from the testing of a chewing gum containing nicotine in a buffered ion-exchange resin (50–53). Developed in Europe, this gum will be available to physicians to dispense by prescription in the United States this year. The rationale for the gum is that it provides a noncigarette based source of nicotine so that the smoker may separate the behavioral components of cigarette smoking cessation from nicotine withdrawal. Under physician guidance, the gum can be used for periods up to several months and then discontinued. Plasma nicotine levels produced by hourly chewing of the stronger dosage level of the gum (4 mg) are comparable to those reached with hourly smoking, although the pharmacologic impact of the inhalation route may differ substantially from the oral route, and side effects (dizziness, oral soreness, nausea, stomach ache, hiccups) do occur, although these are often temporary (54, 55). To date, controlled research has demonstrated higher abstinence rates in groups of subjects treated with nicotine gum compared to placebo (50, 52, 53), although these differential effects sometimes vanish by the 1-year followup point (53). Estimation of followup abstinence rates is calculated from initiation of treatment, not from cessation of gum chewing (highly variable), further complicating traditional evaluation concepts. A final, and perhaps most serious problem with the gum studies published up to the present is that some form of behavioral or psychological treatment almost inevitably accompanies the pharmacologic product. Therefore, the majority of smokers may be unable to benefit from pure nicotine pharmacotherapy without additional behavioral instruction, a not too surprising conclusion in light of earlier discussion on the need for coping techniques to maintain abstinence after successful cessation has occurred.

As the leading and most credible figure in the health care world, the physician should be involved in smoking cessation efforts. After all, physicians as a profession have been phenomenally successful in quitting smoking, declining from a prevalence of about 50% in 1950 to about 10% (in California) in 1980 (56). One study showed that smoking physicians feel less comfortable dispensing advice to their patients to quit smoking and, consequently, do so less forcefully (57). However, a sustained effort to provide physicians (and other health care professionals) with effective interventional materials has produced the American Cancer Society's *Physician's Help Quit Kit* and the National Cancer Institute's *Helping Smokers Quit Kit* (57, 58). Given the importance of smoking as the most potent, preventable source of lung cancer, there is no longer an excuse for physicians to leave this effort primarily to other health care professionals.

Conclusion

To summarize, the next generation of smoking cessation programs will focus on developing cost-effective self-help materials with an emphasis on maintenance of abstinence, on targeting and intervening with high-risk segments of the smoking population, on improving our means of reaching population-sized audiences through mass media technology, and on meaningfully involving physicians as agents of smoking change. The particular role the physician can play is broadly defined, depending on interest, time, and self-perceived skill. An alliance of physician and behavioral scientists is needed to define gaps in the physician's understanding of pharmacologic and behavioral components of smoking and smoking cessation, to develop a continuum of helping modes, to illumine physician–patient communication processes, and to optimize presentation formats.

Any conclusions regarding the relative success or failure of lung cancer prevention efforts to reduce smoking prevalence in the general population must simultaneously take into consideration a number of powerful trends. Smoking is becoming less prevalent among adults in this country, but no one individual or societal force can be credited with this outcome. The persistent educational and interventional efforts of the public health movement and branches of our state and national governments, the patient methodologic research and clinical applications of behavioral scientists, the growing availability of commercial programs, the progressive building of an antismoking and smoking control legislative base, and the new increases in taxation all play a role. A child born today will be less likely to smoke for all of these reasons. There are, of course, powerful adverse societal, economic, and intraindividual forces that work to prolong and promote the self-destructive behavior of tobacco use, but such forces are being opposed. The change in lifestyle defined as smoking cessation will result in an eventual decline in lung cancer incidence and mortality.

Acknowledgments

This effort was supported by U.S. Public Health Service Grant Number CA23974 awarded by the National Cancer Institute, Department of Health and Human Services.

References

1. U.S. Department of Health and Human Services. The health consequences of smoking: a report of the surgeon general. Rockville, MD: Department of Health and Human Services, Public Health Service, Office on Smoking and Health, 1982:50179.
2. Newell GR. Overview of cancer prevention. Cancer Bull 1980;32:128–9.
3. U.S. Department of Health and Human Services. The health consequences of smoking for women: a report of the surgeon general. Rockville, MD: Department of Health and Human Services, Public Health Service, Office on Smoking and Health, 1980.
4. U.S. Department of Health and Human Services. National Health Interview Survey. In: Smoking and Health Bulletin. Rockville, MD: Department of Health and Human Services, Public Health Service, Office on Smoking and Health, 1981:50156.
5. National Institute of Education. Teenage smoking: immediate and longterm patterns. Rockville, MD: National Institute of Education, Department of Health, Education, and Welfare, 1979.
6. U.S. Department of Health, Education, and Welfare. Adult use of tobacco—1975. Rockville, MD: U.S. Department of Health, Education and Welfare, Public Health Service, National Institutes of Health-National Cancer Institute, 1976.
7. Schachter S. Recidivism and self-cure of smoking and obesity. Am Psychol 1982;37:436–44.
8. Gorrod JW, Jenner P. The metabolism of tobacco alkaloids. In: Hayes WJ Jr, ed, Essays in toxicology, Vol 6. New York: Academic Press, 1975:35–78.
9. U.S. Department of Health, Education and Welfare. Smoking and health: a report of the surgeon general. DHEW Publ (PHS) 79-50066. Rockville, MD: Department of Health, Education and Welfare, Public Health Service, Office of the Assistant Secretary for Health, Office on Smoking and Health, 1979.
10. Russell MAH. Tobacco smoking and nicotine dependence. In: Israel Y, Kalant H, Popham RE, Schmidt W, Smart RG, eds, Research advances in alcohol and drug problems, Vol 3. New York: John Wiley and Sons, 1976:1–47.
11. Jarvik ME. The role of nicotine in the smoking habit. In: Hunt WA, ed, Learning mechanisms in smoking. Chicago: Aldine, 1970:155–90.
12. Larson PS, Silvette H. Tobacco—experimental and clinical studies, supplement III. Baltimore: Williams and Wilkins, 1975.
13. Taylor P. Ganglionic stimulating and blocking agents. In: Gilman AG, Goodman LS, Gilman A, eds, The pharmacological basis of therapeutics, 6th ed. New York: Macmillan, 1981:211–9.
14. Ashton J, Marsh JR, Millman JE, Rawlins MD, Telford R, Thompson JW. The use of event-related slow potentials of the brain as a means to analyze the effects of cigarette smoking and nicotine in humans. In: Thornton RE, ed, Smoking behaviour. Edinburgh: Churchill Livingstone, 1978:54–68.
15. American Psychiatric Association. Diagnostic and statistical manual of mental disorders (DSM-III), 3rd ed. Washington, DC: APA, 1980.
16. Krasnegor NA, ed. The behavioral aspects of smoking. NIDA Research Monogr 26. Rockville, MD: U.S. Department of Health, Education and Welfare, Department of Health, Education, and Welfare, Public Health Service. Alcohol, Drug Abuse, and Mental Health Administration, National Institute on Drug Abuse, 1979.
17. Krasnegor NA, ed. Cigarette smoking as a dependence process. NIDA Research Monograph 23. Rockville, MD: U.S. Department of Health, Education and Welfare, Department of Health, Education, and Welfare, Public Health Service, Alcohol, Drug Abuse, and Mental Health Administration, National Institute on Drug Abuse, 1979.
18. Hunt WA, Matarazzo JD. Three years later: recent developments in the experimental modification of smoking behavior. J Abnorm Psychol 1973;81:107–14.
19. Shiffman S. Relapse following smoking cessation: a situational analysis. J Consult Clin Psychol 1982;50:71–86.
20. Marlatt GA, Gordon JR. Determinants of relapse: implications for the maintenance of behavior change. In: Davidson PO, Davidson SM, eds, Behavioral medicine: changing health lifestyles. New York: Brunner/Mazel, 1980:410–52.
21 Griffiths RR, Bigelow GE, Liebson I. Facilitation of human tobacco self-administration by ethanol: a behavioral analysis. J Exp Anal Behav 1976;25:279–92.
22. Horn D. A model for the study of personal choice health behavior. Int J Health Educ 1976;19(2):89–98.

23. Prochaska JO, DiClemente CC. Stages and processes of self-change of smoking: toward an integrative model of change. J Consult Clin Psychol, 1983;51(3):390–5.
24. American Cancer Society. A study of the impact of the 1980 Great American Smokeout, summary report. A national program sponsored by the Gallup Organization, Inc, and analyzed by Lieberman Research Inc. Washington, DC: ACS, January 1981:1–7.
25. Warner KE, Murt HA. Impact of the antismoking campaign on smoking prevalence: a cohort analysis. J Public Health Pol 1982;3(4):374–90.
26. Lichtenstein E. The smoking problem: a behavioral perspective. J Consult Clin Psychol 1982; 50(6):804–19.
27. Fisher EG Jr, Lowe MR, Levenkron JD, Newman A. Structured support and reinforcement of maintained risk reduction. In: Stuart R, ed, Adherence, generalization, and maintenance in behavioral medicine. New York: Brunner/Mazel, 1982.
28. Paxton R. The effects of a deposit contract as a component in a behavioral programme for stopping smoking. Behav Res Ther 1980;18:45–50.
29. Powell DR, McCann BS. The effects of a multiple treatment program and maintenance procedures on smoking cessation. Prevent Med 1981;10:95–104.
30. Lando JA. Successful treatment of smokers with a broad-spectrum behavioral approach. J Consult Clin Psychol 1977;45:361–6.
31. Rosen GM, Lichtenstein E. An employee incentive program to reduce cigarette smoking. J Consult Psychol 1977;45:957.
32. Hughes GH, Hymowitz N, Ockene JK, Simon N, Vogt TM. The multiple risk factor intervention trial (MRFIT): V. Intervention on smoking. Prevent Med 1981;10:476–500.
33. American Cancer Society. National Conference on Smoking *OR* Health, Proceedings. New York: ACS, 1981.
34. Best JA. Mass media, self-management, and smoking modification. In: Davidson PO, Davidson SM, eds, Behavioral medicine: changing health lifestyles. New York: Brunner/Mazel, 1980: 371–90.
35. Dubren R. Evaluation of a televised stop-smoking clinic. Public Health Rep 1977;92:81–4.
36. Dubren R. Self-reinforcement by recorded telephone messages to maintain nonsmoking behavior. J Consult Clin Psychol 1977;45:358–60.
37. McAlister A, Puska P, Koskela I, Pallonen U, Maccoby N. Mass communication and community organization for public health education. Am Psychol 1980;35(4):375–9.
38. Pechacek TF, McAlister AL. Strategies for the modification of smoking behavior: treatment and prevention. In: Ferguson JM, Taylor CB, eds, The comprehensive handbook of behavioral medicine, Vol 3. Extended applications and issues. New York: Spectrum Publications, 1980: 257–98.
39. American Cancer Society. The impact of providing physicians with quitsmoking materials for smoking patients. CA 1981;31:75–8.
40. Davis AL, Faust R, Ordentlich M. Self-help smoking cessation and maintenance programs: a comparative study with 12-month followup by the American Lung Association. Unpublished manuscript, 1982.
41. Danaher BG, Lichtenstein E. Become an exsmoker. Englewood Cliffs, NJ: Prentice-Hall, 1978.
42. Pomerleau OF, Pomerleau CS. Break the smoking habit: a behavioral program for giving up cigarettes. Champaign, IL: Research Press, 1977.
43. Flay BR, Johnson CA, Hansen WB. The USC/KABC-TV smoking prevention/cessation program: preliminary short-term results. Unpublished manuscript, 1982.
44. Griffiths W. Can human behavior be modified? Cancer 1981;47:1221–5.
45. Lichtenstein E, Danaher BG. What can the physician do to assist the patient to stop smoking? In: Brashear RE, Rhodes ML, eds, Chronic obstructive lung disease: clinical treatment and management. St. Louis, MO: C.V. Mosby, 1978:227–41.
46. Pederson LL. Compliance with physician advice to quit smoking: a review of the literature. Prevent Med 1982;11:71–84.
47. Russell MAH, Wilson C, Taylor C, Baker CD. Effect of general practitioners' advice against smoking. Br Med J 1979;2:231–5.
48. Ewart K, Li VC, Coates TJ. Increasing physicians' anti-smoking influence by applying an inexpensive feedback technique. J Med Educ 1983; 8:468–73.
49. Gritz ER, Jarvik ME. Pharmacological aids for the cessation of smoking. In: Steinfeld J, Griffiths W, Ball K, Taylor R, eds, Proceedings of the Third World Conference on Smoking and Health. DHEW Publ (NIH) 77-1413. Washington, DC: U.S. Department of Health, Education and Welfare. Public Health Service, 1977;575–91.

50. Raw M, Jarvis MJ, Russell MAH. Comparison of nicotine chewing-gum and psychological treatments for dependent smokers. Br Med J 1980;281:481–2.
51. Russell MAH, Raw M, Jarvis MJ. Clinical use of nicotine chewing-gum. Br Med J 1980;280:1599–602.
52. Jarvis MJ, Raw M, Russell MAH, Feyerabend C. Randomised controlled trial of nicotine chewing-gum. Br Med J 1980;285:537–40.
53. Fagerstrom K-O. A comparison of psychological and pharmacological treatment in smoking cessation. J Behav Med 1982;5:343–51.
54. McNabb ME, Ebert RV, McCusker K. Plasma nicotine levels produced by chewing nicotine gum. JAMA 1982;248:865–8.
55. Armitage AK. The role of nicotine in the tobacco smoking habit. In: Thornton RE, ed, Smoking behaviour. Edinburgh: Churchill Livingstone, 1978:229–59.
56. Enstrom JE. Smoking cessation and mortality trends among California physicians. Br Med J 1983;286:1101–5.
57. American Cancer Society. I Quit Kit. Publ 2028: New York: ACS 1977.
58. U.S. Department of Health and Human Services. Calling it quits. DHHS Publ (NIH) 79-1824. Rockville, MD: Department of Health and Human Services, Public Health Service, National Institutes of Health, 1979.

CHAPTER **24**

Cancer Prevention and the Smoking, Tobacco, and Cancer Program of the National Cancer Institute

JOSEPH W. CULLEN

[a]Division of Resources, Centers, and Community Activities, National Cancer Institute, National Institutes of Health, Bethesda, Maryland 20205

ABSTRACT

The National Cancer Institute (NCI) has a multifaceted cancer prevention program. It spans a continuum of research activities seeking to elucidate the mechanisms of cancer induction at each step of the cellular process from initiation to transformation of normal cells to malignant cells. The program carries out studies in toxicology, epidemiology, pharmacology, education, behavior change, and information dissemination. With the advent of its newest division, the Division of Resources, Centers, and Community Activities (DRCCA), more emphasis is now being placed on applied prevention and interventions in defined populations. In the area of smoking prevention and cessation research, particular emphasis is being placed on adolescent prevention, the role of physicians as interveners, the use of the media, issues for black and Hispanic populations, and the value of self-help strategies. This chapter provides an overview of NCI prevention activities, stressing particularly new program initiatives in smoking tobacco-related research.

Key Words: **Smoking, interventions, cancer, population studies**

The National Cancer Institute (NCI) is one element in a complex of bureaus, institutes, and divisions housed within the National Institutes of Health. The NCI is actually the largest element within this complex. It is a bureau and has an operating budget of slightly under $1 billion for fiscal year 1983. Figure 1 depicts

[a]Division renamed November 25, 1983, to the Division of Cancer Prevention and Control.

Lung Cancer: Causes and Prevention.

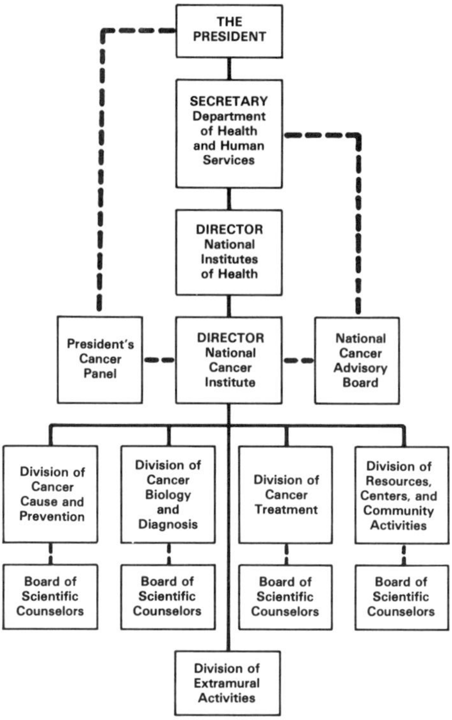

Figure 1. NCI organization and advisory structure.

its organizational structure, including those operating units related to cancer prevention.

The Division of Cancer Cause and Prevention

Essentially two of NCI's five divisions are dedicated to the prevention of cancer. The first established of these divisions is the Division of Cancer Cause and Prevention (DCCP). That division is responsible for planning and conducting the Institutes's program of coordinated research on cancer causation and prevention. The DCCP supports both intramural laboratories and extramural programs that seek to elucidate the mechanisms of cancer induction at each step of the cellular process from initiation to transformation of normal cells to malignant cells. Investigators pursue fundamental studies on chemicals, viruses, and physical agents using the disciplines of cellular and molecular biology, immunology, biochemistry, chemistry, and microbiology as well as epidemiologic studies of human populations to identify risk factors predisposing to various cancers. (On November 25, 1983, the DCCP became known as the Division of Cancer Etiology.)

The overall purpose of these studies is to provide information for preventing, interrupting, or reversing the initiated or transformed cell prior to the development of clinical disease. Figure 2 outlines DCCP's organizational elements.

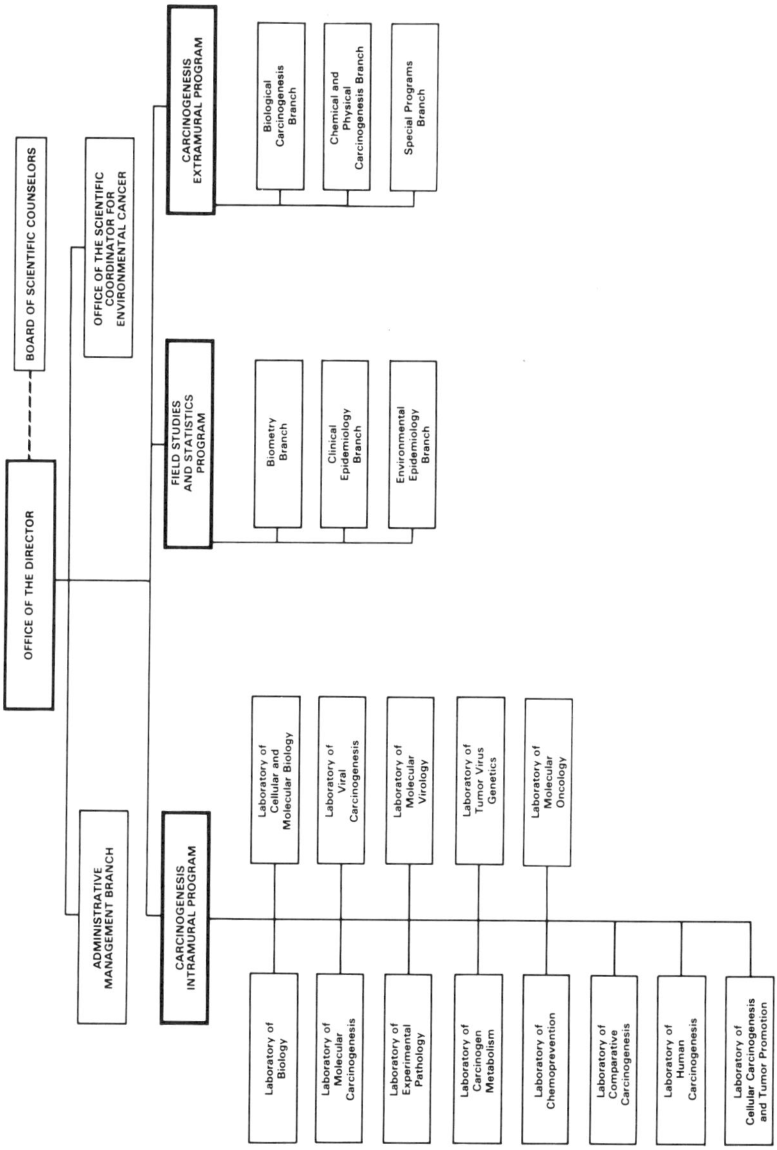

Figure 2. Division of Cancer Cause and Prevention.

The Field Studies and Statistics Program (soon to be renamed the Epidemiology and Biometry Program) (1) plans, directs, coordinates, and evaluates intra- and extramural programs of epidemiologic, statistical, and mathematical research and automatic data processing services for all NCI research programs; (2) establishes program priorities, allocates resources, integrates the projects of various branches, evaluates program effectiveness, and represents program area in management and scientific decision-making meetings within the Institute; (3) through intramural and contract activities, administers research in biometry and epidemiology and the development of mathematical models and statistical methodology; and (4) advises the director of the division and supports the activities of the National Cancer Advisory Board and other scientific advisory committees. The Biometry Branch is responsible for the Surveillance, Epidemiology, and End Results (SEER) Program, which measures the cancer incidence, mortality, and patient survival through a series of population-based registries. This branch also develops various models for a variety of laboratory experiments and conducts analytical studies of suspected factors associated with the risk of developing cancer. The Clinical Epidemiology Branch develops new concepts about cancer etiology from bedside observations of cancer patients, conducts studies of the late effects of childhood cancer, and operates a clinic dealing with the genetics of human cancer. The Environmental Epidemiology Branch consists of several sections concerned with occupational studies to help identify chemical and physical carcinogens; epidemiologic studies to clarify the role of dietary fat, fiber, micronutrients and other nutritional factors; and case control studies of particular cancers to pursue key etiologic leads, as well as demographic and geographic surveys of cancer mortality and incidence in the United States.

The Carcinogenesis Intramural Program plans, implements, and administers the Institute's program of general laboratory research on cancer causation by chemical, physical, and biologic (viral) factors, and on the pathogenesis and prevention of various cancers. The program is comprised of 13 laboratories, four of which have been fully operational for less than 2 years. In the Laboratory of Human Carcinogensis, which carries out biochemical epidemiology studies, laboratory workers identify carcinogen–DNA adducts in human specimens using monoclonal antibodies to the carcinogen-damaged DNA and study the metabolic balance between activation and deactivation of various chemical carcinogens. The Laboratory of Cellular Carcinogenesis and Tumor Promotion studies the role of tumor promoters and their effects on epithelial cells. The Laboratory of Comparative Carcinogenesis is involved in comparative studies of initiation and promotion and mechnisms of action of genotoxic and nongenotoxic carcinogens. The Laboratory of Molecular Oncology is involved in studies on genetic elements required for malignant transformation.

The Carcinogenesis Extramural Program contains three principal elements: the Biological Carcinogenesis Branch is concerned with biologic factors as possible etiologic factors or cofactors in cancer and their control and the management of extramural resource contracts for biologic products; the Chemical and Physical Carcinogenesis Branch maintains an extramural research program on chemical and physical carcinogenesis and maintains resource contracts providing primarily chemical carcinogens and their metabolites and retinoids; the Special Programs Branch consists of an extramural basic and applied research program in biometry, epidemiology, nutrition, and smoking and health.

The Division of Resources, Centers, and Community Activities

The second of the two prevention-oriented divisions within NCI is the Division of Resources, Centers, and Community Activities (DRCCA). This division was renamed on November 25, 1983, to the Division of Cancer Prevention and Control (DCPC).

In Figure 3 the organization and program units of DRCCA are highlighted according to its three program areas: Cancer Control Science, Centers and Community Oncology, and Prevention. This division houses the congressionally mandated cancer control program. Therefore, most of its organizational units are dedicated to reducing cancer incidence, morbidity, and mortality.

The mission of this division is quite broad given the multicomplex of programmatic elements within it. The division (1) plans and conducts basic and applied research and development, technology transfer, demonstration, education, and

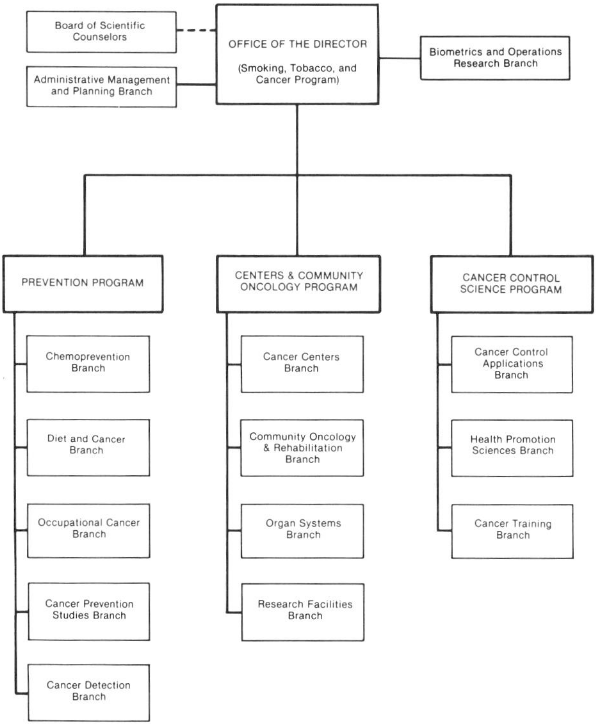

Figure 3. Division of Resources, Centers, and Community Activities.

information dissemination programs to expedite the use of new information relevant to the prevention, detection, and diagnosis of cancer care of cancer patients throughout the country; (2) plans, directs, and coordinates the support of research on cancer prevention and control at cancer centers, community hospitals, and through organ systems programs; (3) supports cancer research training, clinical education, continuing education and career development in cancer prevention and control; (4) administers programs for the support of construction, alteration, renovation, and equipping of extramural research facilities; and (5) coordinates program activities with other divisions, institutes, or federal and state agencies and establishes liaison with professional and voluntary health agencies, cancer centers, labor organizations, cancer organizations, and trade associations.

Programmatically within the division the Cancer Control Science Program develops, supports, and monitors applied research directed toward facilitating the widespread use of proved health promotion and other cancer prevention and management techniques by health professionals, patients and their families, and the general public; monitors basic and clinical research activities to identify new interventions to reduce cancer rates in populations, and facilitates research on their application; provides training opportunities for health professionals in order to create a national cadre of highly skilled individuals capable of identifying, researching, and/or applying cancer prevention and management interventions; establishes program priorities, allocates resources, integrates the projects of the various branches, evaluates program effectiveness and represents the program area in management and scientific decision-making meetings within the Institute; and provides programmatic and consultative support to other divisional, institute, governmental, and private sector organizations that facilitate the application of proved cancer control interventions in populations.

The Centers and Community Oncology Program plans, directs, coordinates, and evaluates the application of successful research advances and practical cancer control interventions in the general population; establishes program priorities, allocates resources, integrates the projects of the various branches, evaluates program effectiveness and represents the program area in management and scientific decision-making meetings within the Institute. Through the extramural funding of specialized and/or broad multidisciplinary centers devoted to basic and/or clinical research, this program advances the knowledge and understanding of the causes, mechanisms, diagnoses, and treatment of cancer; supports or administers an extramural research program aimed at promoting knowledge, technology, and information on cancer patient treatment and continuing care toward improving cancer patient management in community settings; and assists the extramural research efforts through support of the improvement, renovation, and construction of research facilities.

The Prevention Program plans and conducts intramural and extramural research programs directed toward the development, evaluation, demonstration, and promotion of cancer prevention, detection, and diagnosis. This research includes but is not limited to the identification of persons at increased risk of cancer, methods of screening and detection of cancer, and intervention aimed at reducing cancer risk, dietary manipulation, or administration of agents that may inhibit aspects of the carcinogenic process; identifies and disseminates new research findings that are of importance for prevention, early detection, or diagnosis of cancer; and establishes program priorities, allocates resources, integrates the projects of the various branches, evaluates program effectiveness, and represents the program area in management and scientific decision-making meetings within the Institute.

Figure 4 depicts the process of cancer control schematically. The emphasis in cancer control is placed on human interventions in defined populations. This emphasis is necessary because of NCI's congressional mandate to guarantee that the fruits of basic and laboratory studies are systematically evaluated on an ongoing basis for the applicability of the research results for the public health and cancer control. It is the purpose of DRCCA to provide that linkage, the bridge (some refer to it as technology transfer) between basic science and health care. The process is not a magical one. It pursues, as does any scientific method, an orderly sequence of systematic investigation from hypothesis development to controlled testing and evaluation. Cancer control is defined as "the reduction of cancer incidence, morbidity, and mortality through an orderly sequence from research on interventions and their impact in defined populations to the broad systematic application of the research results."

The thrust of the program is to move promising basic research findings through the cancer control phases from the most basic of these phases, the generation of hypotheses (I); through the development and testing of methods to carry out cancer control research as well as measure its impact (II); through controlled trials to establish efficacy and cause and effect relationships (III); to the implementation of the controlled trial methodologies in defined populations where the characteristics of the populations studied are homogeneous enough from which to generalize to large target populations and where denominators of the outcomes in question, particularly cancer incidence, morbidity, and mortality are known rates (IV), and ultimately to the demonstration of the research results in target populations (V). During the conduct of carrying out this logical sequence of activities, it is often necessary to return to earlier phases to fill in research gaps related to the cancer control progress [eg, whereas thousands of case-controlled

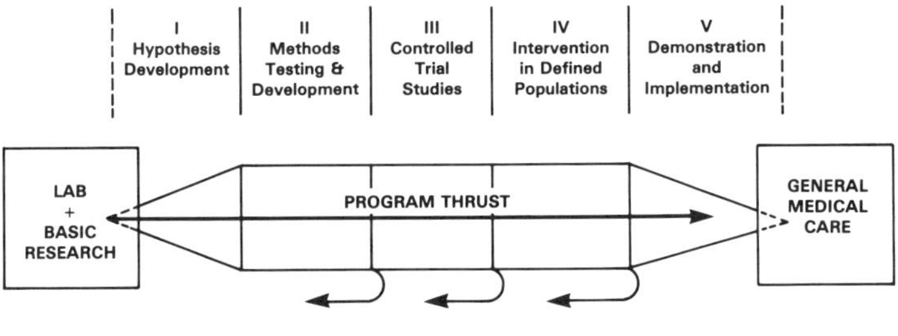

Figure 4. Cancer control science research logic.

studies have linked cigarette smoking with cancer (phase III), only a few studies establishing efficacy through controlled trials are available to produce satisfactory reductions in smoking behavior]. Further hypothesis testing and methods development are required to achieve that end more effectively. (For a more complete description of the cancer control phases see Ref 1).

The Smoking, Tobacco, and Cancer Program

The NCI's Smoking, Tobacco, and Cancer Program (STCP) spans a broad spectrum of scientific inquiry and applications from basic and laboratory research, epidemiology studies, to the prevention and control of smoking and the use of tobacco through interventions and educational demonstrations. More specifically, in this spectrum there are toxicologic studies to determine the promoting and carcinogenic effects of constituents in both the particulate and the gaseous phases of cigarettes; biologic studies to identify individuals at unusually high risk for the development of smoking-related cancers; epidemiologic studies to assess health effects attributable to changing smoking and tobacco habits; biobehavioral studies aimed at understanding dependence on smoking and tobacco use; controlled sociobehavioral trials and interventions in defined populations; and finally demonstrational programs using informational and educational techniques aimed at the professional and lay publics.

Figure 5 depicts the basic program model utilized by NCI in the STCP. Both prevention and cessation are end points with laboratory, epidemiology, and human intervention studies integral to both.

Laboratory and Epidemiology Research

The basic laboratory and epidemiology research components of STCP are carried out through DCCP. Current research in these categories includes the following:

Evaluation of Short-Term Bioassays for Carcinogens as Desirable Adjuncts to Lengthy Mouse Skin Painting Procedures.

The sebaceous gland supression test was found to be a valuable screening technique. Recently, the development of an inbred Syrian golden hamster model promises a new skin bioassay that is sensitive and reproducible. These animals already have shown a sensitivity to laryngeal cancer through exposure to inhaled

NCI SMOKING, TOBACCO, AND CANCER PROGRAM	
Prevention	Laboratory
	Human Intervention
	Epidemiology
Cessation	Laboratory
	Human Intervention
	Epidemiology

Figure 5. Basic program model.

tobacco smoke. This model offers the possibility of a sensitive, rapid, and reproducible skin bioassay system that may be applicable to other suspected carcinogens as well as tobacco smoke condensate.

Research Identifying Carcinogens in Cigarette Smoke.

A reproducible gas chromatography–thermal energy analyzer (GC–TEA) method has been developed and, to date, four tobacco-specific *N'*-nitrosamines have been identified. These are *N'*-nitrosonornicotine (NNN), 4-(methylnitrosamino)-1-(3-pyridyl)-1-butanone (NNK), *N*-nitrosoanatabine (NAT), and *N'*-nitrosoanabasine (NAB). Three of these, NNN, NNK, and NAB, induce benign and malignant tumors of the respiratory tracts of mice and rats. It has been shown that NNN and NNK induce tumors in the upper respiratory tracts of hamsters and that NNK is the most active of the tobacco-specific nitrosamines that also include adenoma and adenocarcinoma of the lung in hamsters.

The same method was used for the quantitative determination of *N*-nitrosodiethanolamine (NDELA) in tobacco, tobacco smoke, and chewing tobaccos. The biologic activity of NDELA was determined in Syrian golden hamsters by skin painting, swabbing of the oral cavity, and subcutaneous injection. Independently of the form of application, NDELA induced carcinomas of the nasal cavity, papillomas of the trachea, and tumors of the larynx in some animals. The higher tumor yield induced by painting the oral cavity, compared to the yield induced by skin painting, indicates that NDELA uptake through the oral cavity in hamsters is greater than intake through the skin. Present evidence indicates that diethanolamine is a major precursor for NDELA in tobacco and tobacco smoke. Diethanolamine is used as a solubilizer for maleic hydrazide, the major sucker-growth inhibitor for United States tobacco crops.

Fractionation of Tobacco and Tobacco Smoke

Fractionation of tobacco and tobacco smoke has resulted in the identification of cocarcinogens and tumor promoters in the neutral and weakly acidic fractions of cigarette smoke condensate. Of these, cyanophenols, catechol, and 3- and 4-methylcatechol have proved to be carcinogens. A semivolatile basic subfraction extracted from cigarette tobacco has been shown to be mutagenic. This subfraction may contribute significantly to the flavor of tobacco smoke.

Tobacco Carcinogenesis

In the area of tobacco carcinogenesis, homogenized leaf curing coupled with a crystallization procedure has enabled the extraction of fraction I and II proteins from tobacco. These extraction procedures have been shown to remove precursors of tumorigenic smoke products resulting from pyrolytic reactions. Sebaceous gland suppression tests on mouse skin have confirmed the lower tumorigenicity of condensate generated from the extracted tobaccos.

Chemical Analysis of Whole Smoke

Chemical analysis of whole smoke from commercial cigarettes has continued in order to assist in the interpretation of results of epidemiologic studies. During the past year, over 120 domestic brands of cigarattes have been processed. Emphasis has been given to the new "low-tar" and ultra "low-tar" cigarettes, which have been analyzed for tar, nicotine, carbon monoxide, hydrogen cyanide, nitrogen oxides, and acrolein content. The profiling of the vapor phase of whole smoke constituents continues to show a quantitative similarity in these constituents among cigarettes with widely different tar deliveries. The one exception occurred with a nontobacco cigarette, which yielded a higher carbon monoxide content than did tobacco cigarettes.

Low-Yield Reference Cigarette

A cooperative study has been initiated with the U.S. Departement of Agriculture for the development of a Low-Yield Reference Cigarette (LYRC). The 1980 U.S. Surgeon General's Report indicated that one of the chief research needs is a study of reduced tar and nicotine cigarettes by routine and frequent surveillance of current and new cigarettes for specific chemical constitutents and their biologic activity. The LYRC is a cigarette containing specific, known amounts of tar and nicotine. It will be used as a reference, or standard, against which commercial cigarettes can be compared. It will be developed, produced, and provided to researchers involved in studies of smoking and health so that they can compare commercial cigarettes to a widely accepted "standard" cigarette. The physical and chemical (tar and nicotine) specifications for the LYRC have been established, and the cigarette is now available for use by investigators.

Nicotine and Cotinine Levels

The concentrations of circulating levels of nicotine and cotinine were determined in beagle dogs exposed to cigarette smoke. Rates of appearance and washout for each substance were determined to established dose–time relationships in this animal model and to suggest methods of quantifying smoke-related components in other model systems. These trials provide the basis for better definition of dose levels and should prove useful in future inhalation experiments in both humans and animals.

The effect of nicotine aerosol formulation on nicotine uptake has been studied in the beagle dog model. Analysis of pulmonary uptake of nicotine in acidic, neutral, or basic media has shown that the rate of uptake is independent of acidity/basicity in the range tested (pH 5–9). This is the first study to examine the effect of pH on pulmonary uptake of nicotine.

Epidemiology Studies

Among the epidemiology studies, preliminary analyses of data from six cities in five European countries show similarities to the United States data in most smoking practices and related factors. However, some differences were observed among the European centers themselves and between European centers and United States centers. For example, increasing risks as a function of daily cigarette consumption were observed for France, Germany, Italy, and the United States, but not for other centers. Also United States respondents smoked significantly more cigarettes a day than did the European respondents, but the latter smoked cigarettes to a shorter butt length and inhaled more frequently than did United States respondents.

Projects in DCCP to be given priority in addition to those already cited as ongoing priorities include:

1. In the inhalation bioassay category, studies of the effects of high tar/high nicotine versus low tar/low nicotine on the respiratory and cardiovascular systems in the beagle animal model. These studies will be the last of the series of inhalation bioassays designed to determine the relevance of cigarette smoke and nicotine to smoking-related diseases and lung cancer. Pathologic examinations and analyses of histologic specimens from predetermined multiple sites within the tracheal bronchial tree of each beagle were completed in 1982.
2. Identification of individuals at risk of developing tobacco-related disease. Animal studies investigating alterations in body fluids associated with disease and tobacco use may assist in identifying smokers at unusually high risk of tobacco-related diseases.
3. Studies to determine the exact contribution of nicotine, including the identification of its metabolic and pyrolytic products, to smoking-related diseases. Nicotine has been shown to be the only controlled variable in tar that is inconsistently related to the rate of tumor incidence in test animals. However, in other studies, nicotine itself proved not be a carcinogen. The relationship between carcinogenic activity of smoke condensates and their nicotine content may be explained in part by the conversion of nicotine to tobacco-specific nitrosamines or to the cooccurrence of nicotine and some other unidentified carcinogen. Tobacco products made from the lamina of plants grown on high levels of nitrate fertilizer contain more nicotine and show higher levels of volatile nitrosamines following combustion.

As the tar and nicotine levels of cigarettes are reduced, smokers may alter their smoking behavior in an unconscious attempt to extract more of the pharmacologically active materials in the smoke. It is therefore possible that in addition to nicotine, the smoker may increase the intake of other constituents, such as carbon monoxide, nitrogen oxides, and hydrogen cyanide. Earlier studies have counted numbers of cigarettes smoked per day, or lengths of cigarettes smoked, but have recorded no data regarding actual intake of smoke constituents by the smoker. Planned studies will produce data about amounts of specific materials extracted by smokers who inhale and exhale quickly, puff and hold their breath, etc.

Human Intervention Studies

Referring back to the model depicted in Figure 5, all of the applied prevention research is administered by DRCCA. This research emphasizes (a) controlled intervention trials to establish cause and effect relationships (eg, reducing smoking incidence rates in youth consequent to a structured health education program in school settings); and (b) interventions in defined populations (eg, reducing smoking incidence rates in an adolescent population where demographic characteristics are known and from which generalizability of the results allow for broadened dissemination to target populations with the same characteristics using the same methodologies).

Toward this end DRCCA is conducting six workshops to identify opportunities for intervention trials and defined populations studies. The content areas and rationale for these workshops are as follows:

The Role of Youth Education in Smoking Prevention and Cessation

The acquisition of smoking behavior is primarily an adolescent phenomenon. Studies have shown that initial or experimental smoking is found to occur in early junior high years (2). It also recognized that school curricula provide a mechanism for reaching virtually the entire population of youth. Recent prevention studies have produced some promising methodologic and substantive findings which indicate that smoking is significantly decreased (at least over a 1–2 year period) in those children and youth receiving smoking prevention programs (3, 4).

In this country 4000 children start smoking cigarettes every day, and the age at which young people begin to smoke is steadily dropping. The percentage of 12- to 14-year-old females who smoke increased eightfold in the last decade (5).

Preventing the initiation of smoking in youth is the highest priority of the STCP (see chapter 17 also). While youth are still tractable and because they are all approachable in a formalized setting such as the school, the program will concentrate heavily on this intervention approach.

The Role of the Physician/Dentist in Smoking Prevention and Cessation

Physicians and dentists are in a unique position to (a) influence their patients to quit smoking or to (b) become prevention agents, particularly in relation to young people who are about to or have just begun to smoke. They possess prestige and credibility as sources of health-related information (6). Health professionals are models of health for the public.

Given the large numbers of patients that physicians and dentists treat each year and given the circumstances under which these individuals interact, a teachable moment presents itself; this interaction requires empirical testing to determine whether an effective and practical intervention can be forged. In a recent study of the effectiveness of general practitioners' advice to quit smoking among British physicians involving over 2000 smoking patients, Russell et al (7) reported a 5.1% 1-year abstinence rate among patients as a result of a very simple and temporally modest intervention. Although on the surface the percentage of smokers remaining abstinent appears small, the cumulative effect of a program involving thousands of physicians would be considerable.

The Role of Self-Help in Smoking Prevention and Cessation

The majority of the 33 million Americans who have stopped smoking between 1964 and 1982 have done so without the assistance of an organized smoking cessation program. Because many individuals are resistant to participating in formal programs and because the cost effectiveness of a self-help approach has considerable face validity, DRCCA has solicited interest in research to examine the characteristics of people who quit through self-help in comparison to those who ask for or require professional assistance. Capitalizing on 3 years of data gathered from these studies, DRCCA will evaluate the feasibility of employing this strategy in human intervention trials.

The Role of Mass Media in Smoking Cessation and Prevention

In the past few years there has been an accelerated outpouring of research studies examining the impact of the mass media on health knowledge, attitudes, and behaviors. A recent comprehensive review of the media and health scientific literature examining the theoretical perspectives and the basic persuasion strategies indicates that mass media campaigns can produce modest influence on the health orientations of the audience (8). Furthermore, considering the large number of adults who have stopped smoking since the U.S. Surgeon General's first report on smoking in 1964 together with the informational and educational campaigns since that time, any forward plan to reduce smoking and tobacco use prevalence should consider the utilization of mass media for smoking prevention and cessation.

The Value of Smoking Prevention and Cessation Interventions in Minority Populations

Most national data indicate that the prevalence of cigarette smoking among blacks exceeds that of whites (because of the high smoking rates of black males rather than of black females). In 1976, 50.5% of black males were smokers compared to 41.2% of white males. However, smoking rates have been declining for both black and white males. In 1965, 10.8% of black males smoked compared to 51.5% of white males. Meanwhile, the prevalence has decreased only slightly for white females (34.2% in 1965 versus 31.8% in 1976) and has been stable for black females (34.4% in 1965 versus 35.1% in 1976).

In contrast to these findings, a more recent nationwide survey of 750 black Americans sponsored by the American Cancer Society found that cigarette smoking was about equally common among blacks (39%) and whites (38%) (9).

In addition to rates described in national surveys of smoking behavior, there have been more elaborate studies involving more restricted samples. Warnecke's study of an urban black female population shows a much higher rate for black female smokers (49%) (10). The large difference may result from the nature of the sample (urban smoking rates are higher than rural).

Whereas some data are available to describe the smoking rates of blacks in comparison to other groups, much less information examines the smoking context—either psychological or social—of the black smoker. Basically, two domains contribute to the environment of the black smoker. The first is occupational setting; the second is prevalence of certain diseases. Because blacks are disproportionately represented in blue collar occupations, they are additionally at risk to the diseases associated with blue collar occupations, such as lung cancer.

The American Cancer Society survey found that blacks were more interested than whites in giving up smoking (30% compared with 24%), and that blacks also felt it would be less difficult than whites (39% compared with 22%).

Hispanic populations in the United States are not only multicultural in origin, they are substantially increasing as a minority subset of the United States population. As in the case of many other ethnic and minority groups, little is known about the health practices of the Hispanic people, including their smoking rates, patterns, and behavior. Similar to the work being carried out with blacks, considerable emphasis will be placed on earlier cancer control phase studies.

Information and Dissemination

The National Cancer Act Amendments of 1974 require that the "Director of the National Cancer Institute (NCI) shall provide and contract for a program to disseminate and interpret on a current basis for practitioners and other health professionals, scientists and the general public, scientific and other information respecting cause, prevention, diagnosis and treatment of cancer."

NCI disseminates information in three categories:

1. Scientific information used and produced by investigators.
2. State of the art information for use of health professionals and the public.
3. Administrative and program information used by NCI and other organizations within the National Cancer Program.

The Office of Cancer Communications (OCC) is a major source of information for the public (including cancer patients and people at risk of developing cancer) and a substantial source for health professionals. It carries out traditional communications support activities for NCI. Within the National Cancer Program, it assumes the role of coordinator of cancer communications and develops new initiatives to help meet responsibilities stemming from the Act to provide the public and health professionals with useful information about cancer.

Among the many programs within the OCC are a number of information and disseminatiom activities related to smoking education. Through its Information Projects Branch, OCC is engaged in a number of projects intended to help smokers who want to quit, either directly or through health professionals; to assist school officials and others interested in education to develop smoking cessation programs for youth; to develop approaches to utilize the workplace and education materials aimed at high-risk minority audiences; and to stimulate smoking-related efforts through the print and audiovisual media. These activities are being developed and implemented in cooperation with other public and private health organizations so that these smoking programs can contribute to an overall coordinated effort.

The following projects related to smoking are under way for health professionals:

1. "Helping Smokers Quit" kit. Intended for use by physicians with patients who want to quit smoking, these kits have been prepared and distributed to more than 150,000 physicians and other health professionals. The availability of the kits is promoted by direct mail, presentations at medical conventions, and print advertisement and editorial coverage in medical and dental newsletters.
2. "Let's Help Smokers Quit" kit. This kit was designed by the American Dental Association and OCC for use by dental professionals (dentists, hygienists,

and assistants) with patients who want to quit smoking. The kit is an adaption of the "Helping Smokers Quit" kit developed for physicians. The focus of this program is oral health care, effects of smoking on periodontal disease, and smoking's cosmetic effects.

3. "Helping Smokers Quit" program. The American Pharmaceutical Association and the NCI are working together to design a smoking cessation program for pharmacists' use in counseling patients who would like to quit smoking.
4. *The Smoking Digest.* The *Digest* was published in 1978 for program planners, leaders, and activists. It summarizes and examines recent information on attitudes about smoking cessation techniques, smoking information campaigns, smoking legislation, and the tobacco industry.
5. Smoking Programs for Youth. To fill a gap in the existing literature on smoking education for young people, OCC has prepared a comprehensive state of the art report. An offshoot of *The Smoking Digest,* this booklet discusses the issues related to adolescent smoking and summarizes policies, curricula, and counseling programs related to smoking prevention/cessation in primary and secondary schools.
6. Promotion of the "Helping Smokers Quit" kit to minority physicians.
7. Translation and Promotion of "Clearing the Air." The NCI pamphlet "Clearing the Air" is a compilation of methods and techniques for giving up cigarettes. OCC has actively promoted its availability in lay and professional publications with Hispanic and black readership. In addition, the booklet and a supporting poster have been translated into Spanish, with appropriate adjustments in format and graphic design, and widely promoted.

References

1. Greenwald P. New directions in cancer control. Johns Hopkins Med J 1982;151:209–13.
2. McAlister A, Perry C, Maccoby N. Adolescent smoking: onset and prevention. Pediatrics 1979;63:650–8.
3. Perry C, Killen J, Telch M, Slinkard LA, Danaher BG. Modifying smoking behavior of teenagers: A school-based intervention. Am J Public Health 1980;70:722–5.
4. Evans RI, Rozelle RM, Maxwell SE, et al. Social modelling films to deter smoking in adolescents: results of a three-year field investigation. J Appl Psychol 1981;66:339–414.
5. U.S. Department of Health, Education and Welfare. The Health Consequences of Smoking. U.S. DHEW Pub (PHS) 79-50065. Washington, DC: U.S. Government Printing Office, 1979.
6. Smoking behavior and attitudes of physicians, dentists, nurses, and pharmacists. MMWR 1977;6:23.
7. Russell MAH, Wilson C, Taylor C, Baker CD. Effect of general practitioner's advice against smoking. Br Med J 1979;2:231–5.
8. Atkin C. Research evidence on mass mediated health communications campaign, In: Nimmo D, ed; Communications yearbook III. NJ: Transaction Books, 1979:518–31.
9. American Cancer Society. A study of smoking behavior among black Americans. New York: Evaxx, Inc, 1983.
10. Warneke RB, Graham S, Rosenthal S, Manfredi C. Social and psychological correlates of smoking behavior among black women. J Health Soc Behav 1978;19:397–410.

CHAPTER **25**

Lung Cancer and Smoking: Reflections and Unresolved Issues

ERNST L. WYNDER and MARC T. GOODMAN

American Health Foundation, 320 East 43rd Street,
New York, New York 10017

ABSTRACT

It is clear that the main emphasis on reducing the high risk of lung cancer must continue to be directed toward cessation of smoking. We present evidence of what can and should be done in this regard for the youth, what can be accomplished in terms of health education to the public and smoking cessation programs to current smokers as well as the possibilities and opportunities that may reside in low-yield cigarettes. Preventive strategies need also be applied to specific occupational groups known to increase the risk of lung cancer.

In adults, education programs have been relatively successful for educated white males. We need to do more for lower socioeconomic men, and for women as a group. Among the issues still to be resolved, in terms of etiology, before we can make preventive suggestions is that of nutrition. There can be no greater challenge in preventive oncology than to reduce tobacco-related cancer rates in men and prevent their further rise in women. As Pasteur said, a scientist needs to discover and apply the discovery with equal energy. In the case of lung cancer, most of our energies need now to be concentrated on application.

Key Words: **Lung cancer prevention, Kreyberg lung types, Alton Ochsner, Evarts Graham, Know Your Body (KYB), smoking cessation, smoking prevention, low tar yield cigarettes**

Alton Ochsner deserves much credit as one of the first to propose the concept that cigarette smoking is etiologically related to lung cancer. He gave me personal encouragement when, together with Evarts Graham, I first began to interview lung cancer patients about their personal histories and environmental exposures. In fact, Alton permitted us to interview his patients in New Orleans,

Lung Cancer: Causes and Prevention.

cases that were part of the initial epidemiologic report we published in 1950 (1). In 1983 Washington University in St. Louis celebrated Evarts Graham's 100th birthday. Alton Ochsner no doubt affected Graham's thinking about the etiology of lung cancer and so was also likely to have influenced Graham's early views of my investigations. I am therefore pleased to acknowledge Alton Ochsner's influence on the early part of my scientific career. This volume focuses on two areas; the etiology and the prevention of lung cancer.

Etiology

Knowledge of the etiology of lung cancer in 1983 remains essentially unchanged since 1950. Cigarette smoking is the principal cause for Kreyberg I lung cancers and, to a lesser extent, for Kreyberg II cancers in both men and women (Figure 1). There are a number of occupations, particularly those that are asbestos related, that increase the risk of lung cancer, especially among smokers. However, the effect of occupational exposure on the overall risk of lung cancer is certainly less than 10% in men, and even smaller in women, as reviewed by Blot (Chapter 4) in this volume.

The high rate of lung cancer in southern Louisiana as compared to northern Louisiana, as presented by Correa, et al in this volume (Chapter 6), probably can be explained by differences in smoking habits. In the presence of a carcinogen as potent as tobacco smoke it is necessary to control for its effect through careful stratification. Before the risk of environmental exposures, such as smoke from forest fires or work in cane fields, can be assessed and regarded as additional risk

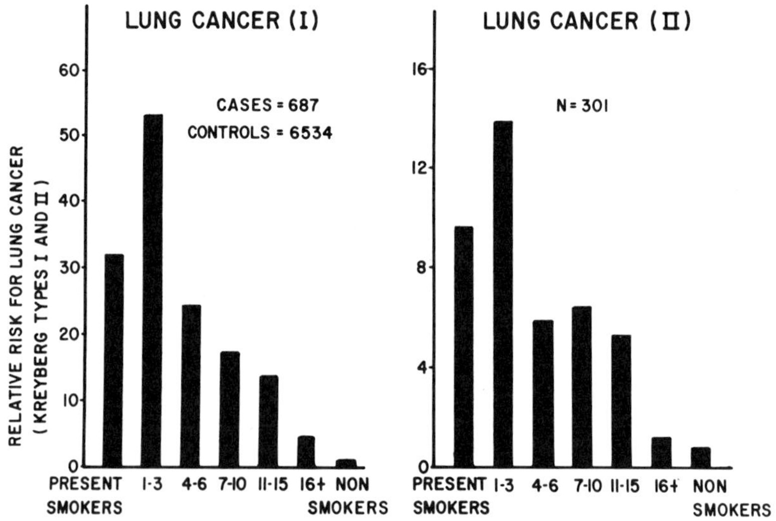

Figure 1. Comparisons of relative risk for lung cancer for present smokers, ex-smokers, and nonsmokers. Ranges on abscissa designate number of years since cessation of cigarette smoking. (17).

factors, possible confounding variables to be addressed should include age of onset, number of cigarettes smoked per day, and types of cigarettes smoked.

Some of the unresolved issues in the etiology of lung cancer are nutritional deficiencies (Vitamins A, C, and E, selenium) and excesses (cholesterol); changing ratio of adenocarcinoma to epidermoid carcinoma; the significance of low-tar-yield cigarettes, smoking compensation, and sidestream tobacco inhalation. The various studies on passive inhalation, reviewed by us in Table 1, contain inconsistencies that do not permit us at the present time to establish a causal association between passive inhalation and lung cancer. Hirayama (2) has suggested that the small room size and the greater proximity of Japanese couples compared to their American counterparts may account for the positive finding in Japan and the lack of association found by Garfinkel in the United States (3). Obviously, sidestream smoke and mainstream smoke contain many of the same carcinogens in the particulate and gaseous phases. Lung cancers in nonsmokers, both male and female, are principally adenocarcinomas located in the periphery of the lung. The question is whether enough of these carcinogens, particularly in the volatile component of the smoke, get deep enough into the lung to induce carcinogenesis. Respirable smoke particulates are unlikely to reach the periphery of the lung in any appreciable amounts. On the other hand, gaseous components are more likely to reach the deeper part of the lung. Preliminary data from the American Health Foundation's investigation of lung cancer in nonsmokers have shown no consistent trend of higher sidestream smoke exposure among cases when compared with nonsmoking controls (Table 2). Occupational factors may be responsible for some of the male cases, particularly those with Kreyberg type I lung cancer. We are now conducting a retrospective case-control study based upon a more detailed questionnaire, which elicits information on exposure to sidestream smoke in childhood, and as adults, at home, at work, in public areas, as well as in transportation. The question of passive inhalation and its role in lung cancer etiology remains at present open ended.

There have been some reports of an apparent increase in adenocarcinoma of the lung in male smokers. Because histology may be associated with etiology as well as prognosis, it is important that pathologists differentiate between the histologic types of lung cancer, as emphasized in this volume by Berg (Chapter 9) so that changing patterns in lung cancer incidence can be assessed.

The Role of Green and Yellow Vegetables

Hirayama (4) presents evidence that eating green and yellow vegetables reduces the risk of lung cancer in both active and passive smokers. Peto et al (5) summarize the existing evidence that deficiencies in retinoids and β-carotene may increase the risk of lung cancer. He suggested that clinical trials be carried out to test the hypothesis that certain vitamins and minerals reduce the incidence of certain cancers, including those of the lung. Table 3 summarizes the evidence to date linking nutritional deficiencies with lung cancer etiology. The area of

Table 1. Summary of studies of lung cancer in nonsmokers[a]

Author; type of study; population	Number of cases	Histology	Findings	Comments
Hirayama, T, 1981; prospective; Japanese nonsmoking wives aged 40+.	174 deaths in married nonsmoking women with lung cancer among 91,540 nonsmoking married women.	Out of a sample of 23 cases, 17 were adenocarcinoma.	Nonsmoking wives of heavy smokers had RR[b] of 2.08. Risk was higher (4.57) in agricultural families when husbands were aged 40–59 at enrollment.	Exposure index was based on husband's smoking habits.
Garfinkel, L, 1981; analysis of data from two prospective studies; ACS[b] population Dorn study of veterans.	195 deaths from lung cancer among male nonsmokers; 564 deaths from lung cancer among female nonsmokers (ACS). 168 lung cancer deaths among nonsmokers (Dorn).	Microscopic confirmation of dx[b] in 69% of cases in first 6 years of ACS study. Among lung cancer cases with confirmed histology, 33% of male and 49% of female nonsmokers had adenocarcinoma compared to 18% of male and 30% of female smokers (Garfinkel L. personal communication, 1983).	No significant increase in lung cancer risk seen in nonsmoking wives of smoking husbands compared to nonsmoking wives of nonsmoking husbands.	Exposure index was based on husband's smoking habits.

Trichopoulos D, et al, 1981; case/control; female Caucasian residents of Athens (19).	40 female nonsmokers with lung cancer other than adenocarcinoma or terminal bronchiolar.	14 cases were histologically confirmed; 19 were cytologically confirmed; 18 were clinically confirmed.	RR of lung cancer associated with having a husband who smokes <1 pack per day was 2.4; RR associated with having a husband who smokes >pack/day was 3.4 (χ^2 for linear trend = 6.45; $p < 0.02$).	Exposure index was based on smoking habits of husbands and former husbands.
Chan WC, Fung SC; Case/control; Hong Kong Chinese (20).	There were only two nonsmokers out of 208 male lung cancer cases; 84 nonsmokers out of 189 female lung cancer patients.	15 of the 84 female cases were squamous or epidermoid cancer; 38 were adenocarcinoma; 15 had no histologic verification.	Among nonsmoking females the proportion of cases whose spouse smoked was slightly lower than that of controls (34 out of 84 or 40.5% vs 66 of 139 or 47.5%). Among nonsmoking females, there was no significant difference in the proportion of cases who used kerosene fuel in cooking compared to controls.	It is unclear what question was used to get inhalation because in an earlier paper (21), the question is given as "Are you exposed to the tobacco smoke of others at home or at work?" whereas here reference is made only to "smoking habits of spouses." No information is given on how many subjects were married.

[a]Source: Reference 22.
[b]RR = Relative Risk; ACS = American Cancer Society; dx = diagnosis.

Table 2. Histologic type of lung cancer in never smokers and smokers[a]

	Males		Females	
	N	%	N	%
Never smoked				
Kreyberg type I	13	35.1	20	20.6
Epidermoid/squamous	13	35.1	16	16.5
Large cell/giant cell	0		4	4.1
Kreyberg type II	20	54.1	72	74.2
Adenocarcinoma	16	43.2	60	61.9
Alveolar	4	10.8	12	12.4
Mixed (Kreyberg I and II) and undifferentiated/anaplastic	4	10.8	5	5.2
Total	37		97	
Smokers[b]				
Kreyberg I	1187	63.1	341	52.3
Kreyberg II	600	31.9	279	42.8
Mixed (Kreyberg I and II) and undifferentiated/anaplastic	95	5.0	32	4.9
Total	1882		652	

[a]Source: Reference 22.
[b]A more detailed breakdown by histologic type is not presented for smokers because this information was not coded. For the smokers this information was retrieved manually.

nutrition and lung cancer represents a challenge to investigators because of the interactive effects of cigarette smoking, socioeconomic status, and nutritional intake, and the inherent difficulty in obtaining reliable dietary histories.

Dyer, et al (6) published preliminary data linking hyperlipidemia to lung cancer. This association is supported indirectly by a recent case-control survey by Hinds et al (7), who found a positive association between increased intake of fat and cholesterol and the incidence of lung cancer. Although overloading of macrophages by cholesterol may be one explanation, further comment on the matter requires confirmation of these data, especially of Dyer's findings.

Prevention

Future conferences on lung cancer should focus on preventive measures such as smoking prevention in youths and adults, chemoprevention, and the nature of less harmful cigarettes. The main emphasis clearly should be directed toward the preventing the adoption of smoking behavior in children. International studies

Table 3. Nutritional carcinogenesis

Carcinogens	Natural additives, contaminants
Initiators	
Promoters	
Accelerators	
Deficiency	Macro/micronutrients
Excess	Calories, macronutrients

indicate that the frequency of smoking among children is proportional to the smoking habits of the adult population (8). Adults need to be role models for their children. Parents in particular should recognize this responsibility. Special health promotion programs, such as our Know Your Body (KYB) health education program, should be part of every school curriculum from grades 1 to 12 (9). The program should be more than didactic. It should address all major risk factors for cancer and heart disease and be evaluted for its cost-effectiveness each year. The Know Your Body children receive, as a case in point, a Health Passport. The curriculum, interwoven into the school's day to day activities, is taught by the teachers. The teachers also are screened and participate in the health promotion effort. The program involves the parents through KYB newsletters addressed to them, and through educational messages brought home by the children. We have data indicating that parental smoking and milk drinking habits, ie, smoking cessation and switching to skim milk, can be influenced. We must strive to have proper school health education, preferably called health promotion, as an integral part of the curricula of schools throughout the country.

Smoking Cessation

It has been shown that lung cancer declines inversely with the duration and amount of smoking (Figure 2). In the United States, perhaps more than in other countries, there has been a significant increase in the percentage of ex-smokers in both sexes, but particularly in men. The percentage of ex-smokers is not associated only with sex, but also with age, education, and race (Figure 3). This knowledge is important in that antismoking education in general and smoking cessation clinics in particular should focus on populations at the highest risk.

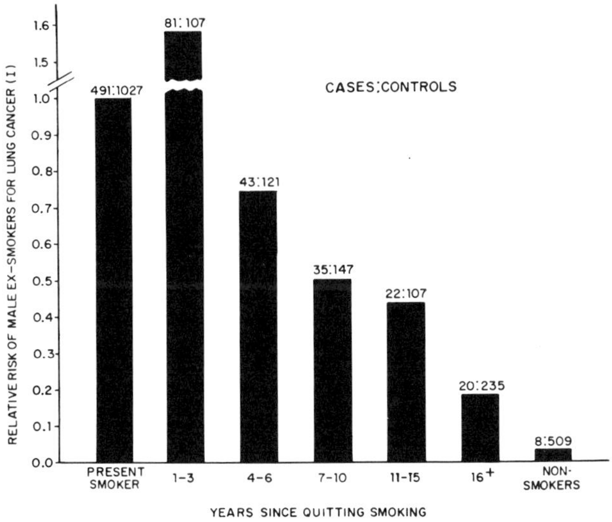

Figure 2. Relative risk of male ex-smokers for cancer of the lung (Kreyberg type I) by years since quitting smoking. (17).

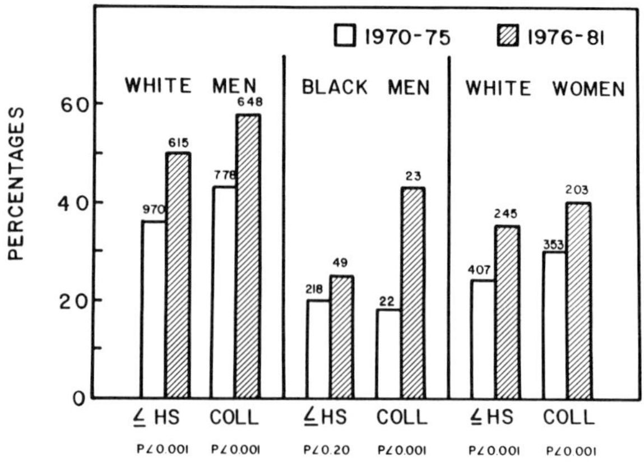

Figure 3. Age-adjusted rates of ex-smokers among ever-cigarette smokers. HS, highschool; Col, college (Unpublished).

Fritz has reviewed the effect of special smoking cessation activities. If every physician would give a short antismoking message to all smoking patients as shown by Russell, the result would be a cost-effective exercise of reducing long-term smoking in a select segment of the population (10). Formal smoking cessation programs, especially with appropriate maintenance support, could reach a 50% success rate for 1 year. Clearly, that is a more efficient (and humane) step for society than carrying out more pneumonectomies or early screening of lung cancer as shown by Fontana in this volume (Chapter 13). It is strongly suggested that every hospital, and certainly every comprehensive clinical cancer center, should provide an ongoing smoking cessation program for all their patients, as well as for the outlying community. The American Health Foundation has trained 70 representatives from various hospitals to conduct such a program (11). The program is best carried out by allied health professionals. Smoking cessation activities must be an integral part of health care services.

The Low-Yield Cigarette

Peto claims in this volume (Chapter 1) that much of the decreasing rate of lung cancer in British men before the age of 50 has resulted in the introduction of filter cigarettes, a concept supported by Lee. We have not noticed such a steep change in the United States, perhaps because the lung cancer rate started to rise earlier in England. In assessing a decline in lung cancer incidence in young males in the United States, it is difficult to separate the effects of smoking cessation from that of filter cigarette use, because, as we have shown, a considerable percentage of ex-smokers exists in this country. The significant decrease in lung cancer rates in British physicians surely results in part from their having stopped smoking in large numbers (12). As with smoking cessation, the smoking of low-yield cigarettes is also affected by education and sex. The characteristics of ex-smokers and people smoking low-yield cigarettes, therefore, are closely interrelated. Long-term filter smokers, that is, those who have smoked such cigarettes for more than 10 years, do have a somewhat lower risk of lung cancer than nonfilter smokers (Figure 4). Because most of these smokers began their smoking "careers" with nonfilter cigarettes, it is too early to judge the risk of lung cancer in a smoker who has smoked filter cigarettes exclusively. This applies especially to smokers of cigarettes with a low-tar yield. Cigarettes delivering 10 mg of tar or less have been smoked by only a small percentage of smokers for more than 10 years (13). It may be some time before the health risk of individuals who began their smoking career with the low-yield cigarette can be determined. Therefore, the challenge to industry is to put greater emphasis on the marketing of cigarettes with smoke contents of a maximum level as has been suggested by Gori (14) and adopted by us in Table 4 (15). A smokeable cigarette could be made that has between 4 and 8 mg of tar and between 0.3 and 0.6 mg nicotine. This is possible both for the smokers to accept and for the manufacturers to produce. When discussing a "less harmful" cigarette, we need to recognize that what may be a less harmful cigarette for lung cancer may not be less harmful for myocardial infarction and chronic obstructive pulmonary disease. Threshold levels of toxicity for various smoke components, ie, tar, nicotine, and gaseous components, are most likely to be quite different for these disease entities.

The question is often raised, "Why work on a less harmful cigarette?" In a society that condones cigarette smoking, as our society is likely to do in the foreseeable future, young people will start the habit, especially those coming from low-income groups, in spite of all our efforts, and some will continue into adulthood because of the apparent "satisfying nature" of cigarette smoking. Those cigarette smokers require our assistance as well. Our task is to monitor the low-yield cigarette epidemiologically (as we are doing), test the safety of new additives, and induce the industry to reduce as far as is practical all the toxic components of

Table 4. The less harmful cigarette: maximum concentrations of some selected toxic agents in the smoke[a]

Toxic component	Maximal proposed concentration
Tar[b]	8 mg
Nicotine	0.6 mg
Carbon monoxide	8 mg
Hydrogen cyanide	100 μg
Benzo [*a*] pyrene[c]	8 ng
Dimethylnitrosamine[d]	5 ng
N′-Nitrosonornicotine	60 ng
Catechol	90 μg
Phenol	20 μg
Acrolein[e]	30 μg

[a]Wynder and Hoffman (15).
[b]Tar = total particulate matter, water, nicotine.
[c]Serves as indicator for tumorigenic Polycyclic Aromatic Hydrocarbons (PAH).
[d]Serves as indicator for volatile nitrosamines.
[e]Serves as indicator for organic cilia toxic agents.

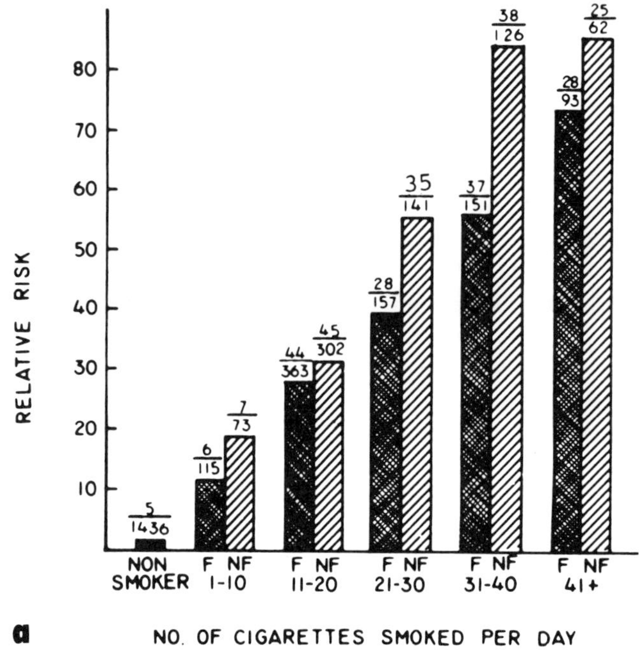

Figure 4(a). Lung cancer (Kreyberg type I) risk in men in relationship to type, filter (F) vs nonfilter (NF) and number of cigarettes smoked. Fractions represent number of cases compared with number of controls in sample (18).

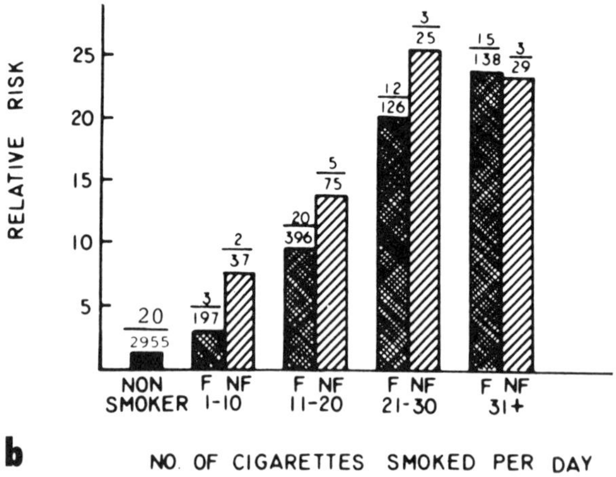

Figure 4(b). Lung cancer (Kreyberg type I) risk in women in relationship to type, filter (F) vs nonfilter (NF) and number of cigarettes smoked. Fractions represent number of cases compared with number of controls in sample (18).

cigarette smoke. We hope that by the end of the decade, the levels of the various components as set forth in Table 4 will have been met by the majority of cigarettes. In setting these levels, we also hope that they are obtained by new Federal

Trade Commission techniques that will consider the manner in which a cigarette is smoked, including the pressure of the lips, and the smoking habits (ie, number of puffs per cigarette and volume of puff) generally used by the smokers of low-yield cigarettes.

Epilogue

Pasteur stressed that scientists must not only discover, but also apply. At times the latter appears to be more difficult. This has certainly been the case as we review the history of smoking and lung cancer. When first reviewing our data, Evarts Graham said to me, "we have only one thing on our side, that is, we are right." And how right he was. It took 14 years before the first U.S. Surgeon General's report was published in 1964 (16). Today, clearly, our attention with regard to lung cancer and other tobacco-related diseases should be increasingly focused on preventive strategies. To succeed, we need to gain societal support, including that of our peers who continue to prefer either basic sciences or clinical medicine. We are, of course, aware of the public apathy toward the existence of an illusion of immortality. There exists a disinterested health care delivery system that essentially pays for the delivery of therapeutic services rather than for preventive care. We are aware of the antagonistic opposition of those who develop products that are harmful to society and who gain from such products. Among all these obstacles, the relative neglect of support from our medical peers causes us the greatest concern. Is not the true art of medicine the prevention of disease? We know, as Graham said in 1949, that our cause is right. We know that some progress has been made, as in the existence of a great number of ex-smokers in the United States as well as in many other countries. There have been some advances in the rather sizeable reduction of tar and nicotine levels of cigarettes and in the ability to launch broad health promotion programs in some of our schools. We are fortunate to have the full involvement of volunteer health organizations, such as the American Cancer Society, the American Heart Association, and the American Lung Association. We also are pleased with the renewed interest in preventive oncology by the Director of the National Cancer Institute and the leadership of the DRCCA of the National Cancer Institute.

One wishes that Drs. Ochsner and Graham could have witnessed the new preventive strategies directed against lung cancer. As great practitioners of the art of surgery, they surely would have received satisfaction that the word "practice" applies and can be conducted in disease prevention as well.

References

1. Wynder EL, Graham EA. Tobacco smoking as a possible etiological factor in bronchogenic carcinoma. JAMA 1950;143:329–36.
2. Hirayama T. Non-smoking wives of heavy smokers have a higher risk of lung cancer: a study of Japan. Br Med J 1981;182:183–5.

3. Garfinkel L. Time trends in lung cancer mortality among non-smokers and a note on passive smoking. JNCI 1981;66:1061-6.
4. Hirayama T. Diet and cancer. Nutr Cancer 1979;1:67-81.
5. Peto R, Doll R, Buckley JD, Sporn MB. Can dietary β-carotene naturally reduce human cancer rates? Nature 1981; 190:201 -8.
6. Dyer AR, Stamler J, Paul O, et al. Serum cholesterol and risk of death from lung cancer and other causes in three Chicago epidemiological studies. J Chronic Dis 1981;34:249-60.
7. Hinds MW, Kolonel LN, Lee J, Hankin JH. Dietary cholesterol and lung cancer risk among men in Hawaii. Am J Clin Nutr 1983;37:192-3.
8. American Health Foundation. Forum: The International Know Your Body Program: Health education and screening for risk factors in children. Prevent Med 1981;10:119-257.
9. William CL, Arnold CB, Wynder EL. Primary prevention of chronic disease beginning in childhood. The "Know Your Body" program: design of study. Prevent Med 1977;6:344-57.
10. Russell M, Wilson C, Taylor C, et al. Effect of general practitioner's advice against smoking. Br Med J 1979;231-5.
11. Bohm E, Powell DR. A ten point practical program to help your smokers quit. Your Patient and Cancer 1982;2:87-100.
12. Doll R, Peto R. Mortality in relation to smoking: 20 years' observations on male British doctors. Br Med J 1976;2:1525-36.
13. Wynder EL, Goodman MT, Hoffmann D. Demographic aspects of the low-yield cigarette: considerations in the evaluation of health risk. JNCI 1984;72 (in press).
14. Gori GB. Low risk cigarettes. a prescription. Science 1976;194:1243-6.
15. Wynder EL, Hoffmann D. Tobacco and tobacco smoke. Oncology 1976; 194:1243-1246.
16. U.S. Public Health Service. Smoking and health. Report of the Advisory Committee to the Surgeon General of the Public Health Service. PHS Publ 1103. Washington, DC: U.S. Department of Health, Education and Welfare, Public Health Service, 1964.
17. Wynder EL, Stellman SD. Comparative epidemiology of tobacco-related cancers. Cancer Res 1977;37:4608-22.
18. Wynder EL, Stellman SD. Impact of long-term filter cigarette usage on lung cancer and larynx cancer risk: a case control study. JNCI 1979;62:471-7.
19. Trichopoulos D, Kalandidi A, Sparros L, MacMahon B. Lung cancer and passive smoking. Intl J Cancer 1981; 27:1 - 40.
20. Chan WC, Fung SC. Lung cancer in non-smokers in Hong Kong. In: Cancer Campaign Vol. 6 Cancer Epidemiology, Grundmann E, Stuttgart: Gustav Fischer, 1982.
21. Chan WC, Colbourne MJ, Fung SC, Ho HC. Bronchial cancer in Hong Kong: 1976-1977. Br J Cancer 1979;39:182 - 192.
22. Kabat GC, Wynder EL. Lung cancer in nonsmoker. Cancer 1984;53:1214 - 1221.

Subject Index

Acrylonitrile, 54
Adenocarcinomas
  cell lines, growth factor and hormone requirements, 256
  females, types of in, 155
  male/female ratios of, 118
  predominance in nonsmoking wives, 194
  relative frequencies, 118
  rises in U.S. of since 1973, 153
  testing and classification, 123-124
  types of in U.S., 119
Adenosquamous carcinoma, 123
Adolescents, prevention of smoking in
  abstract, 219
  and ages at start, 221
  cessation efforts, problems with, 220
  communication-persuasion model, 223
  constraints, 224
  counterarguments, use, 223
  decisions, making of, 222
  discussion periods, 225
  and earlier research, perspectives from, 220-221
  film content, 225
  junior high schools, programs in, 221
  lasting impact of, 226-227
  model of behaviors, 222
  narrators in films, 223
  negative decisions, 223-224
  and perceptions of students, 223
  predisposition, 222
  questions for students, 225
  reinforcement of decision, 223
  saliva specimens, 225-226
  smoking onset rates, effects on of propaganda, 226
  social learning theory, 221-222
  social pressures on children, 221
  time and frequency, 225
  understanding of social influences, 224
  vicariously learned expectations, 221-222
  young children, beliefs of, 221
Alpha radiation (α). *See* Radioactivity and tobacco, *specific isotope*
Air pollution and lung cancer
  abstract, 65
  carcinogens
    aliphatic fractions, 68, 69
    aromatic fractions, 68
    automobile emissions, 69
    azaarenes, 68
    benzo(a)pyrene, 68-69, 70
    epoxides, 69
    incomplete combustion, 67, 68
    iminoarenes, 68
    organics, particulate and vapor, 67
    oxygenated hydrocarbons, 69
    peroxides, 69
    polycyclic aromatic hydrocarbons, 68
    vapor-phase organics, 69
  epidemiological evaluations, 70-71
  geographical studies, 69-70
  mortality rate correlations, 70
  urban factors
    age- and smoking-adjusted mortality ratios, 66
    metropoli, 66, 67
    neighborhoods, 66
    occupational exposures, 66, 67
    risk, 66
    rural, 66
    table, 67
APUD markers, 249, 257
Arginine vasopressin
  and cloning of SCLC, 255-256
  effects on SCLC, 355-356
Arsenic, carcinogen, 9, 48-49
  animal evidence, 49
  carcinogenesis, late stages, 49
  contrast of to zinc, 49
  excess mortality, 48-49
  pesticides, 49
  and smoking, 49
  trioxide form of, 48
Asbestos
  and cigarette smoking, 50
  exposure length, 49
  groups at risk, 49
  hazards of, 10
  and lung cancer, 10, 49
  shipbuilding, 50
  types of mineral fibers of, 50
  World War II workers, exposure of to, 50, 51
Australia, lung cancer rate in, 8
Automobiles, emissions of. *See* Air pollution
Avoidance of various causes of cancer, effects compared, 16

Benzo(a)pyrene, 68-69, 70
  coronene, 69
  reduction in, 68, 69
Beryllium, 54-55

Beta-carotene, 137-138, 178. *See also* Green-yellow vegetables; Vitamin A
Bifurcations in lungs, radiation deposits at, 265, 266, 267, 268, 269, 270
Biotechnology, recent advances in. *See also* DNA; Genes; Viruses
  abstract, 229
  and blastocyst nuclei, 235
  Burkitt lymphoma, 232
  cell membranes, 233
  chromosomal alteration, 235-236
  deletion 3p(14-23), 236
  diagram, 235
  and differentiated cells, 233
  Epstein-Barr virus, 232
  feline leukemia virus, 232
  leopard frog adenocarcinoma, 232, 233
  Lucké tumor herpesvirus, 232, 233
  nuclear transplantation, 233-235
  and oncogenic tumor viruses, 233
  Philadelphia chromosome, 236
  reprogramming pronephric cells to form tumor cells, 234
  temperature shift, effects, 233-234
  testing for functional genes in tumor nuclei, 234-235
  and tumorogenesis, vs. small cell lung carcinoma, 232
  unique banding patterns, 236
  and U.S. mortality rates
    female, 231
    male, 230
  viral infection, and cell membranes, 233
Bischloromethyl ether, 9, 51
  chloromethyl methyl ether, 51
  and oat-cell carcinoma, 51
  and smoking, 51
Blacks. *See also* Epidemiology; *specific type of cancer; specific area studied;* United States
  in cities, 66
  epidemiological studies of, 120
  females, age-adjusted rates, 43, 309
  genetic risk of lung cancer in, 143
  geographical distributions, 41, 42, 44
  human intervention studies in, 309
  increased rates of lung cancer in, 41
  males, age-specific rates of lung cancer in, 42, 309
  quitters, 320
Bombesin, and small-cell lung cancer
  as autocrine regulatory peptide, 256
  and cloning of small cell lung cancer, 255-256
  receptors for, 256
Britain, problems with cigarettes in, 13, 15, 274, 280, 281, 320-321
  average annual consumption, 277
  certifications of deaths, trends, 15
  changes, in cigarette types, 274
  compensation, 276
  popular attitudes to risk of tobacco, 13-14
  tar, 13, 281
  trends, by sex, of risk, 281
Bronchogenic carcinoma, unspecified, 159
Bronchiolar carcinoma, 123, 124

Cadmium, 57
"Cajuns", case-control studies of lung cancer in. *See also* Louisiana
  abstract, 101
  case-control studies, nature of, 102-107
    data in, 105
    location, 105
    questions asked, 106
    recent, table, 106
    results, comparisons, 107
  county maps, distribution of cases, 102
  and lung cancer rates, 101-102
  Mississippi River valley, 102
Canada, lung cancer in, 8
Cancer
  control strategies for, 2
  means of avoiding, percentage effects, 168
Carboxyhemoglobin, 277
Carcinogen inhibition and vitamin A. *See also* Green/yellow vegetables; Vitamin A
  butylhydroxybutyl nitrosamine, vs. 13-*cis*-retinoic acid, 204
  nitrosourea vs. retinoids, 204
  retinoic acid and papillomas, 204
  and squamous metaplasia vs. vitamin A deficiency, 204
  two-step model, 204
  vitamin A vs. methylcholanthrene, 204
Carcinoid, 147, 158
Carcinoma. *See specific type of carcinoma*
Case-control studies. *See also* National Cancer Institute
  industries with more that 25% excess cancer risk, 107
  information, problems of getting, 109
  manufacturing plants, residence near, 108
  other associations, 108
  other factors, 108
  residential exposure and lung cancer risk, 108
  residence, method problems with, 108
Cessation of smoking
  abstinence violation effect, 288
  abstract, 285
  causes, 288
  deaths, 289
  delivery of programs, 289-290
  discussion, 319-320
  effects, 8-9
  Great American Smoke Out, 289
  and motivation, 289
  MRFIT, 289
  percentage of lung cancer deaths due to smoking, 285

precursors, 288
prevalence in U.S. of smoking, 286
quit attempt rates, 286
quit success rates, 286, 289
quitters, age-adjusted rates of among ever-smokers, 320
recidivism, 288
risk reduction, vs. time since quitting, 314, 319
stages, 289
techniques, 289
warnings about smoking, 289
women, 286
Chemoprevention program
components, 199-200
major objectives, 198, 199
model, 199
process, 200
reasons for, 198
research logic and flow
decision points about new substances, 201
diagram, 200
discussion, 200-202
epidemiological studies, 201, 202
human intervention sequence, 201, 202
leads, 201, 202
planning problems, 202-203
stages, 201
substances to be tested, 198
Children. *See* Adolescents
China
cancer rates in, 2
tar in, 18
Chlorinated toluenes, 57
Chloromethyl ethers, vs. smoking habit, and cancer risk, 136
Cholesterol, lung cancer risk studies, 208
Chromium
element, 9
hexavalent vs. trivalent ions, 52
sodium chromate, 52
studies on, 52
zinc chromate, 52
Chromosomes. *See* Genes
Cigarettes. *See also* Tobacco
carcinogens in, 1
importance of vs. pipes, 9
tar reduction in, 1
Cilia, loss of, 280
"Clearing the Air", translations of, 311
Compensation, smoking behavior
by altered manner of smoking, 277-278
and average annual U.K. consumption, 277
carboxyhemoglobin, 277
blood nicotine, 277, 278
factors, 276
by increased consumption, 276-277
lack of connection of with tar reduction, 276
machine smoking, studies by, 277
vs. nicotine delivery, 276
nicotine reduction vs. machine nicotine delivery reduction, 278
problem of, 276
studies, 277
surveys, 276
Conditioning of the young, elements in, 287
Connecticut, lung cancer in
male/female ratio, 118
types, relative frequency, 118
Coping mechanism, use of smoking as, 287
Culture medium, serum-free defined. *See also* HITES
growth factor requirements, 254, 256
problems with serum, 254
and serum-supplemented medium, 254

Demographic distances. *See* Epidemiology
Deletion of 3p chromosome marker, in lung cancer susceptibility, 141, 254
Diethanolamine, 305
Dimethyl sulfate, 57
Directory of Occupational Titles, 87
DNA, analysis of in human lung cancer. *See also* Genes, transforming
aneuploid content of cells, percentages, 253
and B lymphoblastoid cell lines, 254
common deletion, short arm of chromosome, 3, 254
continuous cell culture vs. DNA content, 253
and flow cytometry, results of, 253
multiple aneuploid cell lines, 253
serum-free medium, growth in, 254
survival of patients, vs. DNA content, 253
tumor cells, failure to detect, 253
DNA transfection, 236-239
BL oncogenesis, 237
c-abl oncogene, 237
c-myc oncogene, 237
myc oncogene, 236
new techniques, 237
NIH3T3 cells, 237, 239
oncogenes, varieties of, 237
oncogenic DNA segments, 236
3p deletion, 237
ras retrovirus, 236
reciprocal translocation, 236-237
and restriction fragments from lung carcinoma, 236
Dose-response curves, 8, 177, 275

Elasticity in demand for cigarettes vs. price, 14
Epichlorohydrin, 57
Epidemiologic Analysis with a Programmable Calculator, 177
Epidemiology of lung cancer
adenocarcinomas, 118, 123
adenosquamous carcinomas, 123
age-adjusted rates, problems with, 120
black men, 120

black vs. white, histological distribution of, 120
bronchiolar carcinomas, 123, 124
demographic distances
calculation of, 128-129
and carcinomas, 125, 126, 127
close, table, 126
grade of cancer vs. distance, 126
grade comparisons vs. epidemiological relevance, 125-126
lung cancer types, 125
nature, 125
P values, 126, 127, 128
pleomorphic carcinomas, separation of, 127
use, 125
diagnosis problems, 122
giant-spindle cell carcinomas, 124
leiosarcomas of lung, 123
liposarcomas of lung, 122
lung cancers
confirmed without typing, 121
diagnoses, 100+/year in U.S., 119
logical breakdown and classification of, 123
splitting of smokers apart from nonsmokers, 118
without microscopic confirmation, 121
and Manual of Tumor Nomenclature and Coding, 122
melanoma of lung, 122
and men, squamous cell cancer in, 119
mesotheliomas, coding and assessment of, 122
mucus-secreting adenocarcinomas, 124
and NCI data, 122
nonspecific diagnoses, 120
pulmonary lymphomas, 123
sarcomas, of lung, 123
and SEER, 118, 122
statistical significance, testing of, 127-128
and Third National Cancer Survey, 122
and women, oat cell cancer in, 119
Epidermal growth factor, 256
Epithelium, 266
Estradiol, 254, 256
Etiology of lung cancer, discussion of problems in. *See also specific type of cancer*
depth of inhalation, 315
risk relation to time since quitting, 314
unresolved issues, 315
Etreitate, synthetic retinoid, 208
Europe, lung cancer rates in, 8
Excess annual lung cancer incidence rates, by years of smoking, 3, 4. *See also* Dose response curves

Females. *See* Women
Fiber glass, 58
Filters, 11, 178
Finland, tars in, 17. *See also* Scandinavia
Foundry work, lung cancer risk of
agents causing, 55-56
cohort studies, 55
proportional mortality, 55
France, cigarettes of, 9

Genes, and susceptibility to lung cancer
alveolar cell carcinoma, 144, 146
α_1-antitrypsin, 148-149
aryl hydrocarbon hydroxylase, genetic marker functions, 147-148
inducibility of gene for vs. susceptibility, 148
problems with, 148
autosomal dominant traits, 146
autosomal recessive traits, 147
blood groups, 149
bronchogenic carcinoma, 147
carcinoid, 147
chromosomal abnormalities, 146
excess breaks in, 146
hyperploidy, 146
congenital cystic disease, dominant form, 147
empiric familial risk, 143-144
habits in families, 143-144
heterogeneity, 143
synergism with smoking, 143
and exposure to family-introduced agents, 144
familial aggregates of lung tumors, 146-147
genetic questions, 142-143
hemoglobin Malmö, 147
histiocytoses, 144
host determinants, 144
immune defects, 145-146
alveolar diseases, 145
atypia, 146
dermatomyositis, 146
fibrosis, 145
immunosuppression, 145
and lung cancer, 145
sarcoidosis, 145, 146
scar carcinoma, 146
scleroderma, 145, 146
uranium miners, 145
interstitial pulmonary fibrosis, 147
Kartagener syndrome, 147
malformation of lungs, 147
medullary carcinoma, 147
mesotheliomas, 144
in mice, 148, 149
multiple endocrine neoplasias, 147
multiple leiomyomas, 147
multiple primary neoplasms, 144-145
oat cell carcinoma, 147

pedigrees
and interactions of general susceptibility with external agents, 144
Li-Fraumeni syndrome, 145
pulmonary liposarcoma, 147
summary, 149
twin studies, 143
in U.S.
Cantonese women, 143
Mexican-Americans in Texas, 143
Ohio, blacks in, 143
races compared, 143
southern Louisiana, 142
vitamin A consumption, 143
women, pulmonary adenocarcinoma/squamous cell carcinoma ratio, 142
Genes, transforming, human carcinomas. *See also* DNA
activated transforming genes, 240
B and T lymphocytes, 241
bladder cancers, 240
colon carcinomas, 240, 241
as event in oncogenesis, 240
Kirsten sarcoma virus, 241, 242
lung cancers, 240, 241
lymphoid neoplasms, 240
mammary carcinomas, 240, 241
mice vs. humans, oncogenes in, 240, 241
neoplasia, alterations in, 240
neoplasms from, 239
and NIH3T3 cells, 239, 240
normal DNA, 239
p21 proteins
autokinase activity, 244
cell lines used to study, 243
coding by ras^K, 243
covalent attachment of lipid, 244
immunoprecipitation of, 242, 243
location in cell, 244
mobility of, 243
phosphorylation of, 244
vs. ras^K, 243
preneoplastic alterations, 240
ras^K, organization of
activation mechanism, lung and colon carcinomas, 242-243
antisera, 242
compared to ras^H, 242
gel electrophoresis, 243
and guanine nucleotides, 244
implications of for lung cancer, 243-244
as kinases, 244
molecular weights, 242
monoclonal antibody, 242
normal cells vs. carcinomas, 242
problems with use as sign of lung cancer transformation, 244
restriction endonuclease analysis, 240-241
transformed NIH cells, nature of, 240
transforming genes, identification of
acute transforming retroviruses, 241
cell lines lacking retrovirus homologs, 241
and cellular homologs of, 241
and Harvey sarcoma virus, 241
Kirsten transforming virus, 241
molecular clones, of viral transforming genes, 241
ras^K, lines in, 241-242
Giant-spindle cell carcinomas, 124
Glass. *See* Fiber glass
Graham, Evarts, 313, 314, 323
Green and yellow vegetables. *See also* Japan; Passive smoking; Vitamin A
daily intake vs. lung cancer mortality, in wives, 191
daily vs. nondaily intake, 189, 190, 191, 192, 193
effect on nonsmoking wives vs. husband's smoking and vegetable consumption, 190
and ischemic heart disease mortality rate vs. husband's smoking, 193
and mortality rates from lung cancer vs. husband's smoking, 191
roles discussion, 315, 318
standardized mortality rate, vs. husband's smoking, 192
total consumption of cigarettes vs. vegetable intake, effects, 178

Haviland, Alfred, 74
Hawaii, women in, lung cancers of vs. smoking, 138, 139
Helping Smokers Quit Kit, 293
"Helping Smokers Quit", program and kit, 310
High-risk populations
drug abuse, 290
environment, 290
lifestyle factors, 290
medical problems, 290
National Conference on Smoking *OR* Health, 290
pregnancy, 290
recommendations, 290-291
targeting of, 290
Hispanics, 41, 42, 43, 84, 86, 87, 310
age-adjusted incidence rates, 42, 43
Histological trends of lung cancer, 1973-81
adenocarcinomas, 155
females, 155-56
adenocarcinomas, 155
large-cell carcinomas, 155
NOS, 155-156
histology vs. SEER areas, whites, 1981, 158
males, 155
male/female ratio, 155
malignant carcinoids, 158
NOS, 155, 156
SEER areas
percentage distributions, 156

white females, 157
white males, 156
squamous cell carcinoma, 155
total numbers, 155
HITES medium, cell growth
cells, reactions of, 255
compared with SSM, 255
content, 255
failure to support continuous growth 255-256
growth crisis, 255
origin of cells, 255
selectivity for SCLC cells, 255
Hong Kong, Cantonese women in, lung cancer susceptibility, 141
Hydrocortisone, 254, 256

Iceland. *See* Scandinavia
Immune defects, problems with, 145-146. *See also* Genes, and susceptibility to lung cancer
Incidence of lung cancer vs. cigarette type. *See also* Compensation
abstract, 273
compensation, 276-279
epidemiologic studies
mortality vs. cigarette type, 279
and plasma nicotine levels, vs. unventilated filter cigarettes, 278
tar reduction, and lowered risk, 278, 279
duration of smoking, effects, 275
nicotine, attempts to get, 276
past smoking of high-tar cigarettes, residuum from, 275
percentage of patients with atypical nuclei, 280
percentage of patients with basal cell hyper-plasia vs. cigarettes, number smoked, 280
percentage of patients with lesions and absent cilia, 280
tar, content of, 275
tar deliveries
in developed countries, 274
in developing countries, 275
tar reduction, expected benefits from, 274-276
U.K., changes in smoking in, 1955-81, 274
Industrial processes, possible association with lung cancer. *See also specific industry*
construction, 59
discussion, 59
fishing, 59
painting, 59-60
pesticide applications
chlordane, 60
cohort studies, 60
heptachlor, 60
2,4,5-T, 60
petroleum refining, 60-61
contact with petroleum, 61
excess incidence, 61
rates, 61
and smoking, 61
sugar cane farming, 61
Inhalation, by smokers, 315. *See also* Bifurcations; Radioactivity and tobacco
Insulin, 254, 256
International Classification of Diseases for Oncology, 117
Ischemic heart disease, 179, 183, 193, 194. *See also* Passive smoking

Jaagsiekte, sheep disease, 149
Japan, lung cancer in. *See also* Green and yellow vegetables; Passive smoking; Vitamin A
abstract, 175
active smoking vs. lung cancer risk, 177-178
filter vs. nonfilter, 178
age at start of smoking, vs. smoking-standardized mortality, 177
beta-carotene, 178
dose-response curve, number of cigarettes ever smoked, 177
green and yellow vegetables, 178
lung cancer deaths, trends, 176
lung cancer mortality rates in, 180, 181
risk drop vs. smoking drop, 178
risk vs. green and yellow vegetable consumption, 178
smoking rates, 176
study methods, 176-177
and wife's exposure by husband's smoking, 175

Kirsten sarcoma virus, 23. *See also* Viruses
Know Your Body, 319
Kreyberg I lung cancer, 314, 315, 322
risk in men vs. cigarette number and type, 322
Kreyberg II lung cancer, 314, 315, 322
risk in women vs. cigarette type and number, 322

Large audiences
curriculum and children, 291
evaluation, 291
quit rate, 291
reaching, 290
Lead compounds, 58. *See also* Radioactivity and tobacco
Leiosarcomas, 123, 127
Leiomyomas, 147
"Let's Help Smokers Quit", 311
Li-Fraumeni syndrome, 141
Liposarcomas, 122, 127

Louisiana, lung cancer in. *See also* Cajuns
areas studied, 75
cancer reported, 75
cancer study in
areas, 110
Cajun, definition of, 109-110
Cajun vs. non-Cajun, different foods of, 113
Cajun, probability of being, 110-111
employment of, 111-112
foods eaten by Cajuns, 111-112
hand-rolled cigarettes, 111, 112
methods, 109
odds ratios by degree of Cajun background, 111
smoking, Cajun white males, 112
summary, 113-114
"yes" answers, by age and race, 111
class vs. risk, 77
discussion, 73
diseases, studies about, 80-81
and types of cancer, 81
drinking water, 78, 79
interviews, 75
living near industrial plants, 78, 79
nutrition, 79-80
fresh fruits and vegetables, 79, 80
and pack-years, 80
occupation
discussion, 77-78
occupational exposures, odds ratios, 78
pertinent occupations, odds ratios of, 77
pack-years vs. risk, 76
rates, historical, 74
river deltas, cancer concentration in, 74
sex and race, 76
smoking style vs. risk, 76
suspect materials, 78
Low-risk populations, lung cancer in. *See* Nonsmokers and low-risk populations, lung cancer in
Low-tar cigarettes. *See* Lung cancer incidence vs. cigarette type
Low-yield cigarettes, 320-321, 323
and challenge to industry, 321
components of smoke, 321, 322
drop in cancer in Britain, 320-321
Lung cancer. *See also specific type of cancer*; Epidemiology
bronchofiberscope for diagnosis of, 163
central location of squamous cell carcinomas, 162
cure rates, 2, 162
early symptoms, 162
hilar regions, small cell cancers, 162
history, 48
impact on U.S., 45
other factors, 9
rates, 2, 161, 162
sputum cytology testing, 162-163
three-day pooled sputum test, Mayo Clinic survey, 163
types, 162
x-rays for diagnosis, 162, 163
Lung clearance time, smoking effects on, 265
Lymphomas, 122, 123, 240

Mainstream smoke, 194. *See also* Passive smoking
Males. *See* Men
Mayo lung project, screening for lung cancer. *See also* Screening programs
five-year survival rate, 161
and lung cancer risks and numbers, in U.S., 161-162
other programs, 163-164
rates, methods for, 161
recommendations of, 163
resectable percentages, 161
starting of survey, 163-164
Melanomas, 122
Men, lung cancer and mortality in
Cajuns, 112
in cities, 66
diagnosis, age at, 89, 90
human intervention studies of, 309
Kreyberg I, risk of, 322
mortality in U.S., 39, 230
nonsmokers, 132, 134
odds ratios vs. cancer type, 93
passive smoking, 187
quitters, 320
Scandinavia, 22, 23
70-year-olds, persisting risk in, 5, 6
squamous cell carcinoma, 119
Mesotheliomas, 35, 43, 44, 56, 122, 144
discussion, 44
incidence trends, whites, 43
Metaplasias, 204, 208, 266, 269. *See also* Radioactivity and tobacco
4-Methylnitrosoamino -1-(3-pyridyl)-1-butanone, 305
Miners
lung cancer in 19th century Europe, 48
uranium, 145
Miscertification of lung cancer deaths, 10
Mormons, age-adjusted incidence rates, vs. non-Mormons, 132-134, 137
Mortality figures, trends of in U.K. and U.S.
analysis, problems with, 281-282
daily number of cigarettes, 280
England and Wales
female risk, 281
male risk, 281
men vs. women, 280, 281
number of years smoked, 280
power laws, 280
relative risk, hypothetical population, 280

U.K., other factors in, 281-282
U.S., 161-162, 280, 282
trends, 282
Mortality rates
and cigarette type, 279
and green and yellow vegetables, 190-194
and Japan, study of lung cancer in, 175-178
nonsmokers, 132, 133
passive smokers, 182, 185, 186, 188
U.S., 34-38, 104, 161-162
Mustard gas, 52
Myocardial infarction, risks of by smokers, 11

National Cancer Institute
abstract, 297
Biological Carcinogenesis Branch, 300
Carcinogenesis Extramural Program, 300
Carcinogenesis Intramural Program, 300
Chemical and Physical Oncogenesis Branch, 300
Chemoprevention program, 197-198. *See also* Nutrition; Vitamin A
Division of Cancer Cause and Prevention
Biometry Branch, 300
Clinical Epidemiology Branch, 300
Field Studies and Statistics Program, 300
reasons for, 298
SEER program, 300
structure, 299
Division of Cancer Prevention and Control, 197
Division of Resources, Centers, and Community Activities
Cancer Control Science Program, 302
Centers and Community Oncology Program, 302
diagram, 301
functions, 301-302
phases of research, 303-304
Prevention Program, 302-303
research logic of, 303
Environmental Epidemiology Branch, 300
expenditures of, 297
human intervention studies
age of onset, 308
black females, 309
black males, 309
functions, 307-308
Hispanics, 310
mass media role, 309
number of children who start daily, 307
self-help role, 308-309
physician, role of in intervention, 308
youth education, 308
Information Projects Branch, 310
Laboratory of Cellular Carcinogenesis and Tumor Promotion, 300
Laboratory of Comparative Carcinogenesis, 300
Laboratory of Human Carcinogenesis, 300
Laboratory of Molecular Oncology, 300
Office of Cancer Communications, 310
organization, 297-298
Smoking, Tobacco, and Cancer Program
bioassay models, 304-305
carcinogens in smoke, 305
cotinine, 306
epidemiologic studies, 306-307
fractionation of tobacco and smoke, 305
functions, 304
low-yield reference cigarette, 306
nicotine, 306-307
not as carcinogen, 307
uptake, independence of from pH, 306
nitrosamines, 307
priority projects, 307
program model, 304
tobacco carcinogenesis, 305
whole smoke, chemical analysis, 305-306
SEER program. *See also* SEER
areas of, 154
classification, 154
confirmation rate, 154
and MOTNAC, 154
Special Programs Branch, 301
Neoplasias, 147, 239, 240
New York Times, The, 15
New Zealand, lung cancer rates in, 8
Nickel
dusts, 52
element, 9
refining process, 52-53
Nicotine, 9, 276-279, 286-287, 306-307. *See also* Cigarettes; Passive smoking; Radioactivity and tobacco; Tar
as addicting drug
association of with other stimuli, 287
dependence syndrome, 287
as drug, effects, 286
number of compounds in smoke, 286
reaching of brain by, 286
in blood, 277-278
effects, 306-307
gum containing, as placebo for quitter
and plasma levels, 292
quitting, help to, 292-293
transport enhancement by alkaline smoke,
possibility of, 9
N-nitrosoanatabine, 305
N'-nitrosoanbasine, 305
N-nitrosodiethanolamine, 305
N'-nitrosonornicotine, 305

Nonsmokers and low-risk populations, lung cancer in
ACS cohort, 132
age-adjusted lung cancer vs. religion, 133
age-adjusted mortality rates, U.S., 132
discussion, 131
factors to adjust for, 135
females, studies in, 133-134
histological types in, 318
and lung, mucosal lining of, 131-132
method of smoking, 133
Mormons, 132-134
nonsmokers, lack of rise of lung cancer in, 134
number of cigarettes per day, 133
persisting risk, 133
Seventh-Day-Adventists, age-adjusted rates compared to general population, 134
sex, 132
summary of studies of cancer in, 316-317
smokers, histological cancer types in, vs. those of nonsmokers, 318
in veterans, 132
U.S., 1914 population, 132
NOS (not otherwise specified) carcinomas, rise in U.S. since 1973, 153
Nutrition, use to prevent lung cancer. *See also* Chemoprevention; Green and yellow vegetables; Vitamin A
case/control epidemiological studies, 205-206
cohort epidemiological studies, 206
descriptive epidemiological studies, 205
factors of, and carcinogenesis, 318
metaplasia scores, 208
retinoids, 208
retinol, 206, 207, 208
serum/plasma vitamin A, patients vs. controls, 207
stored blood, cancer risk studies, and vitamin A in, 207-208
vitamin A use and benefits, 205, 206, 207

Oat cell carcinoma, 51, 147, 153, 162. *See also* Small Cell lung cancer
rise in females, 119
rise in since 1973, U.S., 153
Occupations, and lung cancer rates in non-smokers. *See also* Industrial processes; *specific industry*
asbestos, 135
bis-chloromethyl ethers, 135-136
uranium, 135
Ochsner, Alton, 313, 314
Old age, reporting problems in, 10
Oncogenes, 236, 237, 239. *See also* Genes; Viruses
Oncogenesis. *See* DNA transfection; Genes; Viruses
Oxford Textbook of Medicine, 14

Packs per day vs. years of consumption, 8. *See also* dose-response curves
Pack-years, 76, 80, 94
Paper industry, risks in, 107
Passive smoking. *See also* Japan, lung cancer in; Sidestream
active vs. passive smoking, effects compared, 186-188
and lung cancer mortality, 188
numbers of women, 186, 187
relative risks, females, 187
relative risks, males, 187
age-specific mortality rate, wives, by husband's smoking habits, 182
age-standardized mortality rate vs. smoking habits of husband, 179
beta-carotene, 194
cancers other than lung, vs. husband's smoking and mortality of wives, 185
and carbon monoxide, 194, 195
death causes, various, in women, by husband's smoking habits, 183
green and yellow vegetables, 187, 190
hazards, 194
histology of cases, 194
vs. age of husband, 137, 180
vs. husband's drinking habits, 182
and ischemic heart disease, vs. husband's smoking habits, 179, 183
mainstream inhalation, 194
mortality rates, non-lung cancer, wives, vs. age, occupation, and smoking of husband, 185-186
nasal sinus cancer, 194-195
nutrition, in passive smokers, 187
vs. occupation and age of husband, 181
sidestreams, exposure to
entry of, 194
home, 188
workplace, 188
study design, 179
vs. wife's age group, 180
women, by smoking habits of husbands, 136, 137
and work of husband, 137
Pasteur, Louis, 313, 323
Persistence of risk after quitting, 5, 6, 133, 275, 314
Pesticides, 49, 60
Petroleum, 60-61
Physician, role of. *See also* National Cancer Institute
abstinence rates, 292
helping roles model, 292
problems with, 291
Physician's Help Quit Kit, 293
Pipe smokers, Sweden, 9
Pleomorphic cancers, 127
Polonium. *See* Radioactivity and tobacco
Polycyclic aromatic hydrocarbons

and chimney sweeps, 53
skin, 53
steel workers, 53
Prevention, discussion of issues in, 318-319. *See also* Adolescents; National Cancer Institute; Quitting and quitters
Price increases of tobacco as deterrent, 2-3

Quitting and quitters, 286, 289, 293, 310, 314, 320. *See also* Cessation of smoking

Radioactivity and tobacco
and amount of exposure to radon, 54
bifurcations in lungs, metaplasias at, 265
reasons for, 265
clearance time of particles, mean, 265
cumulative dose at bifurcations of smokers dying of lung cancer, 263
lead-210 (isotope), insoluble, 263, 266-268, 269
and bifurcations, deposits at, 266, 267
decay of to polonium-210, 269
deposition in metaplastic cells, 267
dose of alpha radiation from, 267
residence time, 266
stagnant particles and mucus at bifurcations, 266
and tracheal tree, deposition in, 267
lung clearance, impairment of mechanisms of, 265
passive smoking
bifurcations, 270
and polonium-210, 270
and radon daughters, 270
and phosphate fertilizer for tobacco crops, 263-264
polonium-210 in smoke
and alpha radiation dose to epithelium, 266
deposition in lungs, 265-266
elimination rates and means, 266
in sidestream, 266
smokers, levels of in, 266
volatilization of, 265
radiologists, hazards to, 54
radium, 263-265, 268
breakdown of, 265
decay series, 264
radon and its decay products
affinity of for surfaces, 268
air levels of, 268
alpha radiation from, 48, 54
and lead-214, 268
and smoke particles, 268, 269
radiation dose, 268
rates of death, 53, 54
and smoking, 54, 263ff.
tobacco, concentration of isotopes by, 263-264
trichomes, 263
tumor induction
alpha particles, lower limit of for, 269
alpha particles, paths of in cells, 269
and bifurcations, 269
cells close to alpha source, 269
metaplasia, 269
Radium-226. *See* Radioactivity and tobacco smoke
Radon. *See* Radioactivity and tobacco smoke
Ras^{K}. *See* Genes, transforming
Research flow and logic, 200-203
Resectability, 161, 169, 170
Retinoids. *See* Vitamin A
Retinol. *See* Vitamin A
Retroviruses, 240-241
Reynolds, R.J., 15
Risks of lung cancer. *See also* Mortality rates; *specific form of disease*
and age of starting, 5
background and excess, 4
and death rate at age 60, 5
delay, 50-year, in 70-year-old men, 5, 6
nonsmokers, 4
smokers, 4
in town vs. country, 6-7
trends in U.S. comsumption of cigarettes, 6
Rubber manufacturing, 56
rates of risk, 56
Russia, cigarettes of, 17, 18
tar in, 18

Sales of cigarettes and tobacco, control of
Britain, antismoking messages in, 16
elasticity of demand, 14
murder rates, compared to, smoking deaths, 15, 16
propaganda against smoking, 14-15
and public perception of risks
Britain, 16
U.S., 15
radiation, hazards of compared to those of smoking, 15
road accidents, 15, 16
shock messages, 15-16
taxes, 13-14
death rate drop, 14
effects, 14
tobacco, lack of scare about, 15
Scandinavia, lung cancer vs. smoking habits in countries of
age-adjusted rates, lung cancer, 22, 24
trends in, 24
age-specific curves, 23
area-specific smoking indices vs. lung cancer incidence indices, 28
birth cohort analyses, 24
cancer registries of, 22
daily smokers, pattern, 25
Finland
age-adjusted rates, 27

legislation in, 26
lung cancer in, 22-23, 27
percentages in, 25, 26
projection of lung cancer to 2002, 24-25
standardized incidence rates, 21
study in compared with Norway, 27
Finns, ethnic background of, 22
form of tobacco, 29
life risks of lung cancer, 24
Norway, smokers in, 27-28
occupation and smoking as risk factors for lung cancer
Finnish Cancer Registry, 29
observed vs. expected numbers of cases, male, 30
occupational, formula, 29
standardized incidence rates, 29
study, design, 29
rates, 21
sex ratio, 22, 23
smoking, introduction and spread of, 25
trends, recent, 21
urban vs. rural, 23
variations of incidence, 22, 23
and variation of earlier smoking habits, present effects on lung cancer incidence, 21
Sarcomas, 123
Sarcoidosis, 145, 146
Screening programs, features of. *See also* National Cancer Institute; SEER
acceptability of screening, 166-167
benefits, tangibility of
cost/benefit ratio, 171
cancer of concern, 164
cancers hidden from x-rays, 167
control group, keeping untested of, 167-168
detection rate of
advanced/unresectable cases, 170
five-year survival rate, 170
four-monthly screened group, 169, 170
postsurgical stage, AJC system, 170
resection, 169, 170
vs. test, 169
types, 169
ease of use, 165
high-risk groups, concentration on, 166
localization and rapid treatment, 168
MLP
design, 166
discussion, 171-173
factors, negative, 172
followup period, 171-172
present status, 172
tests, application of, 172-173
MLP/Mayo clinic, experience of, 165
preclinical phase, nature, 164-165
randomized, successful, 168-169
backdating, 169
MLP, 169
reliability, 167
safety in, 167
table, 165
X-ray exposure, amounts of, 167
SEER. *See* Survival, Epidemiology, and End Results
Selenium, 255, 256
Sera for cell culture. *See* Culture medium, defined; HITES
Sidestreams, 188, 194, 266. *See also* Japan; Passive smoking
Silica, 58
Silicosis, 58
Small cell carcinoma
incidence in men, 159
treatment for, 158-159
Small cell carcinoma lines, soft agarose in vitro cloning, human specimens
bone marrow, 251
cell lines, use for drug testing, 252-253
as chemotherapy guide, 250-251
clonogenic assay, 252
colony rate per viable 100,000 cells, 251, 252
confirmation methods, 251-252
cytopathologically negative specimens, 251
dihydrofolate reductase, gene for, 253
double minute chromosomes, 253
drug sensitivity testing, 252
growth factor and hormone requirements, 256
materials and methods, 251
and methotrexate resistance, 252-253
multiple vs. single drugs, 252
vs. non-small cell, colony rates compared, 252
signs of small cell lung cancer, 251
specimen sources, 251
tumor colony formation rate, 251
Small cell lung cancer cell lines, use in in vitro lung cancer studies
abstract, 247
agarose colonies, 248
amine precursor uptake and decarboxylation (APUD), 249
cell lines, compared to non-small cell lines, 248-249
characteristics of SCLC disease, 247-248
continuous culture, 248, 249
creatine kinase, BB isozyme of, 249, 250
double times, 249
floating aggregates, 248-249
hormones produced by, 249-250
L-Dopa-decarboxylase, 249
major forms of lung cancer, 247-248
media for growth, 248
neuron-specific enolase, 249, 250
predicted deaths from lung cancer, U.S. 1983, 247-248
sources of cell lines, 248
tumors in athymic nude mice, 248

Small cell lung cancer cells, "conversion" to large-cell morphological variants
APUD cell markers, loss of, 257
deletion, 257
mix of small cells with large cells, vs. survival of human patient, 257
radiation survival curves of cells, 257
rates observed of conversion, 257
and relapse, chemotherapy after, 257
transformation associated with radiation, 258
variant lines, nature of, 257
Smoke, chemical analysis and content of, 286, 305, 306. *See also* Nicotine; Tar
Smoking Digest, The, 311
Social factors encouraging smoking, 287
Squamous cell carcinomas, 142, 155, 162. *See also* Oat-cell carcinomas; Small-cell lung cancer
cell lines, growth factor and hormone requirements, 256
Surface membrane protein phenotypes, lung cancer lines, 233, 258
distinguished from non-small cells, 258
Surgeon General's reports, 3
Survival, Epidemiology, and End Results (SEER)
areas, 156-157
histological trends, 158
materials and methods, 34
men, rates found in, 300
and National Cancer Institute, 300
Survival rates, 161, 170, 257
Surveys, summary about, 3

Talc, 58-59
Tar, 10-13, 16-18, 274-276. *See also* Nicotine
levels
discussion, 16, 17, 18
government measures of, 18
reduction of
British consumption, males, 13
British trends, 13
effect of on number of smokers, 11
expected changes in lung cancer risks, 11
filter vs. plain, mortality compared, 12
Finland, 12
means of, 11
natural trends, early middle age, discussion, 12
preneoplastic lesions, drop in America, 12-13
reductions in delivery, 10
smoker behavior, 11. *See also* Compensation
study problems, 11-12
Teenagers. *See* Adolescents
Texas, lung cancer causes and studies in
abstract, 83
areas studied, 84
ascertainment problems, 87-88
Hispanics, 84, 86, 87
males vs. females, 85
period of, study, 84, 85
results, hospital reports, 87-97
adenocarcinomas, 92-93
age at diagnosis, female, 89, 90
age at diagnosis, male, 89, 90
age and sex vs. cancer type, 92
alcohol, 89, 90
asbestos, 96
and cancer type, 92
cases vs. controls, cigarette and alcohol use, 90
cigarette use, amount, 89, 90
discussion, 97-98
employment, 93, 94, 95, 96
females, 95, 96
males, 95
ex-smokers, 89, 90
industrial odds rates, 96
living with smoker, 89, 90
lung cancer ascertainment, 88
odds ratios, cancer type, female, 93
odds ratios, cancer type, male, 93
odds ratios, passive smoking, 91, 92
odds ratios, smoking variables, 91
pack-years vs. type of cancer, odds ratios, 94
passive smoking, 90-91
percentages, 87-88
population factors in, 88
residence time, 88
Third National Cancer Survey, 34
Tobacco. *See also* Cigarettes; Nicotine; Radioactivity and tobacco; Tar
control of, 2
curing of, 9
and less common cancers, 3
Transferrin, 255, 256

United Kingdom. *See* Britain
United States
cancer rates in, 2
lung cancer rate of mortality. *See also* Blacks; Hispanics; Men; Women
age-specific, white females, 39
age-specific, white males, 39
area-specific, whites, 40
Atlanta, 40
discussion, 38-39
females, white, 1970-75, 103
Louisiana, 40
males, white, 1970-75, 103
mortality vs. time trends, white females, 104
mortality vs. time trends, white males, 104
by race, 40, 41, 42, 43
by sex, 41

recent increases of lung cancer in
factors, 34
incidence trends, variables in, 37
increase, rates of by sex, 33, 34
male/female ratio, 33
malignancies, invasive, 35
mesotheliomas, nonmalignant, 35
mortality, determination of rates, 34-35
New Orleans, recent rates, 33
1983 estimate, 34
nonwhite males, 33
numbers in U.S., recent, 33
populations surveyed, 34
rates and data, determination of, 34
recent mortality trends, 7
whites, incidence and mortality, females
age vs. geography, 38
age-specific death rates, 37
birth cohorts, 35, 36
whites, incidence and mortality, males, 33, 35-36
age-adjusted, 35
age-specific death rates, 36
and geography, 38
Uranium, 135, 145

Vinyl chloride, 55
Viruses
Epstein-Barr, 232
feline leukemia, 232
Harvey sarcoma, 241
Kirsten transforming, 241, 242
Lucké tumor, 232, 233
oncogenic, 233
ras, 236
retroviruses, 241
transforming genes of, 241
Vitamin A vs. lung cancer. *See also* Carcinogen inhibition; Green and yellow vegetables
and age, 213
anticancer nutrients, other, 216
beta-carotene, 212, 215
body mass index, 215
correlation coefficients, 214
death rates in areas of Louisiana, 211-212
and green and yellow vegetables, 215
intake vs. area, 213, 214
intake vs. risk, 138
and lack of vitamin A, effects, 212
malnutrition indexes, 216
methods, 212-213
race, 213
retinol, 212, 213, 215
serum levels vs. mortality, 211, 213, 215-216, 217
and smoking, 215
surveys, 212
Ten-State Nutrition Survey, 212

Welding, 56
chromium compounds, 56
mesothelioma, 56
Women
age-adjusted average SEER incidence rates, U.S. 1970, 43
Cantonese, 141, 143
in cities, 66
diagnosis, age at, 89, 90
drinking of husband, 182
and green and yellow vegetables, 190-194
human intervention studies in, 309
Kreyberg II, 322
mortality, U.S., 39, 231
nonsmokers, 133-134
oat-cell carcinoma, 119
odds ratios vs. cancer type, 93
passive smoking, 136, 137, 179, 183, 185, 187
pulmonary adenocarcinoma/squamous cell carcinoma ratio in, 142
quitters, 286, 320
Scandinavia, 22, 23
World, prevalence of lung cancer in, 2

X-rays, 162, 163, 167